Principles of Neuromusculoskeletal Treatment and Management

A Guide for Therapists

Nicola J. Petty MSc MCSP MMPA MMACP
Principal Lecturer, School of Health Professions, University of Brighton, Eastbourne, UK

With a contribution by

Ann P. Moore PhD GradDipPhys FCSP DipTP CertEd FMACP
Professor of Physiotherapy and Head of Clinical Research Centre for Health Professions, University of Brighton, Eastbourne, UK

Foreword by

Gwendolen Jull MPhty GradDipManipTher PhD FACP
Associate Professor and Reader, Department of Physiotherapy, University of Queensland, Brisbane, Australia

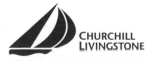

CHURCHILL
LIVINGSTONE

EDINBURGH   LONDON   NEW YORK   OXFORD   PHILADELPHIA   ST LOUIS   SYDNEY   TORONTO   2004

CHURCHILL LIVINGSTONE
An imprint of Elsevier Limited

First published 2004

ISBN 0 443 07062 8

British Library Cataloguing in Publication Data
A catalogue record for this book is available from the British Library

Library of Congress Cataloging in Publication Data
A catalog record for this book is available from the Library of Congress

Notice
Every effort has been made by the author and the Publishers to ensure that the descriptions of the techniques included in this book are accurate and in conformity with the descriptions published by their developers. The Publishers and the author do not assume any responsibility for any injury and/or damage to persons or property arising out of or related to any use of the material contained in this book. It is the responsibility of the treating practitioner, relying on independent experience and knowledge of the patient, to determine the best treatment and method of application for the patient, to make their own evaluation of their effectiveness and to check with the developers or teachers of the techniques they wish to use that they have understood them correctly.

 your source for books, journals and multimedia in the health sciences
www.elsevierhealth.com

The
publisher's
policy is to use
**paper manufactured
from sustainable forests**

Printed in China

Principles of Neuromusculoskeletal Treatment and Management

For my brother, Richard K.H. Petty

For Churchill Livingstone:

Publishing Director, Health Professions: Mary Law
Project Development Manager: Claire Wilson
Project Manager: Gail Wright
Senior Designer: Judith Wright
Illustration Manager: Bruce Hogarth
Illustrations by: Dartmouth Publishing

Contents

Foreword

There has been an enormous increase in the research concerned with identifying and furthering our understanding of the pathophysiology of neuromusculoskeletal disorders. We are learning more and more about the potential impairments in the articular, muscular and nervous systems in persons with musculoskeletal pain as well as their possible functional and psychosocial sequelae. Importantly, there is increasing knowledge about the physiology and psychology of pain. The physical impairments and changes in the pain system can be of variable extent and complexity, and each patient presents with a unique combination of pathophysiological features. There can be no 'recipe' approach to the management of musculoskeletal disorders.

Thus it is quite challenging to write a text that reflects and tries to integrate this vast amount of knowledge to present material in an informative way which can satisfy, challenge and give direction to clinicians in the field of musculoskeletal therapy. Nikki Petty has gone a long way towards meeting this challenge in presenting a text which focuses on providing the information from the basic and applied clinical sciences to underpin the principles essential for effective clinical reasoning in the assessment and management of patients with musculoskeletal disorders. The text first presents the structure of the clinical assessment and highlights the thought processes or clinical reasoning required for effective, interpretative and safe diagnosis and management. This forms the foundation for subsequent chapters, which focus on the knowledge base in the basic and applied clinical sciences in each system, which is necessary for effective problem solving in the management of patients with musculoskeletal pain syndromes. Considerations of patients and their context and the possible influences on assessment and management are also presented.

Changes can occur in each of the articular, muscular, nervous and psychological systems of patients with musculoskeletal pain syndromes but, as highlighted in this text, there is interdependence of the systems both in function and dysfunction; as well, the impairments in each system can be on multiple levels. The challenge for the clinician is to try to unravel the puzzle presented by the patient. The problem solving process is not confined to the initial assessment but is a progressive process during management. It is necessary to carefully monitor the responsiveness of patients, their pain and functional limitations as well as the physical impairments to a chosen intervention. Thus treatment is never static and the plentiful examples provided in the text illustrate the process of changing and modifying treatments in response to the changes in the condition of patients during treatment and their goals.

A tremendous amount of knowledge has been presented in this text, and it provides practitioners with sound principles on which to base their management of patients with musculoskeletal disorders. It should also stimulate further questions on both the mechanisms of musculoskeletal pain and the mechanisms of effect of our treatments, for with increasing knowledge comes the realization of the many factors that we still do not yet fully understand. For example, evidence has been presented of problems of motor control in the muscle system in association with musculoskeletal pain syndromes but at the moment we do not fully understand whether these changes are as a result of pain and/or pathology, protective of pain and pathology or if they are predictive of pain and pathology. Furthermore, the text presents treatment alternatives but why is one patient responsive to a particular therapeutic approach while a seemingly similar patient is not responsive?

This is an exciting era in the field of assessment and management of musculoskeletal pain states. Understanding the principles behind the assessment and management of musculoskeletal pain states as detailed in this text should stimulate the thought processes of clinicians to better manage their patients and to influence future directions of research into musculoskeletal diagnosis and rehabilitation.

Gwendolen Jull

Preface

The aim of this book is to make explicit the underlying principles behind the treatment and management of patients with neuromusculoskeletal disorders. The text has been written for therapists at both undergraduate and postgraduate level.

Therapists at all levels can have difficulty in mastering the principles of patient treatment and management in this field. There can be a tendency to replicate textbook descriptions instead of adapting techniques to suit the needs of individual patients. In addition, the patient as a person can sometimes be forgotten in the drive for technical mastery of hands-on skill. Expert clinicians, however, are those who have excellent communication, technical and clinical reasoning skills. This text discusses the theory and principles that underpin those skills.

The knowledge base of neuromusculoskeletal management is continually evolving and provides an exciting and dynamic field in which to work. While there exists a large body of theoretical knowledge, there is still a lot that is not known and not understood. A recent postgraduate course was entitled 'The Amazing Nervous System', which is a great title; the neuromusculoskeletal system, like the rest of the human body, truly is amazing and 'wonderfully made' (Psalm 139 v14).

I hope that this book will be a useful resource for both undergraduate and postgraduate therapists, as they study this amazing neuromusculoskeletal system.

Eastbourne 2003   Nicola J. Petty

Acknowledgements

I would like to thank the many colleagues and friends who have been involved in the production of this book.

For those involved in the early stages, I would like to thank Ann Moore for her involvement in planning the book; Duncan Arnold for providing some insightful comments on the proposed content; Jon Wright and Fiona Jones for their patience, encouragement and support when things were not going well; and Gaynor Sadlo for listening and helping me organize my time better.

In the middle stage, I would like to thank John Boxall, Liz Bryant, Bernhard Haas, Alan Hough, Claire Jenner, Nicky Pont, Marion Trew and Graham Watts for some timely conversations, snippets of information, computer help or articles.

I would like to thank the staff at Queenwood Library and the British Library for their superb service in processing my hundreds of requests for articles. Thank you to all my generous colleagues at the School for their support and inter-library loans. I would also like to thank Mary Law, Dinah Thom and Claire Wilson at Elsevier for their support and patience.

In the final stage, I would like to thank Guy Canby, Helen Fiddler, Ann Moore and Colette Ridehalgh for reading and providing helpful comments on chapters of the book. Special thanks go to Chris Murphy for reading almost the entire book in the space of three weeks. Many thanks to Colette Ridehalgh and Clair Hebron for the painstaking job of writing a case study for the assessment chapter. Thanks also to Lynne Caladine and Andy Johnston for their comments on some of the preliminary pages.

I would like to thank some particular friends who have encouraged, supported and advised me throughout this three-year project, amounting to around 1500 hours, through almost all of which my cat, Cracker, has been asleep! In particular, I would like to thank Brian and Jackie Arnott, Neil and Judith Barnett, Bernie Brennan, Janet Curtis, Mark and Catherine Dancey, Sarah Davies, April Hedges and Pamela Oakley. Finally, to my mother and father for their constant love and support.

Glossary

Creep: increase in deformation over time under a constant force.

Force: that which changes, or tends to change, the state of rest or motion of matter. Measured in Newtons (N).

Hysteresis: loss of energy (difference between energy expended and energy regained) when a force is applied and then removed. The energy 'lost' is in the form of heat, and the consequence is that the viscoelastic tissue does not return to its original length.

Hypothesis: a proposition made as a basis for reasoning, without the assumption of its truth (Oxford English Reference Dictionary, 1996)

Muscle power: rate of doing work: work divided by time, or force multiplied by velocity. Measured in watts (W).

$$\text{power} = \frac{\text{work (or force} \times \text{distance)}}{\text{time}}$$

or

$$\text{power} = \text{force} \times \text{velocity}$$

Muscle strength: ability to generate force. Measured in Newtons (N) or torque.

Plasticity: 'the ability of cells to alter any aspect of their phenotype, at any stage in development, in response to abnormal changes in their state or environment' (Brown & Hardman 1987). Can also be defined as a change in form due to an alteration in function: 'formfunction' (Kidd, Lawes & Musa 1992).

Stiffness: the resistance to movement felt by the therapist.

Strain: deformation (change in dimension) in a structure due to an externally applied load.

Stress: load or force, per unit area, that develops within a structure due to an externally applied load.

Symptoms: any sensation felt by the patient, including pain, ache, pulling, pins and needles, numbness and crawling.

Torque: moment of force. Calculated by force multiplied by the shortest distance between the line of force and the axis of rotation.

Work: product of force and distance through which it acts. Measured in Joules (J).

$$\text{work} = \text{force} \times \text{distance}$$

REFERENCES

Brown MC, Hardman VJ 1987 Plasticity of vertebrate motoneurones. In: Winlow W, McCrohan CR (eds) Growth and Plasticity of Neural Connections. Manchester University Press, Manchester, p 36–51

Kidd G, Lawes N, Musa I 1992 Understanding Neuromuscular Plasticity, a Basis for Clinical Rehabilitation. Edward Arnold, London, p 69

1

Introduction

The aim of this book is to make explicit the underlying principles behind the treatment and management of patients with neuromusculoskeletal disorders. Vital to any textbook is the arrangement of information – which has to be as user-friendly as possible. It is hoped that the organization chosen will enable readers to find their way easily around the text.

This present chapter aims to help the reader understand how the information has been laid out by giving a brief résumé of what is contained within each chapter. Chapter 2 aims to bridge the gap between the previous text on examination and assessment (Petty & Moore 2001) and this new textbook on treatment and management. Two case studies are provided within this chapter to make explicit the clinical reasoning process involved in the examination and assessment – as well as the treatment and management – of patients.

Chapter 3 provides key information on anatomy, biomechanics, physiology and movement of joint structures and, on the basis of this summary of joint function, then classifies and discusses common clinical presentations of joint dysfunction. Using this classification of dysfunction, Chapter 4 then provides the principles underpinning treatment. This arrangement of a chapter on function and dysfunction followed by a chapter on treatment is used for muscle in Chapters 5 and 6, and for nerve in Chapters 7 and 8.

The chapters on function and dysfunction of joint, nerve and muscle assume that the reader already has a basic understanding of anatomy, biomechanics and physiology. Relevant aspects of these subjects are discussed in order to explain the underpinning of joint, nerve and muscle treatment, as well as the overall management of patients.

In this text, a 'joint treatment' is defined as a 'treatment to effect a change in joint'; that is, the intention of the clinician is to produce a change in joint, and therefore it is described as a joint treatment. Similarly, where a technique is used to effect a change in a muscle, it will be referred to as a 'muscle treatment' and where a technique is used to effect a change in nerve, it will be referred to as a 'nerve treatment'. Thus, techniques are classified according to which tissue the clinician is predominantly attempting to affect.

The treatment of an individual patient is not simply the physical treatment of joint, muscle and nerve. The patient is a person with mind and spirit, as well as body, as is the clinician. This potent combination creates a complex therapeutic relationship which defies a simple cause and effect analysis of our therapeutic interaction. Chapter 9, written by Professor Ann Moore, is of paramount importance. It discusses these issues and provides an overview of the principles of managing patients with neuromusculoskeletal disorders.

Thus, a reader who would like to learn more about the principles of treatment and management of patients with joint disorders would be advised to read Chapters 2, 3, 4 and 9, with muscle disorders Chapters 2, 5, 6 and 9, and with nerve disorders Chapters 2, 7, 8 and 9.

In terms of content, it may be helpful to make some general comments here. Information that is given in anatomy, biomechanics physiology and pathology textbooks is general information. A brief exploration of scientific journals will quickly reveal the enormous variation between individuals. Anatomy journals, for example, describe variations in joint architecture, muscle attachments and nerve pathways, demonstrating the uniqueness of individuals. Anatomy textbooks, therefore, describe what is generally true, but not what is particularly true, for any one individual. This has important implications for clinical practice. Each individual patient presenting for treatment may not have the anatomical structure that has been described in the text-

books. The same might be said of biomechanics, physiology and pathology texts. The content of this textbook is no different: it provides general information on joint, nerve and muscle function and dysfunction, and may not be directly applicable to an individual patient.

Much of what is known about the neuromusculoskeletal system of the human body is presumed on the basis of what is actually known from animals. A considerable amount of research has been carried out on animals and has provided valuable information about function and dysfunction of the neuromusculoskeletal system. Animal research is used explicitly throughout this text to explain function and dysfunction of joints, nerves and muscles. While, generally speaking, it can be assumed that the findings would be similar in the human body it cannot be assumed that the findings would be identical.

Our knowledge of the neuromusculoskeletal system is far from complete. Research often focuses on one area, which is then assumed to reflect other similar areas. For example, the quadriceps muscle group has been used to investigate the principles of muscle strengthening, and the cat knee joint has been used to investigate the behaviour of joint afferent activity during movement. The research provides knowledge of one area, and indirect knowledge of other similar areas. So, for example, the behaviour of joint afferent activity in the cat is presumed to be similar to that of man, and is presumed to reflect afferent activity in other joints. These are logical and reasonable assumptions to make, but we must be aware that we are making these assumptions.

The result is that we have a general understanding of joint, muscle, nerve function and dysfunction. This is often based on specific areas of research on animals, with the assumption that similar findings would occur in humans.

One final point is that research articles are used widely within the text to support or refute arguments. Details of the research carried out, and a critical evaluation of the research, is not provided in the text as this would limit the flow of the arguments. Readers are encouraged to read these articles so that their own understanding is enhanced.

REFERENCE

Petty N J, Moore A P 2001 Neuromusculoskeletal
    examination and assessment, a handbook for therapists,
    2nd edn. Churchill Livingstone, Edinburgh

2

Assessment

The word 'assessment' is used to denote the analysis, or interpretation, of the examination findings by the clinician. At the patient's first appointment, the subjective and physical examination is used, in part, to gather information about the patient. Assessment is the interpretation of this information and is used to guide the clinician in the treatment and management of the patient. Assessment is, in essence, the problem-solving and decision-making process involved in clinical practice and it can be referred to as clinical reasoning. Assessment and treatment are used together in every appointment the patient has with the clinician and can be depicted as shown in Figure 2.1. Only through assessment can the clinician decide on meaningful treatment, and the quality of treatment given will be directly related to the quality of assessment. To quote Maitland et al (2001, p. 53): 'assessment is the keystone of effective, informative treatment'. The subject of clinical reasoning as well as expertise is an expanding field and the reader is referred to two excellent texts: Higgs & Jones (2000) and Jenson et al (1999).

Throughout the subjective and physical examination, the clinician obtains information about the patient. With every piece of information, the clinician will make immediate judgements. Such judgements may or may not be correct. While a high level of expertise may enable a clinician to make correct judgements, and as a consequence provide effective and efficient care of the patient, there is also the possibility of error, leading to ineffective and inefficient care. An analogy may help to clarify this point. The process of examination and assessment is very similar to the work

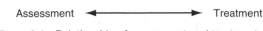

Figure 2.1 Relationship of assessment and treatment.

of a police detective. Let us assume that a man has been murdered. Statistically, the wife is the most likely murderer. On questioning the woman, the lack of an alibi and the fact that she had just had an argument with her husband, may be sufficient evidence for an inexperienced detective to consider her guilty. Once this hypothesis has been made, the detective continues the investigation, looking for information to support the hypothesis, and either not recognizing, or ignoring, the evidence that would negate this hypothesis. In other words, the detective believes that the woman is guilty and is seeking evidence to support this belief. The unfortunate possibility is that this woman may be wrongly convicted of murder. In contrast, an experienced detective acknowledges the lack of an alibi and the argument with the husband, and treats these aspects with suspicion by following this line of enquiry, but does not make the error of believing that these two pieces of information prove that the woman is guilty. This detective seeks out all the other possibilities, however unlikely. Every avenue must be fully explored, and substantial amounts of evidence must be collected to prove the guilt and, as importantly, to disprove the guilt, of every possible suspect. The assumption that the detective must make is that everyone is guilty until proven innocent. Coming back to the clinical situation(!), the clinician collects information to identify a lateral ligament sprain of the knee, for example, and collects information to clarify that the pain in the knee is not coming from the spine or hip, and that it is not a muscle problem or a tibiofemoral or patellofemoral joint problem. In this way, during the examination the clinician explores all possible structures that could be a source of the patient's symptoms, and only once these structures have been seriously and fully explored can the clinician decide that they are not a source of the patient's symptoms. Jones (1994) refers to this as the clinician developing 'multiple diagnostic hypotheses' and an 'evolving concept of the patient's problem'.

The amount and nature of the evidence required to dismiss a structure as a possible source of the patient's symptoms is the very essence of clinical reasoning judgements, clinical mileage and clinical expertise. The clinical presentation of some patients will, of course, be very straightforward. For example, a patient may be referred following a colles fracture and 3 weeks of immobilization, and the patient simply needs local rehabilitation of the forearm, wrist and hand; or a patient may be referred with a simple lateral ligament sprain of the ankle and, again, straightforward rehabilitation is all that is necessary. The requirement in these examples may require little hunting around by the clinician to identify the cause of the patient's symptoms. Indeed, for an acute injury such as a sprained ankle early treatment, not examination (on the first day of attendance), would be the priority. There are, however, a large number of patients who do not have a straightforward presentation. In these situations it is imperative that the clinician has a clear and logical strategy for identifying the source of the patient's symptoms. This chapter attempts to make this strategy explicit.

The initial appointment will usually consist of a subjective examination and a physical examination and these have been more fully described in the previous text (Petty & Moore 2001).

It cannot be emphasized enough that the subjective examination is a critical part of the overall examination. The clinician needs to develop a rapport with the patient that will, among other things, enable them to obtain an accurate and comprehensive understanding of the patient's problem. In order to do this the clinician needs a high level of skill in communication, which includes verbal, non-verbal and listening skills, as well as a thorough understanding of what needs to be asked and why. By the end of the subjective examination the clinician should know:

- what physical examination procedures need to be carried out
- how the physical procedures should be carried out, in terms of symptom production
- of any precautions or contraindications to the physical examination or, later on, with treatment

- what other factors, that might be contributing to the patient's symptoms, need to be examined.

This information helps the clinician to plan the physical examination and this can be formalized using a physical examination form (Fig. 2.2).

The subjective examination clarifies the relative importance of various possible structures that could be a source of the patient's symptoms. For example, a clinician may decide that the patient has a local problem around the knee and that this region is all that needs to be examined in the physical. In this case, clarifying that the patient has no symptoms in the lumbar spine, sacroiliac joint or hip region may provide sufficient evidence to satisfy the clinician that these regions do not need to be examined in the physical. If this evidence is going to be so influential as to completely negate physical examination of these regions, the clinician must be certain that they have been fully explored. For example, to

	Symptom	Symptom	Symptom	Symptom
Is it severe?				
Is it irritable?				
Will you move: -short of production? -point of onset/increase in resting symptoms? -partial reproduction? -total reproduction?				
How will you reproduce symptom: - repeat? - alter speed? - combine? - sustain? - other? (state)				

Are there any precautions or contraindications? Yes No State
What other factors contributing to the patient's symptom(s) need to be examined?

Figure 2.2 Physical examination planning form.

enquire casually of the patient whether they have any pain in these regions is totally inadequate. If this is done, the patient may quietly dismiss a slight ache or stiffness they have been feeling and respond negatively, thus giving the clinician inaccurate information. The physical examination may then focus on inappropriate testing procedures. Rather than a casual enquiry about pain in these regions, it is suggested that the clinician asks the patient, in a deliberate way, 'do you have any pain or stiffness here (lumbar spine, or sacroiliac joint or hip)?', 'nothing at all?'. Having obtained and double-checked the answer, and on some occasions triple-checked the answer, the clinician can now be satisfied that the patient has been given every opportunity to tell them about even the slightest symptom in that region which may be relevant to the patient's problem. Inexperienced clinicians will be surprised how often the patient initially will negate any pain in an area, but when this is checked again, will say 'yes, actually it does sometimes ache a bit'.

The subjective examination will not readily separate out geographically close structures; for example, the clinician may suspect that a patient with pain over the lumbar spine, posterior superior iliac spine and over the groin has a lumbar spine, sacroiliac and/or hip problem. Information about the behaviour of the symptoms, functional limitations, 24-hour behaviour, recent history etc., will probably not clarify for the clinician how much they need to explore the lumbar spine, sacroiliac joint and hip region. The structures lie so close together that movement in one region will produce movement in the other region, and so distinctions are not easily made. The same is true of the cervical spine, scapula-thoracic and shoulder regions. However, where a patient has back pain, and knee or foot pain, or neck pain, and elbow or hand pain, a clearer distinction may be able to be made between the regions. For example, a patient may have had neck pain for 20 years, neck movements feel slightly sore with no pain in the wrist, and the neck pain may have remained the same since the wrist was injured. The wrist pain may have come on recently, simple active wrist movements producing the pain; this scenario would suggest two

separate problems and the clinician could decide to look only at the wrist region on the first attendance. Any hint, however, in the subjective (or physical) examination that the wrist pain is being referred from the cervical spine will require examination of the spine.

The reason why this aspect of the subjective examination is reiterated here is that it is this decision that decides the physical examination procedures to be carried out, and is therefore a vital decision in the overall examination process. Once the testing procedures are decided, the physical examination simply requires the clinician to carry out those tests. Of course, the tests need to be evaluated, and modifications to the physical examination may need to be made. This point is made very well by Jones & Jones (1994) who state that 'the physical examination is not simply the indiscriminate application of routine tests'. Following the physical examination, the clinician is able to discuss with the patient the plan for treatment and management. A basic planning form may be useful, for some clinicians, to clarify their examination findings (Fig. 2.3).

The previous examination and assessment book (Petty & Moore 2001) described the clinical reasoning and assessment process within the step-by-step subjective and physical examination processes. Each aspect of the subjective and physical examination was explained in a bottom-up approach. This text uses a top-down approach, that is, the information is organized according to final decision making prior to starting treatment. It is hoped that, taken together, the two textbooks will provide an explicit account of the clinical reasoning process that leads to the treatment and management of patients with neuromusculoskeletal dysfunction.

DEVELOPING HYPOTHESES

Following completion of the subjective and physical examinations of a patient, the clinician must decide on a number of hypotheses (Jones & Jones 1994). These include:

* source of the symptoms and/or dysfunction. This includes the structure(s) at fault and the mechanism of symptom production

What subjective and physical reassessment asterisks will you use?

Subjective	Physical

What is your treatment plan for the:

Source of symptoms	Contributing factors

What are your goals for discharge?

Figure 2.3 Treatment and management planning form.

- factors contributing to the condition, be they environmental, behavioural, emotional, physical or biomechanical factors
- precautions or contraindications to physical examination and/or treatment
- prognosis of the condition
- plan of management of the patient's condition.

Clinicians may find it helpful to complete the more in-depth clinical reasoning form of the overall management of the patient, shown in the Appendix, to help them identify these categories of hypotheses.

Developing each of these hypotheses requires the clinician to consider information from various aspects of the subjective and physical examination findings. There is never one piece of information from the subjective examination, or one test from the physical examination, that will fully develop any one of the above hypotheses. Rather, it is the weight of evidence, from a number of aspects from the subjective examination and physical examination, that enables the clinician to make a hypothesis. Ideally, all aspects of the subjective and physical examination findings should come together, logically, to formulate a hypothesis; that is, the clinician should 'make features fit' (Maitland 1991 p. 58). Where this is not possible it may prompt the clinician for alternative explanations; for example, perhaps there is a serious pathology underlying the patient's problems which may require medical investigation. The information from the subjective and physical examinations, which may inform each category of hypothesis, is given below.

Source of the symptoms and/or dysfunction

The priority of day one examination is to identify the source of the patient's symptoms. The word 'source' is used here in the widest sense of the word, whether there is an affective, physical, central or autonomic cause. The ability to identify the source of the patient's symptoms may, however, not be possible. For example, a patient with an acute injury may not be able to be fully examined; in this situation the examination will occur over a period of time as the acute state settles.

There are two underlying assumptions used in the identification of the source of the symptoms. The first is that if the patient's *exact* symptoms are reproduced when a structure is stressed, the symptoms are thought to arise from that structure. The word 'exact' means that the quality or 'feel' to the patient is the symptom they are complaining of, which is wholly or partially reproduced by a test. The difficulty with this, of

course, is that there are no functional movements or physical testing procedures which stress individual structures. Active hip flexion, when climbing stairs for example, involves hip joint movement, isotonic activity of the muscles around the hip, alteration in length of the femoral and sciatic nerve, posterior pelvic tilt, knee flexion etc. It is therefore difficult to identify, with any movement, which structure is at fault and producing the patient's symptoms. Similarly, in the physical examination, hip flexion in supine alters the:

- lumbar spine (moved into flexion)
- sacroiliac joint (moved with posterior pelvic rotation and a shear force due to the weight of the thigh)
- hip joint (moved into end-range flexion)
- extensor muscles of hip and knee flexors (lengthened)
- sciatic nerve (lengthened).

If posterior thigh pain is produced on hip flexion overpressure, the clinician cannot be certain which of the above structures is producing this pain. Further testing, and in particular differentiation testing, is necessary to try to tease out which of the above structures is provoking the pain; for example, adding knee extension would increase the length of the sciatic nerve and hamstring muscle group and increase the longitudinal force through the femur to the hip joint. Further differentiation could be achieved by the addition of ankle dorsiflexion, which would increase the length of the sciatic nerve without changing hamstring length or altering hip joint compression. If symptoms are increased with knee extension and dorsiflexion, this would suggest the sciatic nerve as the source of the symptoms; if symptoms are not altered with dorsiflexion this implicates the hamstring muscles or the hip joint. Isometric testing of the hamstring muscles and muscle palpation may then help to implicate the hamstring muscle group. In addition, negative physical testing procedures would be required to negate the other possible structures at fault, that is, the lumbar spine, sacroiliac joint, hip joint and other posterior hip muscles.

The second assumption, in identifying the source of the symptoms, is that if an abnormality is detected in a structure, which theoretically could refer symptoms to the symptomatic area, then that structure is suspected to be a source of the symptoms. For example, if a patient has pain over the inner aspect of the forearm, wrist, and into the little and ring finger, the C8 and T1 nerve roots would be suspected as a source of the symptoms because this is the dermatome area of these nerve roots. Clearly, further examination of the cervical spine would be needed to confirm or refute this.

Having identified the underlying assumptions, the information from the subjective and physical examinations, which informs the hypothesis category of source of symptoms, will now be discussed. Where relevant, reference will be made to the in-depth clinical reasoning form (Appendix). Finding the source of the patient's symptoms may require information from the following:

Body chart

It is critical for the clinician to obtain accurate and comprehensive information for the body chart. This information includes the area, quality, depth, type and behaviour (in terms of intermittent or constant) of symptoms, as well as the all-important aspect of the relationship of symptoms. The body chart thus includes:

1. Area of symptoms. Structures underneath the area of symptoms, or structures which are known to refer to the area of symptoms, are automatically considered to be a possible source of the symptoms (question 1.1 of the clinical reasoning form, shown in the Appendix). A patient who complains of lateral elbow pain must be asked whether there is any pain or stiffness in the cervical spine, thoracic spine or shoulder, as these regions can refer pain to the lateral aspect of the elbow. Patients with neurological symptoms are more likely to report distal symptoms (Austen 1991, Dalton & Jull 1989).

2. Quality of the symptoms. The quality of symptoms for patients with and without neuro-logical deficit are similar (Austen 1991, Dalton & Jull 1989).

3. Depth of symptoms, although – like quality – this can be misleading (Austen 1991).

4. Abnormal sensation – paraesthesia for example – indicates a lesion of the sensory nerves. A knowledge of the cutaneous distribution of the nerve roots and peripheral nerves enables the clinician to distinguish the sensory loss due to a root lesion (dermatome pattern) from that due to a peripheral nerve lesion.

5. Constant versus intermittent symptoms. For example, constant unremitting pain, along with unexplained weight loss, would suggest malignancy as a possible source of the symptoms. Where symptoms are constant the clinician will explore, in the physical examination, movements that *ease* the patient's symptoms. These may then be used to treat the patient.

6. Relationship of symptoms. This is an extremely useful piece of information to guide the clinician to a hypothesis of the source of the symptoms. Symptoms are related when they come on at the same time and ease at the same time. If right neck pain and right lateral elbow pain come on at the same time, and ease at the same time, this would suggest that the cervical spine may be a source of both symptoms. If the patient has only one symptom at any one time, neck pain without elbow pain, and elbow pain without neck pain, this would suggest that there may be two separate problems – perhaps at the cervical spine, producing the neck pain, and a structure around the elbow, producing the elbow pain.

Sometimes, clinicians may ask the patient: 'do you think the symptoms are related?'. This can be a useful initial question to ask the patient as it may reflect their understanding of the symptoms and the condition. The question does not, however, provide accurate information as to the behavioural relationship of the patient's symptoms. The patient may think they are unrelated because:

a. they don't know that forearm pain can come from the spine

b. there is quite a different timescale in the history of the onset of each symptom

c. they don't think their neck ache is relevant
d. they really want you to understand that it is the forearm that bothers them, and that is why they have come for treatment.

Because of these alternative ways of understanding this question it is not helpful in determining the relationship of symptoms.

Simplicity is often the best strategy for obtaining accurate and meaningful information: asking the patient 'when the neck pain comes on, do you get the forearm pain?' and confirming a negative answer with 'so you have the forearm pain without any neck pain?'.

Behaviour of symptoms

Aggravating factors. The clinician asks the patient about their functional abilities and the effect of these activities on the symptoms. The clinician then analyses these movements to determine which structures are being stressed, and to what degree. Obviously, as has been mentioned earlier, each movement will stress a number of structures; the clinician therefore identifies the relative stress on each structure. The structure most stressed would be the most likely structure at fault, and the structure least stressed would be the least likely structure at fault. However, all structures stressed in any way, however minimal, could still be the source of the symptoms, and therefore the clinician cannot completely rule them out.

In addition to functional activities, the clinician asks the patient about theoretically known aggravating movements and postures, for structures which could be a source of the symptoms. For example, a patient may have one symptom, lateral elbow pain. This pain may be referred from the cervical or thoracic spine, from the shoulder region, or from the elbow region; it could be joint, nerve or muscle. The clinician gathers evidence to support or refute each of these regions as a source of the lateral elbow pain. The following questions provide some examples of the types of question that could be asked:

* 'Are there any neck/thoracic/shoulder/elbow/hand movements that you are now

unable to do?' These areas would be asked individually.
* 'Do you have any pain or stiffness in your neck?'
* 'Does turning your head to look over your shoulder produce any of your elbow pain?'
* 'Does sitting reading or looking up at the ceiling produce any of your elbow pain?'
* 'Do you have any pain or stiffness twisting (such as when reversing the car)?'
* 'Do you have any pain when you cough or sneeze?'
* 'Do you have any pain or stiffness lifting your arms above your head?'
* 'Do you have any pain or stiffness when you put your hand behind your back (when you tuck your shirt in, or do up your bra)?'
* 'Do you have any pain or stiffness on bending or straightening your elbow?'
* 'Do you have any problem twisting your arm (pronation/supination)?'
* 'Do you have any problem gripping?'

If a patient finds that elbow pain comes on only with forearm pronation and gripping it would suggest that there is a local problem and that the spine and shoulder are less likely to be implicated in the lateral elbow pain.

Easing factors. The clinician asks about movements or positions which ease the patient's symptoms. The clinician analyses the position and/or movement in terms of which structures are de-stressed. Again, a number of structures will be affected and the clinician needs to determine the relative de-stress of each structure in order to differentiate between possible structures. Positions and movements which ease the patient's symptoms are particularly useful for patients who have constant irritable symptoms (see precautions/contraindications).

Twenty-four-hour behaviour

If the patient's symptoms wake them at night, as a result of sustaining or changing a position, the clinician needs to analyse the position or movement in terms of the structures being stressed. This helps to determine the possible structures at fault which are giving rise to the patient's symptoms. For example, if the patient has left shoulder pain which wakes them when lying on the left shoulder, this could be due to compression of the shoulder region or it could be the position of the neck on the pillows. If, on further questioning, the clinician considers that the neck is well supported on pillows, and the patient wakes in the morning with no neck pain or stiffness, this might negate slightly the neck as the problem, and by deduction, implicate the shoulder region.

The last part of the subjective examination, the recent history (RH), can give very strong clues as to the source of the symptoms or dysfunction. In traumatic injuries in particular, the mechanism of the injury can help to clarify which structure(s) are at fault. For example, if medial knee pain came after a kick on the lateral aspect of the knee, which forced the lower leg into abduction, the medial structures around the knee would be particularly suspect as a source of the patient's symptoms. In addition, the recent history can help to clarify the relationship of the symptoms; for example, the patient may complain of neck and lateral elbow pain which, up to this point in the examination, may have been considered to be related, with the cervical spine suspected of being a source of both symptoms. However, the history of onset of these two symptoms may suggest otherwise: the patient may have had the neck pain for 10 years, the elbow pain for 2 months, and, when the elbow pain started, no change was felt in the neck pain. While this does not rule out the possibility of the neck as a source of the two symptoms, it would suggest that there may be two separate sources.

A hypothesis as to the source of symptoms and/or dysfunction is thus established from the various aspects of the subjective examination, the body chart, aggravating factors, easing factors, 24-hour behaviour of symptoms and recent history. This information will provide answers for question 1.1, in particular, of the clinical reasoning form (Appendix).

Production of symptoms

A common symptom that patients present with is pain. Pain is defined as 'an unpleasant sensory and emotional experience associated with actual or potential tissue damage, or described in terms of such damage' (Merskey et al 1979). Pain has been classified into nociceptive (mechanical, inflammatory or ischaemic), peripheral neurogenic, central, autonomic and affective (Gifford 1998).

Briefly, these mechanisms of pain can be described as follows:

1. Mechanical nociceptive pain is due to mechanical force on nociceptors, for example, lengthening or compressing tissue which contains nociceptors.

2. Inflammatory nociceptor pain is associated with injury to a tissue, producing an inflammatory reaction. The release of chemicals into the tissues sensitizes the nociceptors and produces pain.

3. Ischaemic nociceptor pain is produced by sustained stretch, or compression of collagenous tissue, or sustained activity of muscle, which alters the physical and chemical environment of the tissue, producing sensitization of nociceptors.

4. Peripheral neurogenic pain is pain arising from a peripheral nerve axon; this may be due to sustained stretch or pressure on an axon, or due to a severed axon.

5. Autonomic pain is due to increased sensitivity of the nociceptors from the secretion of catecholamines (adrenaline (epinephrine) and noradrenaline (norepinephrine)) from the sympathetic nervous system.

6. Affective pain is a result of emotions and cognition (beliefs). Emotion (or affect) affects the way the brain processes information, sensations felt, and the body's physiology and can lead to a perception of pain.

The clinical features of each of these mechanisms are given in Table 2.1. More than one mechanism may co-exist; for example, a patient with severe low back pain may have mechanical and inflammatory nociceptive pain with an affective component driven by the patient's emotional state. The clinician needs to be aware of the features of each mechanism to hypothesize which is responsible for producing the patient's pain.

Table 2.1 Clinical features of pain mechanisms

Pain mechanism	Clinical features
Mechanical pain	Particular movements that aggravate and ease the pain, sometimes referred to as 'on/off pain'
Inflammatory pain	Redness, oedema and heat Acute pain and tissue damage Close relationship of stimulus response and pain Diurnal pattern with pain and stiffness worst at night and in the morning Signs of neurogenic inflammation (redness, swelling or symptoms in neural zone) Beneficial effect of anti-inflammatory medication
Ischaemic pain	Symptoms produced after prolonged or unusual activities Rapid ease of symptoms after a change in posture Symptoms towards the end of the day or after the accumulation of activity Poor response to anti-inflammatory medication Absence of trauma
Neuropathic pain	Persistent and intractable Stimulus-independent pain: shooting, lancinating or burning pain Paraesthesia Dysaesthesia
Autonomic pain: early stage pain associated with:	Cutaneous capillary vasodilation Increased temperature Increased sweating Oedema Trophic changes: glossy skin, cracking nails Feeling of heaviness or feeling of swelling
Chronic stage pain associated with:	Coldness Pallor Atrophy of skin – skin flaking Atrophy of soft tissue Joint stiffness Hair loss
Affective pain	Loneliness Hopelessness Sadness Fear Anger

This information will provide answers for question 1.2 of the clinical reasoning form shown in the Appendix.

At the end of the subjective examination the clinician needs to develop a working hypothesis as to the likely source of the symptoms and/or dysfunction and the pain mechanism (question 1.3 of the clinical reasoning form in the Appendix). Positive and negating evidence, from throughout the subjective examination, needs to be considered. The clinician is then able to plan the physical examination, determining which physical tests need to be carried out in order to clarify the source of the patient's symptoms.

Physical testing includes observation, active movements, passive movements, muscle tests, nerve tests and palpation and accessory movements. It is worth mentioning here that each examination procedure is impure and does not test only what its name suggests. A joint test is not a pure joint test, a muscle test is not a pure muscle test, and a nerve test is not a pure nerve test. For example, isometric muscle testing predominantly tests the ability of a muscle to contract isometrically; however, to do this it requires normal neural input and any accompanying joint movement must be symptom-free. Thus, while isometric muscle testing is predominantly a test of muscle, it is also, to some degree, a test of nerve and joint function. Some further examples to highlight this are given in Table 2.2. The reason that this is emphasized is that it needs to underpin the analysis of physical examination findings. If the clinician assumes that the tests are pure, and that a muscle test tests only muscle, then a positive muscle test may be misinterpreted to be indicative of a muscle problem.

Broadly speaking, the aim of the physical examination is to reproduce all, or part, of the patient's symptoms (if the symptoms are non-severe and non-irritable). If symptoms are severe and/or irritable then the aim of the physical examination is to find movements and positions that ease all, or some, of the symptoms. When a test reproduces or eases the patient's symptoms it implicates those structures being stressed or eased by that test. Analysis of the structures predominantly affected by the test will enable the clinician to narrow down the possible structures at fault. By the end of the physical examination the clinician can use all the evidence from the subjective and physical examinations to develop a hypothesis as to the source of the symptoms and/or dysfunction. The

Table 2.2 Analysis of physical tests

Physical tests	Physical test	Involves/tests
Observation	Static and dynamic postures	Emotional state of patient Entire neuromusculoskeletal system
Active and passive movements	Active physiological movements	Patient's willingness to move Muscle strength and length Nerve input to muscle Motor control Joint function
	Passive physiological movements	Patient's willingness to move and be moved Muscle length Joint function
Muscle tests	Isometric muscle test	Patient's willingness and motivation to do this Muscle strength and endurance Nerve input to muscle Joint function
	Muscle strength	Patient's willingness and motivation to do this Muscle strength and endurance Nerve input to muscle Joint function
	Muscle control	Movement control of brain Muscle function
	Muscle length	Joint function to move Nerve function to movement
	Palpation of muscle	Includes palpation of skin and nerve tissue
Nerve tests	Nerve integrity tests	
	Neurodynamic tests	Muscle function to move Joint function to move
	Palpation of nerve	Includes palpation of skin and muscle
Joint test	Accessory movements	Affects any overlying soft tissues Affects muscles attaching to bone Affects local nerves
	Palpation of joint	Includes palpation of skin and overlying muscle

clinician can arrive at a physical clinical diagnosis that will help to provide a basis for their treatment and management of the patient.

The diagnosis will identify where the symptoms are believed to be emanating from, and will vary with the tissue. For example, if a joint is felt to be the source of the patient's symptoms, the clinician may identify altered accessory or physiological movement. If a muscle is felt to be the source of the patient's symptoms, the clinician may hypothesize that there is a muscle or tendon tear, or a muscle contusion. If a nerve is felt to be the source of the patient's symptoms they may hypothesize a reduction in nerve length or a nerve compression injury. Most of these descriptors provide some guidance for treatment and management, but are quite limited.

Generally, the clinician examines the patient to identify a movement dysfunction. While there are a number of known pathological processes leading to specific signs and symptoms, for instance, a tear of the medial meniscus of the knee, or a lateral ligament sprain of the ankle, a large majority of patients with neuromusculoskeletal dysfunction have signs and symptoms which do not clearly identify a known pathology. Evidence includes the fact that normal age-related changes seen on spinal X-ray are often not related to the patient's signs and symptoms (CSAG 1994). Provocative discography of degenerative intervertebral discs reproduces symptoms in only 20% of patients (Klafta & Collis 1969). Moreover, provocative discography of a disc protrusion reproduces symptoms in only 30% of patients (Klafta & Collis 1969). Knowledge of pathology and clinical syndromes is, however, valuable to the clinician who is then able to recognize the signs and symptoms that suggest these conditions and, where necessary, refer to a medical practitioner.

The difficulty of linking signs and symptoms to pathology led to the concept of the permeable brick wall adapted from Maitland et al (2001) and shown in Box 2.1. The left-hand column depicts the knowledge and skills that the clinician brings to the therapeutic relationship. The right-hand column depicts the knowledge and skills that the patient brings to the relationship. The world-wide web has given patients easy access to information about their condition, and they may come with some knowledge of anatomy, biomechanics, physiology etc. The interrupted vertical line of 'bricks' between the clinician and the patient is the 'permeable brick wall' which identifies that sometimes the patient's clinical presentation will fit with a known textbook description of a disorder and the clinician is able to see the link between theory and practice. On other occasions the patient's presentation does not fit, the bricks are in the way, and the clinician cannot make 'features fit'. Where a patient presents with a known textbook description of, for example, a prolapsed intervertebral disc, then the wall is permeable, the clinician is able to link the textbook information to the patient's presentation. However, when a patient's presentation does not fit a known documented presentation, then the clinician is unable to make the link. Where this occurs, the concept states that the patient's presentation is true and sure, and is to be believed, regardless of the fact that the clinician is not able to link the presentation to any theoretical framework.

The clinical reasoning process advocated in this and the companion text (Petty & Moore 2001) assumes this model of thinking: the clinician is concerned with movement dysfunction, not pathology. Occasionally it may be possible to identify a known pathology, that is, where the brick wall is permeable, but more often than not the clinician identifies a movement dysfunction, with a hypothesis as to the structure causing the patient's symptoms and factors contributing to the onset and continuation of these symptoms. For this reason the reader is referred to the numerous pathology textbooks available for details of known pathologies and their clinical presentation.

The clinical diagnosis used by the expected reader of this text will be related to movement dysfunction, and treatment will aim to restore that movement. The meaning of the word 'diagnosis' includes 'the identification of the cause of a mechanical fault' (Oxford English Reference Dictionary 1996), and it is this meaning that is used in this text. The patient presents with pain, for example, and the clinician seeks to identify where that pain is emanating from. For this reason other pieces of information are added to the clinical diagnosis to describe the movement dysfunction fully and this often involves simply identifying the positive physical tests. For example:

'A patellofemoral joint problem giving anterior knee pain which is a mechanical nociceptive pain, which is not severe and not irritable. There is a tight lateral retinaculum pulling the patella laterally during eccentric control of knee flexion, which is eased with a medial glide of the patella'.

'A right C4/5 zygapophyseal joint dysfunction giving one area of pain in the right side of the neck and the lateral upper arm, which is an inflammatory and mechanical nociceptive pain and is not severe and not irritable. A component of the pain is thought to be a neural interface, as there is a positive upper limb tension test 2a, biasing the median nerve (ULTT2a). Cervical movements exhibit a regular compression pattern'.

It can be seen that the above descriptions provide a summary of the main findings of the

---

Box 2.1 Permeable brick wall (after Maitland et al 2001, with permission)

The clinician		The patient
	▌	Clinical presentation:
Beliefs	▌	Beliefs
Values	▌	Values
Experience	▌	Experience
Skill	▌	Skill
Anatomy	▌	Anatomy
Biomechanics	▌	Biomechanics
Physiology	▌	Physiology
Pathology	▌	Pathology
Diagnosis	▌	Diagnosis
Theories	▌	Theories
Research findings	▌	Research findings

examination. The descriptions revolve around the physical testing procedures, which are by nature tests of movement. Having said this, there are exceptions, such as identifying a possible torn meniscus, a spondylolisthesis, a prolapsed intervertebral disc, as well as identifying serious pathology that may require medical intervention; these are considered under precautions and contraindications.

Factors contributing to the condition

These factors include environmental, behavioural, emotional, physical or biomechanical factors (Jones 1994). One or more factors may be responsible for the development, or maintenance, of the patient's problem. Environmental factors, such as the patient's work station or their tennis racket, will be identified in the social history of the subjective examination. Behavioural and emotional factors will be identified throughout the subjective and physical examination as the clinician becomes aware of the patient's attitude towards themselves, the clinician, and the condition. Physical and biomechanical factors, such as a short leg, poor posture or reduced muscle length, will be identified from the physical testing procedures carried out in the physical examination. At the end of the subjective and physical examination, the clinician needs to develop a hypothesis as to which, if any, of these factors may be contributing to the patient's problem. This information would inform question 2 of the clinical reasoning form shown in the Appendix. The extent to which these factors are thought to be contributing to the patient's condition will determine when they are addressed in the management of the patient.

Precautions for physical examination and/or treatment

This hypothesis serves a number of purposes. It helps to identify patients who are appropriate for neuromusculoskeletal treatment, whether there are any precautions for examination and treatment, to avoid exacerbation of their condition, and to avoid unnecessary discomfort for

the patient. These aspects will be discussed in turn.

Screening patients for neuromusculoskeletal treatment

The first over-arching purpose is to identify patients who are appropriate for treatment and to screen out those who are not. The clinician determines whether the patient's symptoms are emanating from a mechanical neuromusculoskeletal disorder or whether the symptoms are due to some other disease process. If the symptoms are being produced from a neuromusculoskeletal disorder then treatment is appropriate; if not then neuromusculoskeletal therapy may not be appropriate, and referral to a medical practitioner may be needed. Having identified that the patient is suitable for treatment, the clinician must then decide how the physical examination, and later treatment, needs to be tailored to the patient's presentation.

Precautions for examination and treatment

Information from the subjective examination provides vital information on any precautions to joint and nerve mobilization, and this is summarized in Table 2.3. A brief explanation of the possible causes underlying the finding is given and, where appropriate, the implications for examination and/or treatment. This information would guide the response to question 3 of the clinical reasoning form shown in the Appendix. For further information on the clinical presentation of pathological conditions the reader is referred to suitable pathology textbooks such as Goodman & Boissonnault (1998) and Grieve (1981).

As well as the identifying any precautions for neuromusculoskeletal examination and treatment, the clinician needs to identify, as early as possible, how best to examine the patient. The clinician needs to make every effort to avoid exacerbating the patient's condition, and this is done by identifying the irritability of the symptoms. The clinician also needs to be able to explore fully the patient's neuromusculoskeletal system without provoking unnecessary discomfort for

Table 2.3 Precautions to spinal and peripheral passive joint mobilizations and nerve mobilizations

Aspects of subjective examination	Subjective information	Possible cause/implication for examination and/or treatment
Body chart	Constant unremitting pain	Malignancy, systemic, inflammatory cause
	Symptoms in the upper limb below the acromion or symptoms in the lower limb below the gluteal crease	Nerve root compression Carry out appropriate neurological integrity tests in physical examination
	Widespread sensory changes and/or weakness in upper or lower limb	Compression on more than one nerve root, metabolic (e.g. diabetes, vitamin B12), systemic (e.g. RA)
Aggravating factors	Symptoms severe and/or irritable	Care in treatment to avoid unnecessary provocation or exacerbation
Special questions	Feeling unwell	Systemic or metabolic disease
	General health: –history of malignant disease, in remission	Not relevant
	-active malignant disease if associated with present symptoms	Contraindicates neuromusculoskeletal treatment, may do gentle maintenance exercises
	-active malignant disease not associated with present symptoms	Not relevant
	-hysterectomy	Increased risk of osteoporosis
	Recent unexplained weight loss	Malignancy, systemic
	Diagnosis of bone disease (e.g. osteoporosis, Paget's, brittle bone)	Bone may be abnormal and/or weakened. Avoid strong direct force to bone, especially the ribs
	Diagnosis of rheumatoid arthritis or other inflammatory joint disease	Avoid accessory and physiological movements to upper cervical spine and care with other joints
	Diagnosis of infective arthritis	In active stage immobilization is treatment of choice
	Diagnosis of spondylolysis or spondylolisthesis	Avoid strong direct pressure to the subluxed vertebral level
	Systemic steroids	Osteoporosis, poor skin condition requires careful handling, avoid tape
	Anticoagulant therapy	Increase time for blood to clot. Soft tissues may bruise easily.
	HIV	Check medication and possible side-effects
	Pregnancy	Ligament laxity, may want to avoid strong forces
	Diabetes	Delayed healing, peripheral neuropathies
	Bilateral hand/feet pins and needles and/or numbness	Spinal cord compression, peripheral neuropathy
	Difficulty walking	Spinal cord compression, peripheral neuropathy, upper motor neurone lesion
	Disturbance of bladder and/or bowel function	Cauda equina syndrome
	Perineum (saddle) Anaesthesia/paraesthesia	Cauda equina syndrome
	For patient's with cervicothoracic symptoms: dizziness, altered vision, nausea, ataxia, drop attacks, altered facial sensation, difficulty speaking, difficulty swallowing, sympathoplegia, hemianaesthesia, hemiplegia	Vertebrobasilar insufficiency, upper cervical instability, disease of the inner ear
	Heart or respiratory disease	May preclude some treatment positions
	Oral contraception	Increased possibility of thrombosis – may avoid strong techniques to cervical spine
	History of smoking	Circulatory problems – increased possibility of thrombosis
Recent history	Trauma	Possible undetected fracture, e.g. scaphoid

the patient; this is done by identifying the severity of the patient's symptoms.

Severity of the symptoms

The clinician determines the severity of every symptom. If the symptoms are constant: the symptoms are deemed to be severe if the patient reports that a single movement, which increases this pain, is so severe that the movement has to be stopped. If the symptoms are intermittent: the symptoms are deemed to be severe if a single movement produces symptoms that are so severe that the movement has to be stopped. Severe symptoms will limit the extent of the physical examination. The clinician would, in this situation, aim to examine the patient as fully as possible, but within the constraints of the patient's symptoms. The effect of severe pain on active movements is given below as an example of how a physical test has to be adapted.

Active movements would involve the patient moving to a point just *before* the onset of (or increase in) the symptom, or just *to* the point of onset (or increase), and would then immediately return to the starting position. No overpressures would be applied. This requires the clinician to give clear instructions to the patient. For example, if active shoulder flexion is being examined the clinician may instruct the patient in the following way (emphasis is in italics):

Intermittent severe symptom: 'Lift your arm up in front of you, and *as soon as you think you are about to get your arm pain*, bring your arm down again' or 'lift your arm up in front of you, and *as soon as you get your arm pain*, bring your arm down again'.

Constant severe symptom: 'Lift your arm up in front of you, and *as soon as you think your arm pain is going to increase*, bring your arm down again' or 'lift your arm up in front of you, and *as soon as your arm pain increases*, bring your arm down again'.

For passive movements, the patient may be asked to say as soon as they think they are *about to* feel their symptom (intermittent), or feel it is *about to* increase (constant). In both cases, pain is avoided. Alternatively, the patient may be able to tolerate movement just to the onset (or increase) of the symptom. The clinician would carry out the passive movement and, under the instruction of the patient, take the movement to only the first point of pain – and then immediately return to the starting point. In both situations the clinician must give clear instructions to the patient. For example, for passive shoulder flexion, the clinician may instruct the patient in the following way (emphasis is in italics):

Intermittent symptoms: 'I want to move your arm, but I want you to *tell me as soon as you think you are about* to get your arm pain, and I'll bring your arm down'.

'I want to move your arm, but I want you to *tell me as soon as you get your arm pain*, and I will bring your arm down'.

Constant symptoms: 'I want to move your arm, but I want you to *tell me as soon as you think you are about* to get more of your arm pain, and I'll bring your arm down'.

'I want to move your arm up, but I want you to *tell me as soon as you get more of your arm pain*, and I will bring your arm down'.

The clinician must be able to control the movement and carry it out very slowly. This is necessary in order to avoid overshooting and causing unnecessary symptoms and to obtain an accurate measure of range of movement for reassessment purposes. This process is depicted in Figure 2.4.

Irritability of the symptoms

The irritability of the symptoms is the degree to which the symptoms increase and reduce with provocation. When a movement is performed, and pain is provoked, for example, and this provoked pain continues to be present for a length of time, then the pain is said to be irritable. While in the previous text (Petty & Moore 2001) a period of 2–3 minutes was given, this text gives no definite time period. Any period of time that is required for symptoms to return to their resting level is classified as irritable. In order to avoid a

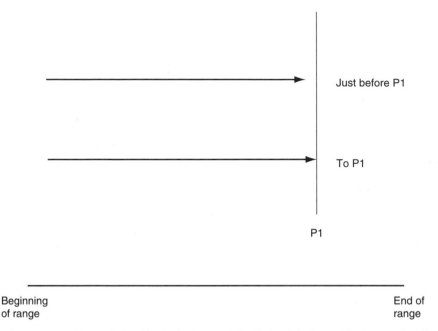

Just before P1

To P1

P1

Beginning
of range

End of
range

Figure 2.4 A passive movement is carried out just prior to, or at, the first point of onset (or increase) of the symptom (P1).

gradual increase in resting symptoms, a time delay will be required between provocative testing procedures. This will increase the appointment time, which may not be possible in a busy department. As well as this, repeatedly provoking symptoms and then waiting for them to settle will add little to the clinician's understanding of the patient's condition. For this reason, an alternative strategy is used whereby movements are carried out within the symptom-free range; irritable symptoms are not provoked at all.

For the examination of active movements for a patient with intermittent symptoms, the patient would move to a point just before the onset of the symptoms and then immediately return to the start position. In this way, symptoms are not provoked and therefore there will be no lingering symptoms. For example, if active shoulder flexion is being examined, the clinician may instruct the patient in the following way (emphasis is in italics):

Intermittent symptoms: 'Lift your arm up in front of you, and *as soon as you think you are about to get your arm pain*, bring your arm down again'.

Constant symptoms: 'Lift your arm up in front of you and *as soon as you think your arm pain is going to increase*, bring your arm down again'.

For passive movements, the patient may be asked to say as soon as they think they are *about to* feel the symptom (intermittent), or feel that it is *about to* increase (constant). In both cases, pain is avoided. The clinician must give clear instructions to the patient. For example, for passive shoulder flexion, the clinician may instruct the patient in the following way (emphasis is in italics):

Intermittent symptoms: 'I want to move your arm, but I want you to *tell me as soon as you think you are about to get your arm pain*, and I'll bring your arm down'.

Constant symptoms: 'I want to move your arm, but I want you to *tell me as soon as you think you are about to get more of your arm pain*, and I'll bring your arm down'.

For irritable symptoms, whether intermittent and constant, it is particularly important that the clinician clarifies after each movement the patient's resting symptoms, to avoid exacerbating symptoms.

Special questions

This section of the subjective examination is concerned with identifying precautions to examination and treatment, and is summarized in Table 2.3. The special questions ask about known pathological conditions of the patient as well as those symptoms which may suggest a pathological condition. The implication of such pathologies and symptoms, on the examination and treatment of the patient, is suggested. Some of this information has been obtained from pathology textbooks, for example Goodman & Boissonnault (1998), and some is simply suggested by the author. The reader should note this limitation.

A patient who feels generally unwell may be suffering from a systemic or metabolic disease. For the presence of malignant disease, but in remission, there are no precautions to examination or treatment. If, on the other hand, there is active malignancy, then the primary aim of the day one examination will be to clarify whether or not the presenting symptoms are being caused by the malignancy or whether there is a separate neuromusculoskeletal disorder. If there is a separate neuromusculoskeletal disorder then there are no precautions to examination and treatment. If the symptoms are thought to be associated with the malignancy then this may contraindicate most neuromusculoskeletal treatment techniques, although gentle maintenance exercises may be given.

A patient who has had a hysterectomy may be at an increased risk of osteoporosis. Recent unexplained weight loss is a common sign associated with malignancy and systemic diseases. The clinician will ascertain whether they have diagnosed a bone disease. Osteoporosis and Paget's disease produce abnormal and weakened bone which would increase the risk of fractures, particularly over the ribs. For this reason the presence of bone disease would contraindicate strong direct forces applied to bone.

A diagnosis of inflammatory joint disease such as rheumatoid arthritis would contraindicate accessory and physiological movements to the upper cervical spine and care is needed in applying forces to other joints. The reason for this is that inflammatory arthritis weakens ligaments, particularly in the upper cervical spine. This increases the risk of subluxation or dislocation of the C1/C2 joint, which may cause spinal cord compression.

A diagnosis of infective arthritis, in the active stage, requires immobilization. For this reason, neuromusculoskeletal therapy is contraindicated.

The presence of spondylolysis or spondylolisthesis would contraindicate strong direct pressure to the subluxed vertebral level as this might increase the subluxation and cause spinal cord or cauda equina compression.

Systemic steroids can weaken the skin and lead to osteoporosis. For this reason the patient requires careful handling and avoidance of tape so that the skin is not damaged. The clinician should be aware that osteoporosis weakens bones and so strong direct forces to the bones may be inadvisable.

Anticoagulant therapy causes an increase in the time for blood to clot. The clinician needs to be aware that this may cause soft tissues to bruise when force is applied.

If a patient has been diagnosed with HIV, their medication may have side-effects that will affect neuromusculoskeletal treatment.

If a patient is pregnant there will be ligament laxity. This may cause a reduction in joint stiffness and an increase in range of joint movement. Excessive forces may be inadvisable.

Diabetes can cause delayed healing and so affect the patient's prognosis. Diabetes is also associated with peripheral neuropathies.

Bilateral pins and needles or numbness in both hands and/or both feet may be due to spinal cord compression.

There are obviously many reasons why a patient may have difficulty walking; of concern here is the possibility of spinal cord compression, an upper motor neurone lesion or peripheral neuropathy. These may be further tested in the physical examination by carrying out neurological integrity tests, including the plantar response.

Disturbance of bladder or bowel function may be due to compression on the cauda equina. Loss of sensation or paraesthesia in the perineum is also suggestive of cauda equina compression.

Dizziness, altered vision, nausea, ataxia, drop attacks, altered facial sensation, difficulty speaking, difficulty swallowing, sympathoplegia, hemianaesthesia, hemiplegia indicate vertebrobasilar insufficiency (VBI), upper cervical instability or disease of the inner ear. A lack of blood supply to the vestibular nuclei in the brainstem causes dizziness, the most common symptom of VBI (Bogduk 1994).

Heart or respiratory disease may preclude some treatment positions; for example, the patient may not tolerate lying flat.

Oral contraception and smoking are each associated with an increased risk of thrombosis. For this reason strong techniques to the cervical spine are inadvisable for patients taking oral contraceptives.

A traumatic onset of symptoms may give helpful clues as to the source of the patient's symptoms as the mechanism of the injury is analysed in detail. There is the possibility of a fracture underlying a traumatic incident; for example, a fall on the outstretched hand may cause a scaphoid fracture which is sometimes difficult to identify on X-ray.

The reader is referred to pathology textbooks for further information on pathological conditions and their clinical presentation. The reader is then encouraged to read an excellent chapter that highlights the challenge of clinical practice to distinguish benign neuromusculoskeletal conditions from serious pathologies (Grieve 1994). Safe clinical practice requires a constant awareness, by the clinician, that what appears straightforward may not be.

Prognosis of the condition

The clinician needs to develop a hypothesis as to whether the patient's condition is suitable for neuromusculoskeletal treatment and management, and the likely prognosis. A large number of positive and negative factors from throughout the subjective examination will inform this hypothesis. These factors include the patient's age, general health, lifestyle, attitude, personality, expectations and attitude towards their condition, towards themselves and towards the clinician, as well as the mechanical versus inflammatory nature of the symptoms, severity and irritability of the symptoms, degree of tissue damage and length of time and progression of the condition. By considering all of these factors, the clinician is then able to provide the patient with a hypothesis as to how long and to what extent the symptoms may be eased with treatment. The prognosis is as specific as possible for the patient. At discharge, it is useful for the clinician to compare the final outcome with the predicted outcome; this reflection will help the clinician to learn and enhance their ability to hypothesize in the future. A hypothesis could, for example, be: 'will restore full range of movement in the shoulder region, and completely alleviate the shoulder pain; neck pain and stiffness will be reduced by 50%'. This information would provide answers for question 5 of the clinical reasoning form shown in the Appendix.

Management

Management can be considered in two phases: the initial appointment on day one and the follow-up appointments.

Initial appointment

The clinician develops a plan as to how to treat and manage the patient and the condition. The first step in this process occurs between the subjective and physical examinations. At this point, the clinician must decide what structures are suspected to be a source of the symptoms and need to be examined in the physical examination. Along with any precautions or contraindications, a plan of the physical examination is developed. The aims of the physical examination are to:

- identify the source of the patient's symptoms
- confirm, if necessary, any precautions or contraindications, for example, identify the presence of spinal cord compression
- further explore, if relevant, any factors contributing to the patient's condition, for example, measure leg length.

In order to identify the source of the symptoms the clinician uses the information from the subjective examination to predict the findings of the physical examination. This includes:

- the structures thought to be at fault
- which tests are likely to reproduce/alter the patient's symptoms
- how the tests need to be performed to reproduce/alter the patient's symptoms; for example, combined movements may be required
- what other structures need to be examined in order to disprove them as a source of the symptoms.

The process then involves putting the possible structures at fault in priority order and planning the physical examination accordingly. The information would provide answers for question 4.1 in the clinical reasoning form shown in the Appendix.

At the end of the physical examination the clinician needs to reflect on all the information from both the subjective and physical examinations and to develop a treatment and management plan. Almost all the information obtained will be used in this process. The information would provide answers for questions 4.2–4.8 of the clinical reasoning form shown in the Appendix.

The physical testing procedures which specifically indicate joint, nerve or muscle tissues as a source of the patient's symptoms are summarized in Table 2.4. At one end of the scale the findings may provide strong evidence, and at the other end they may provide weak evidence. Of course, one may find a variety of presentations between these two extremes.

The strongest evidence that a joint is the source of the patient's symptoms is that active and passive physiological movements, passive accessory movements and joint palpation all reproduce the patient's symptoms, and that following a treatment dose, reassessment identifies an improvement in the patient's signs and symptoms. For example, let us assume a patient has lateral elbow pain caused by a radiohumeral joint dysfunction. In the physical examination there is limited elbow flexion and extension movements due to reproduction of the patient's elbow pain, with some resistance. Active movement is very similar to passive movement in terms of range, resistance and pain reproduction. Accessory movement examination to the radiohumeral joint reveals limited posteroanterior and anteroposterior glide of the radius due to reproduction of the patient's elbow pain with some resistance. Following the examination of accessory movements, sufficient to be considered a treatment dose, reassessment of the elbow physiological movements are improved, in terms of range and pain. This scenario would indicate that there is a dysfunction at the radiohumeral joint – first, because elbow movements, both active and passive physiological, and accessory movements, reproduce the patient's symptoms, and second, because, following accessory movements, the active elbow movements are improved. Even if the active movements are made worse, this would still suggest a joint dysfunction because it is likely that the accessory movements would predominantly affect the joint, with much less effect on nerve and muscle tissues around the area. Collectively, this evidence would suggest that there is a joint dysfunction, as long as this is accompanied by negative muscle and nerve tests.

Weaker evidence includes an alteration in range, resistance or quality of physiological and/or accessory movements and tenderness over the joint, with no alteration in signs and symptoms after treatment. One or more of these findings may indicate a dysfunction of a joint which may, or may not, be contributing to the patient's condition.

The strongest evidence that a muscle is the source of a patient's symptoms is if active movements, an isometric contraction, passive lengthening and palpation of a muscle, all reproduce the patient's symptoms, and that following a treatment dose, reassessment identifies an improvement in the patient's signs and symptoms. For example, let us assume that a patient has lateral elbow pain caused by lateral epicondylalgia, a primary muscle problem. In this case reproduction of their lateral elbow pain is found on active wrist and finger extension, isometric contraction of the wrist extensors and/or

Table 2.4 Physical tests which, if positive, indicate joint, nerve and muscle as a source of the patient's symptoms

Test	Strong evidence	Weak evidence
Joint		
Active physiological movements	Reproduces patient's symptoms	Dysfunctional movement: reduced range, excessive range, altered quality of movement, increased resistance, decreased resistance
Passive physiological movements	Reproduces patient's symptoms; this test same as for active physiological movements	Dysfunctional movement: reduced range, excessive range, increased resistance, decreased resistance, altered quality of movement
Accessory movements	Reproduces patient's symptoms	Dysfunctional movement: reduced range, excessive range, increased resistance, decreased resistance, altered quality of movement
Palpation of joint	Reproduces patient's symptoms	Tenderness
Reassessment following therapeutic dose of accessory movement	Improvement in tests which reproduce patient's symptoms	No change in physical tests which reproduce patient's symptoms
Muscle		
Active movement	Reproduces patient's symptoms	Reduced strength Poor quality
Passive physiological movements	Do not reproduce patient's symptoms	
Isometric contraction	Reproduces patient's symptom's	Reduced strength Poor quality
Passive lengthening of muscle	Reproduces patient's symptom's	Reduced range Increased resistance Decreased resistance
Palpation of muscle	Reproduces patient's symptoms	Tenderness
Reassessment following therapeutic dose of muscle treatment	Improvement in tests which reproduce patient's symptoms	No change in physical tests which reproduce patient's symptoms
Nerve		
Passive lengthening and sensitizing movement i.e. altering length of nerve by a movement at a distance from patient's symptoms	Reproduces patient's symptoms and sensitizing movement alters patient's symptoms	Reduced length Increased resistance
Palpation of nerve	Reproduces patient's symptoms	Tenderness

finger extensors, and passive lengthening of the extensor muscles to the wrist and hand. These signs and symptoms are found to improve following soft-tissue mobilization examination, sufficient to be considered a treatment dose. Collectively, this evidence would suggest that there is a muscle dysfunction, as long as this is accompanied by negative joint and nerve tests.

Further evidence of muscle dysfunction may be suggested by reduced strength or poor quality during the active physiological movement and the isometric contraction, reduced range, and/or increased/decreased resistance, during the passive lengthening of the muscle, and tenderness on palpation, with no alteration in signs and symptoms after treatment. One or more of these findings may indicate a dysfunction of a muscle which may, or may not, be contributing to the patient's condition.

The strongest evidence that a nerve is the source of the patient's symptoms is when active and/or passive physiological movements reproduce the patient's symptoms, which are then increased or decreased with an additional sensitizing movement, at a distance from the patient's symptoms. In addition, there is reproduction of the patient's symptoms on palpation of the nerve, and following neurodynamic testing – sufficient to be considered a treatment dose – an improvement in the above signs and symptoms.

For example, let us assume this time that the lateral elbow pain is caused by a neurodynamic dysfunction of the radial nerve supplying this region. The patient's lateral elbow pain is reproduced during the component movements of the upper limb tension test 2b (ULTT 2b) and is eased with ipsilateral cervical lateral flexion sensitizing movement. There is tenderness over the radial groove in the upper arm and, following testing of the ULTT2b, sufficient to be considered a treatment dose, an improvement in the patient's signs and symptoms. Collectively, this evidence would suggest that there is a neurodynamic dysfunction, as long as this is accompanied by negative joint and muscle tests.

Further evidence of nerve dysfunction may be suggested by reduced range (compared to the asymptomatic side) and/or increased resistance to the various arm movements, and tenderness on nerve palpation.

It can be seen that the common factor for identifying joint, nerve and muscle dysfunction as a source of the patient's symptoms is reproduction of the patient's symptoms, alteration in the patient's signs and symptoms following a treatment dose, and lack of evidence from other potential sources of symptoms. It is assumed that if a test reproduces a patient's symptoms then it is somehow or other stressing the structure at fault. As mentioned earlier, each test is not purely a test of one structure – every test, to a greater or lesser degree, involves all structures. For this reason, it is imperative that, whatever treatment is given, it is proved to be of value by altering the patient's signs and symptoms. The other factor common in identifying joint, nerve or muscle dysfunction is the lack of positive findings in the other possible tissues; for example, a joint dysfunction is considered when joint tests are positive and muscle and nerve tests are negative. Thus the clinician collects evidence to implicate tissues and evidence to negate tissues – both are equally important. The reader is reminded of the earlier analogy of the detective who must collect evidence to prove the guilt or innocence of all possible suspects. The classification of joint, nerve and muscle used in this textbook is summarized in Table 2.5.

The first priority of treatment will be to address the source of the patient's symptoms, and later any relevant contributing factors. The types of treatment for joint, nerve and muscle are summarized in Table 2.6.

Good clinical practice requires that the clinician knows the effects of their treatment. This involves continual assessment of the patient at each attendance, so that the effect of the previous treatment is known, and after the application of each treatment technique within a treatment session. Any significant finding relevant to the patient's problem, in the subjective and physical examinations, is highlighted in the clinical notes by using asterisks (*) for ease of reference. These subjective and physical findings are referred to as 'asterisks' (Maitland 1991) or 'markers'. Rather than fully re-examine the patient at each attendance, the clinician simply checks with the patient any change in these asterisks from the subjective examination, and re-tests the physical asterisks. In this way, the clinician obtains an overview of any change in the patient's condition by looking at the key features of the patient's presentation. Aspects of the subjective findings, which may be used as reassessment asterisks, include:

- information from the body chart
- aggravating factors
- easing factors

Table 2.5 Joint, muscle and nerve dysfunctions

Joint dysfunction	Muscle dysfunction	Nerve dysfunction
Hypomobility	Reduced length	Reduced length
Altered quality of movement		
Symptom production	Symptom production	Symptom production
	Reduced strength, power and endurance	
	Altered motor control	Altered nerve conduction

Table 2.6 Types of joint, muscle and nerve treatment techniques

Joint	Muscle	Nerve
Accessory movement	Strength, power and endurance training	
Physiological (active or passive) movement	Passive or active lengthening of muscle	Passive or active lengthening of nerve
Accessory with physiological (active or passive) movement		
Soft-tissue mobilizations (includes frictions)	Soft-tissue mobilizations (includes frictions)	Soft-tissue mobilizations (includes frictions)
Exercises to enhance motor control and coordination	Exercises to enhance motor control and coordination	Exercises to enhance motor control and coordination
PNF	PNF	PNF
Taping	Taping	Taping
Electrotherapy	Electrotherapy	Electrotherapy

- functional ability
- drug therapy
- 24-hour behaviour.

Aspects of the physical examination will include any abnormal joint, nerve and muscle test.

Follow-up appointments

Following treatment, both within and between treatment sessions, the subjective and physical asterisks may alter. However, they may not change in the same way: some may improve, some may worsen or some may remain the same. The clinician has to make an overall judgement as to whether the patient has improved, worsened or stayed the same. It can be useful, when making this judgement, to consider the weighting of each test.

A change in subjective asterisks would seem to be fairly strong evidence that there has been a change. A patient who is able to increase the time ironing or walking, or is able to sleep better, for example, seems fairly clear, although the response will depend, in part, on the patient's attitude to their problem, to the clinician and towards treatment, which may positively or negatively affect the patient's response. Further questioning of any change is always needed to clarify that it is the condition that has improved and not something else. For example, if sleeping has improved, the clinician checks the details of the nature of that improvement, and whether there is any other explanation, such as a new mattress or a change in analgesia etc. that would explain the improvement.

The change in the physical findings also needs careful and unbiased analysis by the clinician. A test must be carried out in a reliable way for the clinician to consider that a change in the test is a real change. That is, a test must – as far as possible – be replicated within and between treatment sessions so that any change in the test result can be considered a real change. Clearly, some of the tests carried out are easier to replicate than others. For example, a change in an active movement is rather more convincing than the clinician's 'feel' of a passive physiological intervertebral movement (PPIVM). The clinician will do well to evaluate critically their reassessment asterisks and consider carefully how much weight they can place upon them, when they interpret a change.

At each attendance, the clinician needs to obtain a detailed account of the effect of the last treatment on the patient's signs and symptoms. This will involve the immediate effects after the last treatment, the relevant activities of the patient since the last treatment, and enquiring how they are presenting on the day of treatment. Patients who say they are worse since the last treatment need to be questioned carefully as this will often be due to some activity they have been involved with rather than any treatment that has been given. Patients who say they are better also need to be questioned carefully as the improvement may not be related to treatment. If the patient remains the same, following the subjective and physical reassessment, the clinician may consider altering the treatment dose and then seeing whether this alteration has been effective. The process of assessment, treatment and assessment is depicted in Figure 2.5. After, perhaps, the third attendance it may be useful to reflect on the response of the patient to treatment. Suggested prompts are given in question 6 of the clinical reasoning form shown in the Appendix.

The more long-term effects of treatment are determined by comparing the subjective and physical asterisks at a follow-up appointment, with the findings at the initial assessment. The clinician's hypotheses from the initial examination of the patient are often rather tenuous and are strengthened at each subsequent treatment session as the effects of treatment become known. Critical in this process is the reassessment of all joint, nerve and muscle asterisks following a treatment, as this allows the clinician to develop a hypothesis of the relationship between the structures. For example, a unilateral posteroanterior pressure to C4 that improves both cervical movements, and a positive neurodynamic test, would suggest a common source of symptoms and a possible neurodynamic interface problem; where this treatment improves only cervical movements, with no change to the neurodynamic test, it may suggest two separate problems. For further information the reader is referred to the relevant chapter on assessment by Maitland et al (2001).

After the patient has been discharged it may be useful for the clinician to reflect on the overall management of the patient by completing question 7 of the clinical reasoning form shown in the Appendix.

This completes the discussion on assessment. Two case studies now follow to help clarify the development and implementation of treatment and the management of two patients. The case studies are organized such that the left-hand column provides the clinical examination findings of the patient. The right-hand column provides the thoughts and thus the interpretation of the clinician; these are not firm conclusions – they simply provide the on-going generation of hypotheses as the information is revealed. It is hoped that, in this way, the clinical reasoning process will be made very explicit.

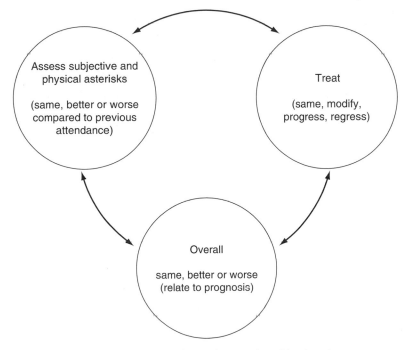

Figure 2.5 Modification, progression and regression of treatment.

REFERENCES

Austen R 1991 The distribution and characteristics of lumbar-lower limb symptoms in subjects with and without a neurological deficit. In: Proceedings of the Manipulative Physiotherapists Association of Australia, 7th biennial conference, New South Wales, p 252–257

Bogduk N 1994 Cervical causes of headache and dizziness. In: Boyling J D, Palastanga N (eds) Grieve's modern manual therapy, 2nd edn. Churchill Livingstone, Edinburgh, ch 22, p 317–331

CSAG 1994 Report on back pain. Clinical Standards Advisory Group. HMSO, London

Dalton P A, Jull G A 1989 The distribution and characteristics of neck-arm pain in patients with and without a neurological deficit. Australian Journal of Physiotherapy 35(1):3–8

Gifford L 1998 Pain. In: Pitt-Brooke J, Reid H, Lockwood J, Kerr K (eds) Rehabilitation of movement, theoretical basis of clinical practice. W B Saunders, London, ch 5, p 196–232

Goodman C C, Boissonnault W G 1998 Pathology: implications for the physical therapist. W B Saunders, Philadelphia

Grieve G P 1981 Common vertebral joint problems. Churchill Livingstone, Edinburgh

Grieve G P 1994 The masqueraders. In: Boyling J D, Palastanga N (eds) Grieve's modern manual therapy, 2nd edn. Churchill Livingstone, Edinburgh, ch 63, p 841–856

Higgs J, Jones M 2000 Clinical reasoning in the health professions, 2nd edn. Butterworth-Heinemann, Oxford

Jensen G M, Gwyer J, Hack L M, Shepard K F 1999 Expertise in physical therapy practice, Butterworth-Heinemann, Boston

Jones M A 1994 Clinical reasoning process in manipulative therapy. In: Boyling J D, Palastanga N (eds) Grieve's modern manual therapy, 2nd edn. Churchill Livingstone, Edinburgh, ch 34, p 471–489

Jones M A, Jones H M 1994 Principles of the physical examination. In: Boyling J D, Palastanga N (eds) Grieve's modern manual therapy, 2nd edn. Churchill Livingstone, Edinburgh, ch 35, p 491–501

Klafta L A, Collis J S 1969 The diagnostic inaccuracy of the pain response in cervical discography. Cleveland Clinical Quarterly 36:35–39

Maitland G D 1991 Peripheral manipulation, 3rd edn. Butterworth-Heinemann, London

Maitland G D, Banks K, English K, Hengeveld E 2001 Maitland's vertebral manipulation, 6th edn. Butterworth-Heinemann, Oxford

Merskey R, Albe-Fessard D G, Bonica J J et al 1979 Pain terms: a list with definitions and notes on usage. Pain 6:249–252

Petty N J, Moore A P 2001 Neuromusculoskeletal examination and assessment – a handbook for therapists, 2nd edn. Churchill Livingstone, Edinburgh

Case study 1

Case study 1 for a patient with arm and hand symptoms.

32-year-old female

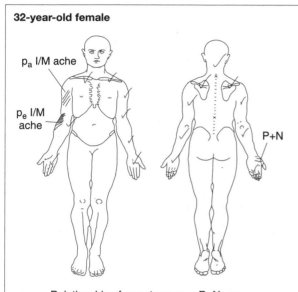

p_a I/M ache

p_e I/M ache

P+N

Relationship of symptoms p_a = P+N = p_e

Clinical reasoning

Area of symptoms suggests that the following structure may be implicated. For upper arm pain: cervical spine (somatic or radicular); shoulder: upper limb nerves or underlying muscles; for forearm pain: cervical spine (somatic or radicular), elbow or superior radioulnar joint, radial or median nerves or underlying muscles. P+N: radial nerve, or radicular referral from cervical spine (?C5, C6)

All symptoms are intermittent; this suggests a mechanical nociceptive pain, but the presence of P+N may suggest a peripheral neurogenic component

Relationship of symptoms

Pe can occur independently of P+N and Pa. P+N occur only in the presence of Pe. Pa occurs with worsening Pe and P+N

The onset of each symptom is linked, which suggests a single source of symptoms i.e. cervical spine nerve root (? C5 or C6) or neurodynamic component

Aggravating factors

Typing for 5 mins Pe, increases after 20 mins and onset of P+N. After 2 hours Pa

Cutting bread (gripping) Pe immediately, P+N occasionally, no Pa

Arm in coat Pe and P+N immediately, no Pa

Cervical spine movements √√
Cervical spine stiffness √√

Arm elevation √√
Lying on shoulder √√

Elbow movements √√
Supination/pronation √√

Identifies source of symptoms as follows: cervical spine (somatic or radicular), shoulder, elbow or superior radioulnar joint, radial or median nerves or underlying muscles

Radial nerve, shoulder, elbow, superior radioulnar joint

Negates cervical spine
Negates cervical spine

Negates shoulder
Negates shoulder

Negates elbow
Negates superior radioulnar

Because of the positive relationship of symptoms, the spine must continue to be suspected as a source of symptoms. However, because gripping does not involve movement of the cervical spine, peripheral structures must be fully examined

Severity

Typing – can continue after onset of symptoms
Cutting bread – can continue
Single movements do not reproduce symptoms

Not severe, as the patient can continue activities which reproduce her symptoms

In terms of the physical examination. Single movements do not reproduce symptoms. It will therefore be necessary to combine active movements in order to reproduce Pa, Pe and P+Ns

Irritability

Typing – eases immediately if ceased within 30 mins
Cutting bread – eases immediately when stops
Arm in coat – eases immediately

Non-irritable, as the symptoms cease immediately unless they are reproduced for a prolonged period of time. Because the examination will not equate with more than 30 mins of typing, this is considered to be non-irritable in terms of the physical examination

24-hour behaviour

Wakes 2x per night with P+N, ?? lying on arm, no Pe or Pa.
No pain on waking
Pain activity dependent during day

Nerve pain can be worse at night, may be either cervical spine radicular or peripheral nerve

Special questions

None of note

No precautions or contraindications

History of present condition

Onset of symptoms approximately 6 months ago. ?? cause. Patient noticed Pe first. Approx 1 month later P+N onset at time of worsening Pe. Noticed Pa about 4 weeks ago during a period of increased typing at work and increase in Pe and P+N. Problem ISQ at present

Provides supporting evidence that all the symptoms are related

Past medical history

Nil of note, no history of musculoskeletal pain

First episode of pain, so good prognosis

Social history

Touch typist, can be typing for up to 8 hours per day

Must assess and educate patient about keyboard positioning to try to prevent future recurrence if appropriate, as this may be a contributory factor

Plan of physical examination

Contradictory evidence was gained from the subjective examination. The relationship of symptoms and the HPC and aggravating factors suggested that there is a single source of symptoms. This, together with the body chart, would implicate the cervical spine. However, the aggravating factors for cervical spine were negative Therefore, when examining the cervical spine it will be necessary to use combined movements

The aggravating factors, together with the body chart, implicate the elbow region and radial nerve as a source of symptoms

Although the aggravating factors could also have implicated the shoulder region, the area of symptoms Pe and P+N and the relationship of symptoms, negate this as a source

The plan for day one is therefore to examine fully the elbow and radial nerve and cervical spine. Clearing the shoulder region is not a priority. Because of P+N a neurological integrity test will be necessary

Physical examination

Observation In sitting

Increased thoracic kyphosis, protracted shoulder girdle and poking chin

Cervical spine active movements

F/LLF/Lrot √√
F/RLF/Rrot √√
E/LLF/Lrot √√
E/RLF/Rrot √√

Active movements

Elbow joint / radioulnar joint

F √√
E √√
Sup √√
Pro √√
F /FAbd/Add √√
E abd √√ .
E Add grinding of joint ++ and reproduction of Pe (20%)

Clinical reasoning

Very poor posture may increase the strain on the neuro-musculoskeletal system. This may be a contributing factor

No symptom reproduction, suggesting that the cervical spine is not a source of symptoms. In order to exclude fully the cervical spine as a source of symptoms it will be necessary to perform accessory movements of the cervical spine, followed by reassessment of asterisks

This suggests that elbow structures are a source of symptoms for Pe. ?? May suggest more radiohumeral than superior radioulnar

Neurological integrity testing

Sensation √√
Myotomes √√
Reflexes √√

Nothing abnormal
Negates cervical radiculopathy

ULTT 2b (radial nerve bias)

Left – Shoulder depression / medial rot / pronation / wrist flexion / elbow extension / Abduction 40 degrees – strong stretch in forearm – reduced with left cervical lateral flexion

Right – Shoulder depression / medial rot / pronation / wrist flexion / elbow extension – 45 degrees Pe and P+N, decreased with right cervical lateral flexion

Suggests a neurodynamic component for production of Pe and P+Ns

Isometric muscle testing

Wrist extension – Pe (20%) – strength 50%
Middle finger extension – Pe (30%)
Wrist flexion √√
Gripping – Pe (50%)

Suggests muscle as a source of symptoms
Suggests that extensor carpi radialis brevis may be a source of symptoms

Cervical spine accessory movements

In neutral √√
In combined positions √√

Negates cervical spine

Reassessment

Active movements of elbow – ISQ
ULTT 2b – ISQ
Isometric muscle tests ISQ

Provides further evidence that the cervical spine is not the source of symptoms or an interface for the neurodynamic component

Palpation of elbow region

Tenderness around the right common extensor origin Pe (10%). No tenderness left

With the result of isometric muscle tests, strongly suggests extensor muscles as a source of symptoms

Accessory movements – elbow

Humeroulnar √√

Radial head ↨ reproduce Pe (20%) IV+

Suggests radiohumeral or superior radioulnar joint as a source of Pe

Radial head ↨ in flexion – no Pe IV+

Suggests more radiohumeral than superior radioulnar as amount of flexion changes response

In ULTT 2b (radial nerve bias) ↨ radial head Pe (50%) and P+N no Pa

Suggests mechanical interface to radial nerve for source of Pe and P+N

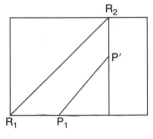

Reassess

E / Add elbow – Pe (10%)

Suggests a local joint component

ULTT 2b Right – Shoulder depression / medial rot/pronation / wrist flexion / elbow extension – 30 degrees Pe and P+N

Provides further evidence that the radial head is a mechanical interface affecting Pe and P+Ns

Isometric muscle testing – ISQ

Suggests a separate muscular component

Impression

There is evidence to suggest wrist extensor muscles, radiohumeral joint and radial nerve local to the elbow. Evidence from the physical examination negates a cervical component

Plan

Clear glenohumeral joint

Because there is no strong evidence from the subjective examination that the glenohumeral joint is not a source of symptoms it will be necessary to clear this in the physical examination D2

Discuss work ergonomics and give advice on alterations as necessary

In ULTT 2b (at P_1) ↨ radial head IV + 3 × (30 secs)

This was the technique of choice because it was the most provocative procedure and on reassessment asterisks improved. Grade IV+ was chosen because it was a resistance problem and in order to achieve the greatest effect it is necessary to work as far into resistance as pain allows

Day 2

Patient reports no change in subjective markers. No soreness after treatment
Discussed work position, patient will contact occupational health for an ergonomic assessment

E / Add elbow grinding of joint – Pe (20%)

ULTT 2b Right – Shoulder depression / medial rot / pronation / wrist flexion / elbow extension – 45 degrees Pe and P+N

No change

Isometric muscle testing – ISQ
In ULTT 2b (radial nerve bias) $\downarrow$ radial head Pe (50%) and P+N no Pa

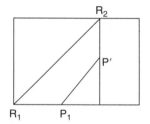

Glenohumeral joint

Combined movements in positions related to – aggravating factors √√

Negates glenohumeral joint

Accessory movements √√
Reassessment of asterisks ISQ

Treatment

In ULTT 2b (at P_1) $\downarrow$ radial head IV+ 3 × (30 secs)

Reassessment

E /Add √√

ULTT 2b Right – Shoulder depression / medial rot / pronation / wrist flexion / elbow extension – 20 degrees Pe and P+N

This suggests that the joint and nerve components are related (for example the radial head and the radial nerve). With a separate muscle component

Isometric muscle testing – ISQ

Day 3

Typing 10–15 mins Pe, P+N after 30 mins no Pa.
Cutting bread ISQ

Increased time before onset of Pe and P+Ns. No Pa.
Indicates an improvement

Arm in coat √√

E /Add √√

ULTT 2b Right – Shoulder depression / medial rot /
pronation / wrist flexion / elbow extension – 30 degrees
Pe and P+N, decreased with right cervical lateral flexion

Isometric muscle testing – ISQ

In ULTT 2b (radial nerve bias) ↓ Pe (30%) and P+N no
Pa

Shows improvement in joint and nerve components, but
muscle component remains ISQ. Will need to address
muscle component separately

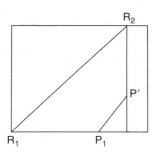

Specific soft-tissue mobilization assessment. Medial
glide in elbow extension most provocative Pe (40%)

Further assessment of muscle component

Treatment

In extension accessory (medial glide). SSTM to common
extensor origin IV+ 3 × (30 secs)

Reassessment

E /Add √√

No change

ULTT 2b Right – Shoulder depression / medial rot /
pronation / wrist flexion / elbow extension – 30 degrees
Pe and P+N

No change

Isometric muscle testing

Wrist extension Pe √√
Middle finger extension (20%)
Gripping (30%)

Improved, and so supports a separate muscle
component

Treatment 2

In ULTT 2b (at P_1) $\downarrow$ radial head IV+ 3 × (60 secs)

The duration of treatment has been increased in an attempt to gain quicker progress. It was felt that this treatment could be progressed despite adding a new treatment technique as the new technique aimed to address the muscle component and the initial technique had not affected the muscle component

Reassessment

ULTT 2b Right – Shoulder depression / medial rot / pronation / wrist flexion / elbow extension Pe and P+N

Isometric muscle testing – ISQ

Plan

Progress both treatments (addressing all components)

Assess effects of active neural/muscle mobilization (ULTT 2b) and if appropriate teach for home exercise

This would enable the patient to continue their own treatment and become less reliant on passive modalities

Ensure that ergonomic advice has been given

Case study 2

Case study 2 for a patient with back and lateral calf pain.

43-year-old male

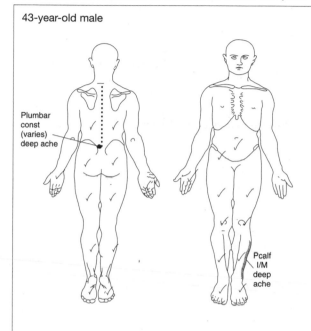

Plumbar
const
(varies)
deep ache

Pcalf
I/M
deep
ache

Clinical reasoning

Area of symptoms suggests the following structures may be implicated. For lumbar pain: lumbar spine or SIJ; for calf pain: referral from lumbar spine or SIJ, low lumbar neurodynamic, L5 dermatome or sclerotome, or L5/S1 nerve root, superior tibiofibular joint, peroneal muscles, common peroneal nerve

Constant but varying lumbar spine pain suggests inflammatory and mechanical component

Relationship of symptoms

Plumbar and Pcalf come on together – they are related

Lumbar spine and calf pain come on together, never separately, suggests that symptoms are related and therefore implicates lumbar spine, SIJ, L5/S1 nerve root, or a neurodynamic component as source of both symptoms

Aggravating factors

Bending forward Plumbar, no Pcalf
Slump sitting: Plumbar immediately and, if knee extended, Pcalf
Sitting upright: no pains
Long sitting: both pains
Standing: no pains
Walking: no pains
Standing on one leg no pains
Turning over in bed no pains

Identifies the source of symptoms as follows:
lumbar spine/SIJ
lumbar spine/neurodynamic component
extension eases lumbar pain
lumbar spine/neurodynamic
extension asymptomatic, negates L5/S1 nerve root
extension asymptomatic, negates L5/S1 nerve root
not SIJ
not SIJ
Because of the positive relationship of symptoms and aggravating factors linking lumbar spine/neurodynamic structures to all of the patient's symptoms, the superior tibiofibular joint and peroneal muscles are removed from the hypothesis of possible structures at fault

Severity

Bending forward – able to stay with pain

Not severe

Irritability

Returning to extension eases pain immediately

Not irritable

easing factors:
lying prone eases both pains

Eased by extension +/– not weight-bearing. Negates L5/S1 nerve root

24-hour behaviour

Not woken, first thing in morning stiff in lumbar spine for 15 mins only

More mechanical than inflammatory

Special questions

Nil of note

No precautions or contraindications

History of present condition

Moving washing machine 10 days ago felt Plumbar as bending over and pushing with left foot in front of right. Next morning on rising felt Pcalf as well as Plumbar. Patient thinks just strained his back and wants some exercises to help reduce his pain

Recent onset with expected inflammatory component. Position of injury suggests neurodynamic component Patient has positive attitude to his problem, appropriate expectations, and is confident of improvement. Relationship again emphasizes relationship of symptoms

Stage (or status) of condition

No change, still has both pains to same intensity

Need to try to produce a change with treatment

Past medical history

Nil of note. No history of LBP, calf pain

First episode of low back pain, so good prognosis. Must educate patient about back pain to get a speedy recovery this time and educate to try to prevent a recurrence in the future

Social history

Services washing machines, full-time job, often having to move machines. Still working. Plays football 2 × a week, not been playing since injury

Must educate patient on moving and handling. Need to make appointments convenient to his work. Need to encourage his return to football. Still at work – good prognostic indicator

Physical examination

Observation in standing: nil of note

Active movements

Identifies source of symptoms as follows:

lumbar:
*flex fingertips to base of patella, Plumbar overpressure
increased Plumbar and produced Pcalf

Lumbar spine/SIJ

with cervical flexion: increased calf pain

With neurodynamic component

with pelvic compression: pain ISQ ext full range no pain
on OP

Not SIJ

lat flex L full range no pain on OP

As expected, negates L5/S1 nerve root
As expected, negates L5/S1 nerve root

lat flex R full range no pain on OP

As expected

rotation L full range no pain on OP

As expected

rotation R full range no pain on OP

As expected

*flex/R lat flex 1/4 range lat flex Poalf OP increased
Plumbar & Pcalf

Lumbar spine/neurodynamic component

flex/L lat flex full range no pain on OP

Movements of flexion, contralateral lateral flexion
suggests a regular stretch pattern

SIJ

Standing flex NAD

Not SIJ

Sitting flex NAD

Not SIJ

Hip flex ipsilateral   NAD

Not SIJ

   contralateral   NAD

Not SIJ

Active movements confirm relationship of symptoms
and a flexion related problem

Neurological integrity

Sensation   NAD

No neurological deficit, negates L5/S1 nerve root

Strength   NAD

compromise

Reflexes   NAD

Neurodynamic tests

*SLR   60 degrees   Plumbar
     70 degrees   Plumbar & Pcalf

plantarflexion eased Pcalf

Neurodynamic component

Accessory movements

Central PA L4 and L5 stiff and tender
Unilateral PA left L4 tender
Unilateral PA left L5 stiff and Plumbar, with cephalad
inclination increased Plumbar

L5/S1 symptomatic level producing both pains

Movement diagram of unilateral PA left L5

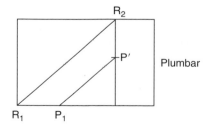

Resistance problem with a little pain. Treatment grade of
movement could be IV or IV+

In lumbar flexion/R lat flex did unilateral PA L5 with ceph inclination: Plumbar, no Pcalf

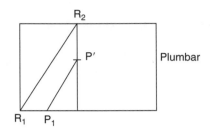

Maximum pain provoked in combined position but calf pain not produced, suggests mechanism of pain production of Plumbar and Pcalf different; perhaps Plumbar mechanical nociceptive, Pcalf neurodynamic. In combined position more pain at L5 than L4: confirms L5/S1 level rather than L4/5

‖ Lumbar flex fingertips 2″ lower PISQ
‖ Flex/R lat flex ISQ
‖ SLR ISQ

On reassessment: some improvement, examination may not have done sufficient to produce a strong therapeutic effect

SIJ

AP/PA/Longitudinal caud/ceph NAD

Not SIJ

‖ Lumbar flex fingertips 2″ below base patella PISQ
‖ Flex/R lat flex ISQ
‖ SLR ISQ

On reassessment no improvement. Final confirmation not SIJ

Source of symptoms:

L5/S1 dysfunction with a neurodynamic component giving rise to mechanical nociceptive pain in the leg and inflammatory nociceptive ache in the lumbar spine

PPIVM reduced flexion/lat flex R & rotation L L5/S1 otherwise NAD

Confirms flexion hypomobility L5/S1. May use rotation/SLR as treatment technique
Explanation of above given to the patient. Discussed and agreed treatment plan

Treatment day 1

Unilateral PA with ceph
Inclination left L5 Grade IV × 1 (1 min)

Try at the most symptomatic level. Grade IV to reduce resistance and increase range

‖ Lumbar flex fingertips 3″ below base patella increased
‖ Plumbar OP increased Plumbar and produced Pcalf
‖ Flex/R lat flex 1/4 range lat flex Pcalf OP increased
‖ Plumbar & Pcalf
‖ SLR ISQ

Slightly further lumbar flexion, pain the same

ISQ

ISQ

Unilateral PA with ceph inclination left L5 Grade IV × 1 (1 min)

Try another repetition

‖ Lumbar flex FT 3″ below base of patella & Plumbar
‖ 'less', OP increased Plumbar and produced Pcalf
‖ flex/R lat flex 1/3 range lat flex Pcalf OP increased
‖ Plumbar & Pcalf but 'less'
‖ SLR ISQ

Less pain now on lumbar flexion

Combined movement improved in range and pain

No change in SLR

Unilateral PA with ceph
Inclination left L5 Grade IV × 1 (1 min)

‖ Lumbar flex FT mid calf increased Plumbar, OP
increased Plumbar and produced Pcalf
Flex/R lat flex 1/2 range lat flex no Pcalf OP increased
Plumbar & Pcalf but 'less than before'
‖ SLR   ISQ

Three repetitions of mobilization treatment has improved
flexion and combined movement of flexion and lateral
flexion. No improvement on SLR, may need to treat neurodynamic component next time

Explained probable cause of back and leg pain and
explained natural history of back pain. Patient motivated
to look after his back

Must try to prevent a re-occurrence
Patient's motivation is excellent; this may help to prevent this acute injury becoming a chronic condition

Day 2

Patient felt less back and calf pain for 2 hours after last
treatment, then ISQ. Has not had to lift at work, on light
duties

Some lasting improvement for 2 hours, good sign that
further treatment will have longer symptomatic relief.
Patient must be looking after back, good

‖ Lumbar flex FT 3″ above base patella increased
Plumbar, OP increased Plumbar and produced Pcalf
Flex/R lat flex 1/3 range lat flex no Pcalf OP increased
Plumbar & Pcalf
SLR   ISQ
‖ Movement diagram of unilat PA left L5

Maintained some improvement in flexion and combined
flex/lat flex range

SLR not changed by treatment yet

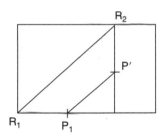

Movement diagram also maintained some improvement

Unilateral PA with ceph inclination left L5 Grade IV+ × 3
(1 min)

Need to progress treatment: increase Grade to a IV+
since pain eased and good response to last treatment

‖ Lumbar flex FT mid calf increased Plumbar, OP
increased Plumbar and produced Pcalf.
Flex/R lat flex 1/2 range lat flex no Pcalf OP increased
Plumbar & Pcalf
‖ SLR   ISQ

Improved range

Improved range and no calf pain now at end of active
range. Still no change, need to treat neurodynamic
component

Unilateral PA with ceph inclination left L5 Grade IV+ × 3 (1 min) in flexion/R lat flex	Fully progress joint treatment
Lumbar flex FT mid calf increased Plumbar, OP increased Plumbar and less Pcalf. Flex/R lat flex 1/2 range lat flex no Pcalf OP increased Plumbar & Pcalf, but less intense SLR ISQ	Progression of joint treatment has improved lumbar spine movements, but has had no effect on neurodynamic component. Need to treat SLR directly
Mobilized SLR with hip flexion movement to approx 60 degrees, producing lumbar spine and some calf pain ×1 (1 min)	Start with a movement that provokes part of the calf pain, don't want to exacerbate the calf pain. If no flare up progress to stronger movement
Lumbar flex ISQ as above flex/R lat flex ISQ as above SLR 70 degrees increased Plumbar, 80 degrees increased Plumbar and produced Pcalf	No effect on lumbar movements SLR improved in range
Repeat SLR treatment as above × 1 (1 min)	
Lumbar flex range ISQ but Plumbar and Pcalf 'less' flex/R lat flex ISQ as above SLR 75 degrees increased Plumbar, 85 degrees increased Plumbar and produced Pcalf	SLR treatment eased calf pain on lumbar flexion No change to combined movement SLR improved in range
Repeat SLR treatment as above ×1 (1 min)	
Lumbar flex slight increase in range and Plumbar & Pcalf 'less' flex/R lat flex ISQ as above SLR 80 degrees increased Plumbar, 85 degrees increased Plumbar and produced Pcalf	SLR treatment increased range as well as reduced calf pain; no change to combined movement Further improvement in SLR range
Patient agreed to do daily SLR stretches (every 2 hours) Explanation given Patient to attend 6 week back care classes in the physiotherapy department	Need to ask patient to continue treatment at home Need to educate patient to prevent a re-occurrence

Day 3

Exercises feel they are 'loosening up the back and leg pains'. Back pain not constant anymore. Much less calf and back pain since last treatment. Able to bend forwards more easily and can slump sitting without just a little calf pain. In long sitting in the bath only has some calf pain, able to straighten left knee down now
Back feels less stiff in morning

The patient is improving at a satisfactory rate. The inflammatory pain in the lumbar spine is settling which is expected as it is 15 days post injury
All original functional difficulties are improving

‖ No resting symptoms
Lumbar flex FT mid calf Plumbar, OP increased Plumbar and produced Pcalf
flex/R lat flex 1/2 range lat flex OP increased Plumbar & Pcalf
SLR   80 degrees Pcalf only movement diagram of
‖ unilat PA left L5

Maintained improvement

Maintained improvement

Improved with home exercises. Doing them correctly and frequently

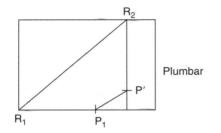

Plumbar

Movement diagram also Improved since last treatment

In flexion/right lateral flexion did unilateral PA with ceph inclination left L5 Grade IV+ × 3 (1min)

Progress treatment by applying PA in the symptomatic combined position

‖ Lumbar flex FT ankle joint, OP produced some Pcalf.
flex/R lat flex full range lat flex OP some Pcalf
‖ SLR 85 degrees Pcalf

Range and pain improved
Range and pain improved
Improved range of SLR

Grade V rotation R manipulation L5/S1

‖ Lumbar flex FT ankle joint, OP no pain.
flex/R lat flex full range lat flex OP some Pcalf, but less
‖ SLR   85 degrees Pcalf ISQ

Some improvement in lumbar spine movements

mobilized SLR with hip flexion movement to approx 60 degrees, producing lumbar spine and some calf pain ×3 (1min)

‖ Lumbar flex FT ankle joint, OP no pain
flex/R lat flex full range lat flex OP slight Pcalf, 'much less than before'
‖ SLR 85 degrees Pcalf, 'less'

SLR treatment improved pain
SLR treatment improved pain

Less pain

Home exercises checked, to continue to do exercises and see in 1 week
Continuing with back care classes

Vast improvement, with home exercises the patient's condition should continue to improve

Day 4

No back or leg pain for last 4 days. Taking care of back and learnt how to move washing machines and generally how to look after back

This may help prevent re-occurrence

Lumbar flex full range and no pain on OP flex/R lat flex full range and no pain on OP SLR full range and no pain on OP movement diagram of unilat PA left L5

Asymptomatic
Asymptomatic
Asymptomatic

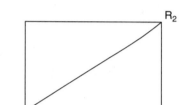

Asymptomatic

Discharged with advice

Must emphasize must continue to look after back if to prevent a re-occurrence

Appendix Clinical reasoning form

At the end of the subjective examination start to complete the form.
At the end of the physical examination answer the questions in **bold**.

1.1 Source of symptoms

Symptomatic area	Structures under area	Structures which can refer to area	Supporting evidence

1.2 What is the mechanism of each symptom? Explain from information from the subjective and **physical examination findings**

	Symptom:	Symptom:	Symptom:	Symptom:
Subjective				
Physical				

1.3 Following the physical examination what is your clinical diagnosis?

2. Contributing factors

2.1   What factors need to be examined/explored in the physical examination?

2.2 How will you address each contributing factor?

3. Precautions and contraindications

3.1   Are any symptoms severe?   Yes   No
      Which symptoms, and explain why

3.2   Are any symptoms irritable?   Yes   No
      Which symptoms, and explain why

3.3 How much of each symptom are you prepared to provoke in the physical examination?

Symptom	Short of P1	Point of onset or increase in resting symptoms	Partial reproduction	Total reproduction

3.4 Will a neurological examination be necessary in the physical?
          yes   no   Explain why

3.5 Following the subjective examination are there any precautions or contraindications?
          yes   no   Explain why

4. Management

4.1 What tests will you do in the physical and what are the expected findings?

Physical tests	Expected findings

4.2 *Were there any unexpected findings from the physical? Explain*

4.3 *What will be your subjective and physical reassessment asterisks?*

4.4 *What is your first choice of treatment (be exact) and explain why?*

4.5 *What do you expect the response to be over the next 24 hours following the first visit? Explain*

4.6 *How do you think you will treat and manage the patient at the 2nd visit, if the patient returns:*

Same

Better

Worse

4.7 *What advice and education will you give the patient?*

4.8 What needs to be examined on the 2nd and 3rd visits?

2nd visit	3rd visit

5 Prognosis

5.1 List the positive and negative factors (from both the subjective *and physical examination findings*) in considering the patient's prognosis?

	Positive	Negative
Subjective		
Physical		

5.2 Overall, is the patient's condition:
      improving   *worsening*   *static*

5.3 What is your overall prognosis for this patient? Be specific

6. After third attendance

6.1 Has your understanding of the patient's problem changed from your interpretations made following the initial subjective and physical examination? If so explain

6.2 On reflection, were there any clues that you initially missed, mis-interpreted, under- or over-weighted? If so explain

7. After discharge

7.1 Has your understanding of the patient's problem changed from your interpretations made following the third attendance? If so explain how

7.2 What you have learnt from the management of this patient which will be helpful to you in the future?

3

Function and dysfunction of joint

In this text, the term 'joint' generally refers to both the intra-articular and periarticular structures.

The function of the neuromusculoskeletal system is to produce movement and this is dependent on each component of the system, that is, normal function of joint, nerve and muscle. This interrelationship is depicted in Figure 3.1, which was a theoretical model originally devised to describe stability of the spine (Panjabi 1992a) but which is applicable to the entire neuromusculoskeletal system. Similarly, the stability of the knee joint has been described as 'a complex systematic sensory-motor synergy which includes the ligaments, antagonistic muscle pair (flexors and extensors), bones, and sensory mechanoreceptors in the ligaments, joint capsule, and associated muscles' (Solomonow et al 1987). This description could equally be applied to all peripheral joints, so while this chapter is concerned with the function of joints, it is important to highlight that the joint does not function in isolation but in a highly interdependent way with muscle and nerve. For a joint to function optimally there must be normal functioning of the relevant muscles and nerves.

Some examples of how joint, nerve and muscle function together to stabilize joints may help to highlight this close relationship. Anatomically, ligament is often not a separate distinctive tissue but blends together with muscle to form a unified stability system (Strasmann et al 1990). For example, in the spine the supraspinous ligament and the superficial part of the interspinous ligament actually form the attachment of longissimus

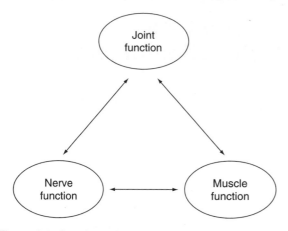

Figure 3.1 Interdependence of the function of joint, nerve and muscle for normal movement (after Panjabi 1992a, with permission). Normal function of the neuromusculoskeletal system requires normal function of joint, nerve and muscle.

thoracis pars thoracis (Adams et al 2002). In the lumbar spine, multifidus blends with the zygapophyseal joint capsule (Yamashita et al 1996), in the shoulder supraspinatus and teres minor blend with the glenohumeral joint capsule and at the knee biceps femoris fuses with the lateral collateral ligament (Williams et al 1995). So, anatomically, ligament and muscle appear to function together.

Stability of a joint is a function of joint stiffness (Panjabi 1992b), and this is provided not only by the joint capsule but also by skin, muscle and tendon. The relative contribution of these tissues has been estimated in the wrist of the cat, with the joint capsule providing 47% of joint stiffness, muscle 41%, tendon 10% and skin 2% (Johns & Wright 1962). In the human lumbar spine, a number of the ligaments are considered too weak to contribute significantly to joint stiffness and are regarded as transducers serving a proprioceptive function (Adams et al 2002, Panjabi 1992a). During lumbar spine flexion and extension, muscle has been found to augment segmental stability (Panjabi et al 1989, Wilke et al 1995). There is substantial evidence throughout the body that stability of joints is enhanced by muscle (Hortobagyi & DeVita 2000, Knatt et al 1995, Louie et al 1984, Louie & Mote 1987, McGill & Norman 1986, Panjabi et al 1989, Perry et al 1975,

Phillips et al 1997, Pope et al 1979, Shoemaker & Markolf 1982, Solomonow et al 1986, Solomonow et al 1987, Walla et al 1985, Wilke et al 1995).

The nervous system underpins this joint stability function of muscle. In the upper limb, stimulation of afferents in the medial ligament of the elbow causes activation of the muscles overlying this ligament (flexor carpi radialis, flexor carpi ulnaris, flexor digitorum profundus and flexor digitorum superficialis, and pronator teres). This is thought to be a protective reflex to avoid excessive ligamentous tension (Phillips et al 1997). In the lower limb, in the anaesthetized cat, passive ankle dorsiflexion causes activation of mechanoreceptors in the posterior joint capsule which produces a reflex facilitation of gastrocnemius and inhibition of tibialis anterior; similarly, passive plantarflexion causes activation of mechanoreceptors in the anterior joint capsule which produces facilitation of tibialis anterior and inhibition of gastrocnemius (Freeman & Wyke 1967a). In lumbar spine, the supraspinous ligament contains mechanoreceptors which, when stimulated, cause a reflex contraction of the multifidus muscle; this is thought to improve spinal stability (Indahl et al 1995, Indahl et al 1997, Solomonow et al 1998). Collectively, this research clearly links the interdependent relationship of joint, nerve and muscle in providing joint stability.

This section has sought to highlight the complex interdependent nature of joint with muscle and nerve. Various aspects of joint function will now be discussed.

JOINT FUNCTION

The following aspects of joint function will be considered:

- classification of joints
- anatomy, biomechanics and physiology of joint
- nerve supply of joint
- classification of synovial joints
- joint movement
- biomechanics of joint movement.

A joint is the junction between two or more bones, and the function of a joint is to permit limited movement and to transfer force from one bone to another (Nigg & Herzog 1999).

Classification of joints

Joints can be classified as either synarthrosis (not synovial) or diarthrosis (synovial) (Norkin & Levangie 1992). Synarthrosis joints are further divided into fibrous and cartilaginous joints (Fig. 3.2).

Fibrous joints can be further subdivided into suture joints, as in the joints of the skull, gomphosis joints, as in the joints between a tooth and the mandible or maxilla, and a syndesmosis joint between the shaft of the radius and ulna (Fig. 3.3). As the name suggests, in each type of joint fibrous tissue unites the joint surfaces and, as a result, only a small amount of movement is possible.

Cartilaginous joints can be further subdivided into symphysis, as in the symphysis pubis and the interbody joint (two vertebral bodies and the intervening disc) in the vertebral column (Figure 3.3), and synchondroses, as in the first chondrosternal joint. In this type of joint, fibrocartilage or hyaline cartilage directly unites the bone and, again, only a small amount of movement is possible.

Diarthrosis or synovial joints are characterized by having no tissue uniting each end of the bone; rather, a joint space exists, thus allowing movement to occur. Synovial joints are characterized by a fibrous joint capsule lined with a synovial membrane, the bone end being covered by hyaline cartilage with a film of synovial fluid. Fat pads lie within the synovial membrane, filling the irregularities and potential spaces within the joint, and ligaments and tendons lie either within

or adjacent to the joint. There may be a meniscus, for example in the knee joint, fibro-adipose meniscoids, for example in the zygapophyseal joints, a labrum, for example in the glenohumeral or hip joints, and bursae within the joint. Figure 3.4 identifies the features of two synovial joints, one with an intra-articular disc and one without.

Anatomy, biomechanics and physiology of joint tissues

Ligaments

Ligaments may be:

- named parallel bundles of the outer fibrous capsule
- intra-articular, as in the cruciate ligaments of the knee, the ligamentum teres of the hip and the intra-articular ligament of the costovertebral joint
- peri-articular, as in the lateral collateral ligament of the knee.

Ligaments consist of 70% water and 30% solids, with the solids made up of 70–80% collagen, 3–5% elastin, and the remainder a ground substance (Akeson et al 1987, Nordin & Frankel 1989). Ligaments attach directly to bone, that is, there is an abrupt well-defined area of attachment, with a clear demarcation of ligament and bone (Woo et al 1988). The ligament in direct attachments has a superficial layer blending with the periosteum and a larger, deep layer inserting directly into the bone via a layer less than 1 mm of fibrocartilage (Cooper & Misol 1970, Woo et al 1988). Sometimes, ligament attaches rather more indirectly, such that there is a more gradual and

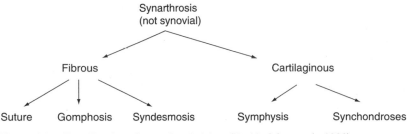

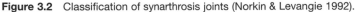

Figure 3.2 Classification of synarthrosis joints (Norkin & Levangie 1992).

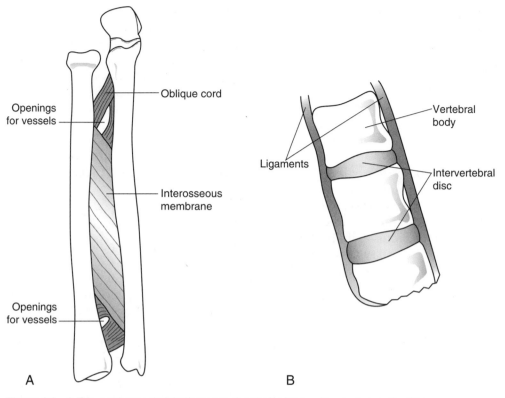

Figure 3.3 **A** The syndesmosis joint between the shaft of the radius and ulna; the fibrous interosseous membrane unites the two bones (from Palastanga et al 2002, with permission). **B** The symphysis joint between the vertebral bodies in the spine (from Palastanga et al 2002, with permission).

less distinct area of attachment (Woo et al 1988). Similar to direct attachments, the ligament has a superficial and deep layer. The superficial layer this time provides the predominant attachment, blending with the periosteum and bone via Sharpey's fibres (Woo et al 1988), while the deep layer attaches directly to the bone.

The collagen fibres in ligament are arranged in parallel bundles which have an undulated or 'crimping' appearance under the microscope (Frank & Shrive 1999) when they are relaxed. The ligament buckles under compression, and so it is only the stretching of ligament with tensile loading that is functionally important (Panjabi & White 2001). The crimping gives some slack to the ligament during minimal tensile loading (longitudinal stretching), and as it straightens out it provides some resistance (Frank & Shrive 1999, Threlkeld 1992). Figure 3.5 demonstrates

the change in fibre alignment during lengthening of a typical ligament.

The strength of connective tissue to tensile loading can be depicted on a force (or load) displacement curve, shown in Figure 3.6. The load or force is plotted against the stretch or deformation. In both load displacement and stress strain curves, the slope of the curve is the modulus of elasticity and is a measure of the 'stiffness' of the ligament (Panjabi & White 2001). It can be seen in Figure 3.6 that very little force is initially required to deform the ligament, a region referred to as the 'toe' region (Threlkeld 1992) or 'neutral zone' (Panjabi & White 2001). Stiffness then increases, so that greater force is required to deform the ligament; this region is referred to as the elastic zone (Panjabi & White 2001). Forces within the elastic zone will result in no permanent change in length; as soon as the force is released the tissue

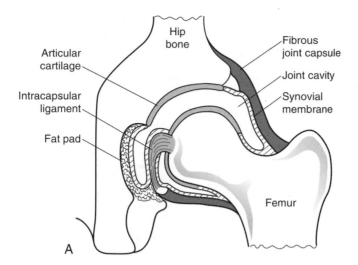

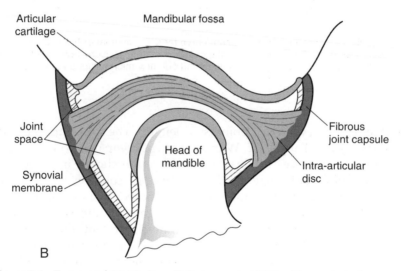

Figure 3.4   Two synovial joints (from Palastanga et al 2002, with permission). **A** Hip joint. **B** Temporomandibular joint with an intra-articular disc.

returns to its pre-load shape and size (Panjabi & White 2001). The neutral zone and elastic zone fall within the normal physiological range of forces and deformation on ligament during everyday activities (Nordin & Frankel 1989).

Towards the end of a joint's physiological range the force and deformation may be sufficient to cause micro-trauma of individual collagen fibres and bundles and to produce a permanent elongation of the connective tissue (Threlkeld 1992). A rough guide to the amount of force required to cause a permanent change in length has been estimated to be between 224 N and 1136 N (Threlkeld 1992), with micro-failure of connective tissue beginning at approximately 3% elongation, and macro-failure at approximately 8% (Noyes et al 1983). The point at which there is permanent deformation is termed the

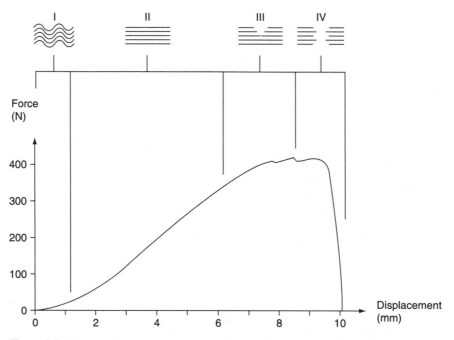

Figure 3.5 A typical force displacement curve for a ligament (after Frank & Shrive 1999, with permission). I = toe region where the collagen is crimped (schematic representation), II = linear region where collagen is straightened out, III = microfailure and IV = failure region.

'yield stress', and the region beyond this point is known as the plastic zone (Panjabi & White 2001). A further increase in force will lead to trauma and eventually failure of the ligament.

The progressive failure of the human anterior cruciate ligament of the knee can be seen in the force displacement curve in Figure 3.7. The early part of the curve relates to clinical testing of the anterior drawer test for the knee. During normal functional activities, forces occur within the physiological loading zone. Greater forces than this result in micro-failure, injury and eventually failure of the ligament. Figure 3.8 depicts various force displacement curves for other ligaments in the body. It can be readily seen that there are quite large variations between ligaments, reflecting differences in function.

If the strength of a ligament is to be compared to another tissue, then a stress strain curve can be drawn, where stress is the force per unit area (measured in Pa or N/m^2) and strain is the percentage change in length (from the resting length). The stress strain tensile properties of ligament compared to bone, cartilage, muscle and nerve are shown in Table 3.1. The stress strain curve of collagen, of which ligament is mostly composed, is shown in Figure 3.6.

Ligaments are viscoelastic, that is, they have time-dependent mechanical properties. These properties affect the behaviour of ligaments to movement and forces and are therefore important principles for clinicians. They can be summarized as:

• elastic nature
• viscous nature
• creep phenomena
• stress relaxation
• load dependent
• hysteresis.

The elastic nature means that ligaments will stretch and return to their original shape like an elastic band. The viscous nature means that ligaments will gradually elongate over a period of

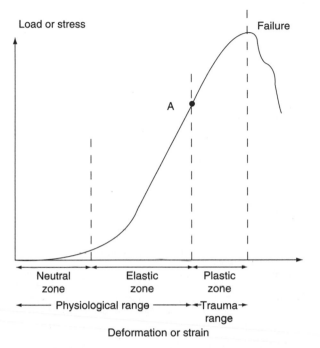

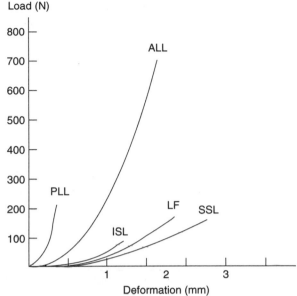

Figure 3.6   Load (or force) displacement curve or stress strain curve of connective tissue (after Panjabi & White 2001, with permission). The physiological range is divided into an initial neutral zone followed by an elastic zone. Further force causes trauma and enters the plastic zone. Point A is the junction between the elastic and temporary displacement, and the plastic and permanent displacement. This point is known as the yield stress and is the minimum stress necessary to cause a residual strain in the material.

Figure 3.8   Load displacement curves for various spinal ligaments (from Panjabi & White 2001, with permission). The slope of the curve of the posterior longitudinal ligament (PPL) is greatest, demonstrating greatest stiffness. Stiffness values gradually lessen with the anterior longitudinal ligament (ALL), interspinous ligament (ISL), ligamentum flavum (LF) and finally supraspinous ligament (SSL).

time, when a constant force is applied. The ability of ligaments to elongate gradually with a constant force (or load) is known as creep and is depicted in Figure 3.9 (Panjabi & White 2001). The magnitude of the force is below the linear region of the load displacement curve. The phenomenon of stress relaxation means that ligaments undergo load (or stress) relaxation. When the deformation is kept constant (Fig. 3.9), the force (or stress) within ligament decreases over time (Panjabi & White 2001).

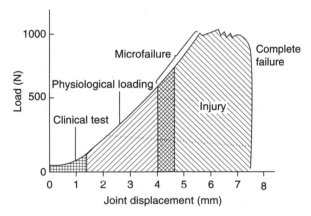

Figure 3.7   Load displacement curve of the anterior cruciate ligament of an in vitro human knee (from Nordin & Frankel 1989, with permission). The force displacement curve during the anterior draw test is depicted in the early toe region, with physiological loading in the linear region, followed by eventual microfailure and complete failure.

Table 3.1   Tensile properties of ligament compared to bone, cartilage, muscle and nerve (Panjabi & White 2001)

Tissue	Stress at failure (MPa)	Strain at failure (%)
Ligament	10–40	30–45
Cortical bone	100–200	1–3
Cancellous bone	10	5–7
Cartilage	10–15	80–120
Tendon	55	9–10
Muscle (passive)	0.17	60
Nerve roots	15	19

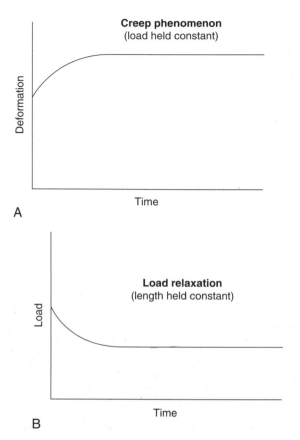

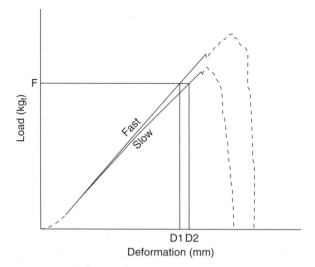

Figure 3.10 Ligament is load-dependent. It can be seen that a given force (F) applied quickly will produce a certain deformation (D1), and if applied more slowly will produce a greater deformation (D2) (after Noyes et al 1974, with permission).

Figure 3.9 Creep and load relaxation (from Nordin & Frankel 1989, with permission). **A** Creep is the increase in deformation that occurs when a constant load is applied over time. **B** Load relaxation is the decrease in stress within a ligament when a constant force is applied over a period of time.

Ligaments share load-dependent properties, that is, the stress-strain (or load-displacement) curve depends on the rate of loading. When the ligament is loaded quickly it will be stiffer and will deform less than when it is loaded more slowly (Fig. 3.10). This is relevant when applying therapeutic force, as a slower rate will result in less resistance and more movement. The additional effect of having load-dependent properties is that the failure point of the ligament will be higher with a higher loading rate; in other words, the ligament will be stronger and less likely to rupture when the force is applied at a faster rate.

Ligaments demonstrate the phenomenon of hysteresis, which is the energy loss during loading and unloading (Fig. 3.11). The unloading curve lies below the loading curve and reflects a greater energy expenditure on loading compared to the energy regained during unloading. This results in a loss of energy known as hysteresis loss (Panjabi & White 2001). It can also be seen that hysteresis produces an elongation of the tissues. If the force applied is less than the yield stress, then the elongation will be temporary, and if it is the same, or greater, than the yield stress the elongation will be permanent.

A ligament is stiffest in its central area and less stiff at its attachment site. So when a ligament is stretched, most lengthening occurs at the site of least resistance, at the insertion site (Woo et al 1988).

The tensile strength of a ligament is increased with exercise. Exercise causes an increase in the cross-sectional area of ligament and an increase in the collagen content (Tipton et al 1970) as well as increased strength at the attachment site of the ligament (Woo et al 1988).

The biomechanical properties of ligaments change with age; ligaments in younger subjects (16–26 years of age) have two to three times greater strength and stiffness than those in subjects of more than 60 years of age (Noyes & Grood 1976). In a younger age group, ligament fails after 44% elongation and a stress of 37 MPa, while in an

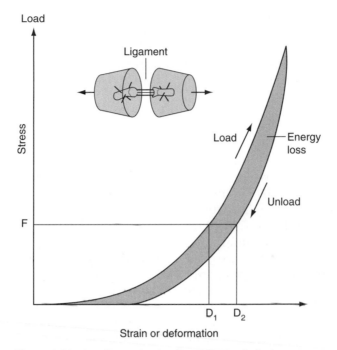

Figure 3.11   Loading and unloading curves to indicate hysteresis (after Panjabi & White 2001, with permission). The shaded area depicts the loss of energy with deformation and is a measure of hysteresis. The unloading curve does not return to the same point on the strain or deformation axis; there is an increase in length as a result of the application of load. For a given force (F) there is a lengthening from the loading curve (D1) to the unloading curve (D2).

older population failure occurs at 30% elongation with a stress of 13 MPa (Noyes & Grood 1976).

Fibrous joint capsules and synovial membranes

The outer layer of a fibrous capsule is composed of dense irregular and regular fibrous tissue and completely surrounds the bone ends, attaching into the periosteum of the bone. Where the fibrous tissue is arranged in regular fashion, in parallel bundles, it is referred to as a named ligament. Fibrous capsules have a poor blood supply but are highly innervated. They are often reinforced by adjacent ligamentous and musculotendinous structures. The inner layer of the fibrous capsule forms the synovial membrane, which is composed of areolar connective tissue and elastic fibres, and is highly vascularized.

Articular cartilage

Articular cartilage is white dense connective tissue covering the bone ends of synovial joints and is between 1 and 5 mm in thickness. The function of articular cartilage is to distribute load and to minimize friction of opposing joint surfaces (Mow et al 1989). It is composed largely of water, chondrocytes, collagen and proteoglycans, and it contains no blood or lymph vessels or nerve supply in normal joints. It obtains nutrients from synovial fluid, and during movement nutrients are pumped through the cartilage (O'Hara et al 1990). The permeability of articular cartilage is greatest on its surface and least in the deeper layers (Shrive & Frank 1999), and depends on the compressive loading (Mow et al 1984). Permeability decreases with increased compressive loading (Mow et al 1989). Cyclic loading of joints, as in walking, has been found to increase the pumping of large solutes such as growth factors, hormones and enzymes into articular cartilage – although it has no effect on the transport of small solutes such as glucose and oxygen (O'Hara et al 1990).

Microscopically, articular cartilage has a layered appearance. The most superficial layer is densely packed with collagen fibrils which are orientated parallel to the articular surface. This arrangement is thought to help resist shear forces at the joint (Shrive & Frank 1999). The middle layer is characterized by the collagen fibrils being further apart, and the deepest layer has fibrils lying at right angles to the articular surface (Fig. 3.12). The collagen fibrils in this layer cross the interface between the articular cartilage and the underlying calcified cartilage beneath, a region known as the tidemark. This arrangement anchors the cartilage to the underlying bone.

The orientation of the collagen fibres in the different layers is considered to enhance the tissue's ability to distribute tensile loading across the articular surface (Askew & Mow 1978). Collagen fibrils are able to resist high tensile forces; the fibres collapse on compressive forces (Fig. 3.13). Most of the water in articular cartilage is closely associated with the collagen fibrils which, together with the proteoglycans, create a fluid-filled matrix that has the mechanical characteristics of a solid object (Mow et al 1989).

Articular cartilage, like ligamentous tissue, is viscoelastic. It therefore has an elastic and viscous nature, displaying creep, stress relaxation and hysteresis, and has a sensitivity to the rate of loading. The behaviour of articular cartilage to compressive and tensile loading is discussed below.

Compressive loading of articular cartilage

The compressive properties of articular cartilage depend on which layer is tested; the deepest layer is the stiffest because of its higher proteoglycan content (Shrive & Frank 1999). The creep response of articular cartilage when a constant compressive force is applied is due to exudation of fluid (Fig. 3.14). The rate of fluid loss reduces over time until the compressive stress within the cartilage equals the applied compressive load so that equilibrium is reached. At this point the compressive load is resisted by the matrix of collagen and proteoglycan.

The stress relaxation of articular cartilage is shown in Figure 3.15. A compressive force is applied to the cartilage until a specific amount of deformation is reached; the force is then held constant. During the initial compression phase the stress within the cartilage increases (to point B), but once the force is held constant, there is a gradual reduction in stress (from point B to point E). Point E indicates the point where equilibrium is reached.

Articular cartilage demonstrates the phenomenon of hysteresis with cyclic compressive loading (Fig. 3.16). The unloading curve lies below

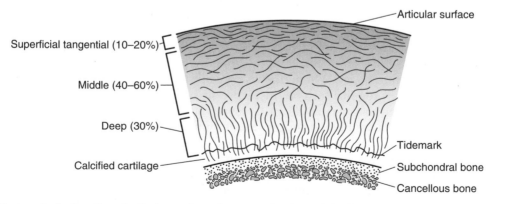

Figure 3.12 Longitudinal section of articular cartilage demonstrating the varied orientation of collagen fibrils in the superficial, middle and deep layers (after Mow et al 1989, with permission).

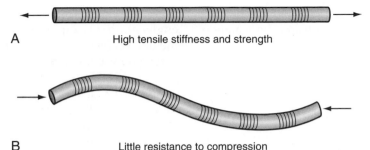

A High tensile stiffness and strength

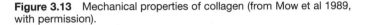

B Little resistance to compression

Figure 3.13 Mechanical properties of collagen (from Mow et al 1989, with permission).

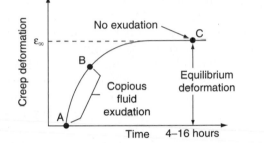

Figure 3.14 Creep response of articular cartilage with a constant compressive load (after Mow et al 1989, with permission).

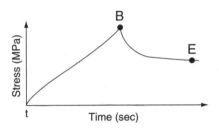

Figure 3.15 Stress relaxation of articular cartilage with a constant rate of compression. Point B is the maximum stress within the tissue, followed by the gradual reduction in stress until equilibrium is reached at point E (after Mow et al 1989, with permission).

the loading curve and reflects a greater energy expenditure on loading than the energy regained during unloading. Hysteresis produces a reduction in cartilage thickness.

The stress strain curve of articular cartilage is dependent on the rate of loading: the faster the rate of loading the stiffer the articular cartilage becomes and the less deformation occurs; with

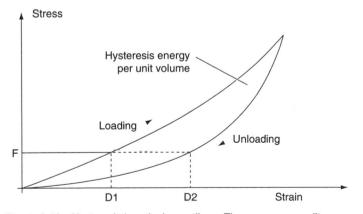

Figure 3.16 Hysteresis in articular cartilage. The energy expenditure on loading is greater than the energy regained during unloading; the area between the curves depicts the energy loss or hysteresis energy (after Shrive & Frank 1999, with permission). For a given force (F) there is a reduction in thickness from the loading curve (D1) to the unloading curve (D2).

slower rates of loading the articular cartilage is more compliant and there is greater deformation (Shrive & Frank 1999).

Synovial fluid

Synovial fluid contains surface-active phospholipid (SAPL), which is adsorbed as the outermost layer of articular cartilage (Hills & Monds 1998). Adsorb is where the articular cartilage holds SAPL to its surface to form a thin film. This film creates, in engineering terms, boundary lubrication, which prevents the adjacent articular surfaces contacting each other and reduces friction during movement, even under high loading (Hills 1989, Hills 1995). SAPL also has been shown to have anti-wear properties (Hills 1995). SAPL has been found to be deficient in osteoarthritic joints (Hills & Monds 1998) and this reduction causes increased resistance to joint movement (Hills & Thomas 1998), a commonly reported clinical phenomenon.

Movement of the joint increases the production of synovial fluid (Levick 1983) and helps to distribute synovial fluid over the articular cartilage (Levick 1984). The flow of synovial fluid into the joint cavity depends, to some extent, on the intra-articular fluid pressure and on the removal of fluid via the synovial lymphatic system (Levick 1984). Intra-articular fluid pressure depends on a large number of factors, including the volume of fluid, rate of change of volume, joint angle, age of the person and muscle action (Levick 1983). Joint movement is also required to remove fluid via the synovial lymphatic system. Lack of movement will reduce the removal of synovial fluid and so will result in an increase in intra-articular volume and pressure. Moderate amounts of movement will increase both the volume of synovial fluid, but also the removal of fluid via the lymphatic system. Excessive movement causes a greater increase in the volume of synovial fluid than the removal of fluid, resulting in increased intra-articular volume and pressure (Levick 1984).

Synovial joint lubrication

A variety of mechanisms are thought to ensure that synovial joints are able to maintain almost friction-free movement under a variety of func-tional activities. The mechanisms are taken from engineering principles of joint lubrication and include boundary and fluid lubrication.

Boundary lubrication Surface-active phospholipid (SAPL) is adsorbed as the outermost layer of articular cartilage (Hills & Monds 1998). This layer prevents the adjacent articular surfaces contacting each other and reduces friction during movement, even under high loading (Hills 1989, Hills 1995).

Fluid lubrication A thin film of lubricant separates the adjacent articular surfaces. There are three mechanisms: hydrodynamic lubrication, squeeze film lubrication, and elastohydrodynamic lubrication. Fluid film lubrication is thought to operate under low loads and high speeds (Nordin & Frankel 1989).

Hydrodynamic lubrication occurs when the articular surfaces do not lie parallel and then one articular surface slides on the other. A wedge of viscous fluid provides a lifting pressure to support the load (Fig. 3.17).

Squeeze film lubrication occurs when the two articular surfaces move towards each other – the

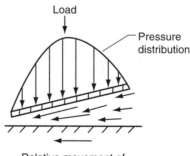

Figure 3.17 Hydrodynamic lubrication (from Nordin & Frankel 1989, with permission).

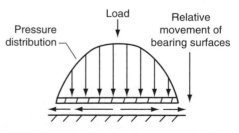

Figure 3.18 Squeeze film lubrication (from Nordin & Frankel 1989, with permission).

fluid pressure between them increasing and helping to support the load (Fig. 3.18).

These two mechanisms are related to the nature of the fluid and the shape and position of the joint surfaces. An additional mechanism is related to the fact that articular cartilage is not rigid and is termed elastohydrodynamic lubrication (Nordin & Frankel 1989). The fluid pressures developed from the above two mechanisms cause deformation of the articular surface, which increases its surface area. This increases the time taken for the fluid to be squeezed out and therefore enhances the ability to withstand load.

Fat pads

Fat pads are generally considered to be space fillers or cushions in synovial membrane, in the potential spaces or irregularities of synovial joints. They may enhance joint lubrication (Williams et al 1995). At the elbow, for example, there are a number of fat pads, including one in the olecranon, coronoid and radial fossae and the trochlear notch (Williams et al 1995). In the lumbar spine, fat pads in the zygapophyseal joints extend through the joint capsule to the superior articular recess where they are displaced during spinal movement (Bogduk 1997).

Menisci and meniscoids

Fibrocartilage menisci are found in the temporomandibular, knee, and sternoclavicular joints. The menisci in the knee joint increase the congruence between the articular surfaces of the femur and tibia, distribute weight-bearing forces, act as shock absorbers and reduce friction (Norkin & Levangie 1992, Palastanga et al 2002). The medial meniscus is innervated (apart from the inner third) by mechanoreceptors and free nerve endings, with greatest density at the anterior and posterior horns (Albright et al 1987). The greater density at the horns is thought to enable proprioceptive feedback at the extreme of joint range (Albright et al 1987). The same arrangement has been found in the temporomandibular joint, with greatest density of mechanoreceptors at the anterior and posterior margins of the intra-articular disc (Zimny & St Onge 1987). Fibro-adi-

pose meniscoids in the zygapophyseal joints are thought to protect the joint by preventing articular surface apposition during movement and by reducing friction (Bogduk 1997).

Bursae

Bursae are sacs made of connective tissue lined by a synovial membrane and filled with fluid similar to synovial fluid. A bursa acts as a cushion to reduce friction. Bursae can be found between skin and bone, between muscle and bone, tendon and bone, and ligament and bone. Some named bursae include the subacromial bursa lying between acromion and the glenohumeral joint capsule and the psoas bursa lying between the tendon of psoas and the pubis and hip joint capsule (Williams et al 1995).

Labra

Two joints in the human body contain a labrum: the glenohumeral joint and the hip joint. They form a fibrocartilagenous wedged-shaped rim around the glenoid and acetabular fossae, respectively. They deepen the articulating socket and may aid lubrication of the joints (Williams et al 1995).

Nerve supply of joints

Most of the components of joints, such as capsule, ligament, articular disc, meniscus and fat pad are innervated; in fact the only structure that is not innervated is the avascular articular cartilage (Messner 1999).

The nerve endings in joint can be classified into four types:

- Ruffini end organs
- Pacinian corpuscles
- Golgi endings
- free nerve endings.

Ruffini end organs

These are encapsulated (covered in a capsule) type I nerve endings that lie around collagen fibres and are stimulated by the displacement of the collagen (Fig. 3.19). They are low-threshold, static and dynamic mechanoreceptors, supplied

A

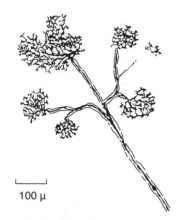

100 μ

B

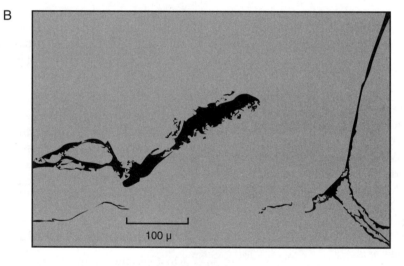

100 μ

C

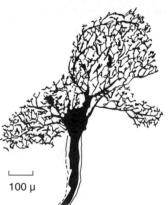

100 μ

Figure 3.19 Three types of nerve ending. **A** Ruffini end organs (type I). **B** Pacinian corpuscles (type II). **C** Golgi endings (type III). (From Skoglund 1956, with permission.)

by A β fibres (or group II afferents). They signal static joint position, direction, amplitude and velocity of joint movement and change in intra-articular pressure (Messner 1999). Activation of Ruffini end organs has been found to directly affect the tone of the overlying muscle (Freeman & Wyke 1967a). Ruffini end organs innervate the posterior capsule of the cat knee joint, almost exclusively, and are extremely sensitive to a change in capsule stretch (Fuller et al 1991). For this reason they are thought to signal the limit of knee extension (Grigg & Hoffman 1982).

Pacinian corpuscles

These are encapsulated, low-threshold, type II mechanoreceptors (Freeman & Wyke 1967b), supplied by A β fibres (or group II afferents) (Fig. 3.19). They are stimulated by dynamic movement, signalling the start and end of a movement, deceleration and acceleration and a change in stress applied to the tissue in which they occur (Messner 1999). Some are stimulated mainly by compression (Clark 1975, Grigg et al 1982), while others are stimulated by tensile loading (Clark 1975, Grigg 1994, Grigg et al 1982). In the cat they are stimulated throughout knee joint movement, particularly during end-range and combined movements (Clark 1975, Krauspe et al 1992). Activation of Pacinian corpuscles directly affects the tone of the overlying muscle (Freeman & Wyke 1967a).

Golgi endings

These are encapsulated, high-threshold type II mechanoreceptors (Fig. 3.19) that signal extreme ranges of movement (Zimny 1988). They are supplied by A β fibres (or group III afferents).

Free nerve endings

Free nerve endings do not have a capsule. There are two types of free nerve ending: type IVa and type IVb (Messner 1999). Type IVa nerve endings are associated with blood vessels and have a vasomotor function. Type IVb nerve endings lie between the collagen and elastic fibres of the connective tissue in which they occur. Both type IVa and type IVb nerve endings signal pain and are therefore classed as nociceptors. The axon may be a myelinated A δ fibre or an unmyelinated C fibre with a lower conduction velocity.

Afferent fibres can be classified according to their conduction velocity as I or A α, II or A β, III or A δ and IV or C fibres (Palastanga et al 2002). These nerve endings have been identified in the limbs, spine, costovertebral joints and temporomandibular joints in both man and animals (Wyke & Polacek 1975). Fresh amputated human knees revealed innervation by a variety of the encapsulated and free nerve endings (Kennedy et al 1982). Encapsulated nerve endings were found in the joint capsule, posterior cruciate ligament and the outer surface of the menisci. Free nerve endings have been found throughout the joint tissues, including the collateral ligaments, joint capsules, synovia, cruciate ligaments, infra-patellar fat pad and the outer surface of the menisci (Kennedy et al 1982). Interestingly, in the cervical spine of man group III nerve endings have not been identified; the zygapophyseal joint contains types I, II and IV nerve endings only (Wyke 1970). Type I is found in the superficial layer of the joint capsule, type II in the deeper layer of the joint capsule and fat pads, and type IV throughout the joint capsule, fat pads and walls of blood vessels (Wyke & Polacek 1975).

The various descriptive names for each type of nerve ending, along with its function, position and afferent nerve is given in Table 3.2.

In the cat, free nerve endings are continuous with group III and IV axons, or afferents (Heppelmann et al 1990). In the cat knee joint group III and IV afferents have a limited response to joint movement, with rather more response to end-range positions (Clark & Burgess 1975, Krauspe et al 1992, Schaible & Schmidt 1983). There is a large variation within any one animal, and also variation according to whether the afferent is in the posterior or medial articular nerve (Clark & Burgess 1975, Grigg et al 1986). While the group III and IV afferents in the medial articular nerve and the group III afferents in the posterior articular nerve respond to movement, group IV afferents in the posterior articular nerve respond only to

Table 3.2 Nerve endings and afferents supplying joints (Albright et al 1987, Freeman & Wyke 1967b, Kennedy et al 1982, Messner 1999, Palastanga et al 2002, Strasmann & Halata 1988, Wyke 1979, Zimny 1988, Zimny & St Onge 1987)

Type of nerve ending	Descriptive name for nerve ending	Function	Position	Afferent nerve
Type I	Ruffini endings Golgi-Mazzoni endings Meissner corpuscles Spray-type endings Basket endings Ball-of-tread endings Bush-like endings	Low-threshold slowly adapting static and dynamic mechano-receptors – signal static joint position, changes in intra-articular pressure and direction, amplitude and velocity of joint movement	Joint capsule (superficial layer) Ligaments Meniscus Articular disc	A β fibre, myelinated, diameter 5–10 μm or group II afferent
Type II	Pacinian corpuscle Krause's Endkorperchen Vater'schen Korper Vater–Pacinian corpuscle Modified Pacini(an) corpuscle Simple Pacinian corpuscle Paciniform corpuscle Golgi-Mazzoni body Meissner corpuscle Gelenknervenkorperchen corpuscle of Krause Club-like ending bulbous corpuscle Corpuscula nervosa articularia	Low-threshold rapidly adapting dynamic mechanoreceptors – signal beginning and end of movement, deceleration and acceleration, change in vibration or stress	Joint capsule (deeper layer) Ligaments Meniscus Articular disc Fat pads Synovium	A β fibre, myelinated diameter 8–12 μm or group II afferent
Type III	Golgi endings Golgi Mazzoni corpuscles	High-threshold very slowly adapting mechanoreceptors – signal extreme ranges of movement or when there is considerable stress	Ligaments Meniscus Articular disc	A β fibre, myelinated diameter 13–17 μm Group II axons
Type IVa	Free nerve terminals	High-threshold, non-adapting pain receptors	Joint capsule (superficial and deep layers) Ligaments Meniscus Articular disc Fat pads	C fibre, unmyelinated, diameter 1–2 μm And thinly myelinated A fibre, diameter 2–4 μm Type III and IV axons
Type IVa	Free nerve endings	High-threshold, non-adapting pain receptors	Articular blood vessels	A δ fibre, myelinated diameter 2–5 μm Group II/III axons
Type IVb	Free nerve endings	Vasomotor function	Articular blood vessels	C fibre, unmyelinated diameter < 2 μm Group IV axons

noxious input, suggesting a nociceptive function (Grigg et al 1986). While group III and IV afferents respond to movement, their sensitivity is low, suggesting a limited role in proprioception and perhaps more of a nociceptor role (Grigg 1994, Schaible & Schmidt 1983). Group III and IV afferents are sensitized in the presence of joint inflammation (Coggeshall et al

1983, Grigg et al 1986, Schaible & Schmidt 1985), suggesting that they may have a proprioceptive function (Ferrell 1980).

Effect of joint afferent activity on muscle

Joint afferent activity directly affects overlying muscle activity. Passive dorsiflexion of an anaesthetized cat ankle joint causes activation of mechanoreceptors in the posterior joint capsule, which produces a reflex facilitation of gastrocnemius motor neurones and inhibition of tibialis anterior (Freeman & Wyke 1967a). Similarly, passive plantarflexion, causes activation of mechanoreceptors in the anterior joint capsule, which facilitates tibialis anterior and inhibits gastrocnemius (Freeman & Wyke 1967a). Thus, when the joint capsule is put on a stretch, the mechanoreceptors cause activation of muscle that would, on contraction, reduce this stretch, and inhibition of the muscle that would increase the stretch. The mechanoreceptors stimulated were slowly adapting type I fibres which are activated during the ankle movement and continue to be active once the movement has stopped, and rapidly adapting type II fibres which are activated only during the ankle movement. The type III fibres in the ankle ligaments and the type IV fibres distributed throughout the capsule, ligaments, fat pad and blood vessels, are not activated during passive ankle movements (Freeman & Wyke 1967a). In the cervical spine, activation of type I, II and IV receptors affects not only the muscles around the neck but also the muscles around the eye and the mandible (Wyke & Polacek 1975).

The mechanism by which joint mechanoreceptors affect muscle, depends on the type of receptor. Type I and II receptors are thought to affect muscle via the fusimotor neurone–muscle spindle loop, whereas type III and IV receptors influence muscle activity directly via the alpha motor neurone (Wyke & Polacek 1975).

The converse has also been demonstrated, that is, that muscle activity can directly affect mechanoreceptor activity (Ferrell 1985). In the cat knee joint, it has been found that, at extreme flexion and extension positions, and with passive movement, mechanoreceptor activity can be influenced (increased or decreased) by muscle contraction around the knee (Ferrell 1985).

Effect of joint afferent activity on pain

Stimulation of the joint mechanoreceptors causes a reduction in transmission of nociceptor activity from the free nerve endings (Wyke 1970). It has

been suggested that it is only type I afferent discharge that effects the transmission of pain (Wyke & Polacek 1975).

From Table 3.2 it can be seen that type I, II and III nerve endings are supplied by A β fibres, while type IV nerve endings are supplied by group A δ and C fibres.

The nerve supply to the skin is also relevant, as this will be involved in any joint movement. Details of skin sensation can be found under nerve function in Chapter 7.

Classification of synovial joints

While all synovial joints share the features described above, they vary a great deal in terms of the shape of the articular surfaces and subsequent movement that occurs.

Joint surfaces can be classified as flat, ovoid and sellar (MacConaill 1966):

- flat is where the articular surfaces are flat, or plane, although no surface is completely flat
- ovoid is where the articular surfaces are wholly concave or wholly convex
- sellar is where the articular surfaces are concave in one plane and convex in another.

Synovial joints are classified as gliding, hinge, pivot, ellipsoidal, saddle and ball and socket (Fig. 3.20):

1. Gliding joints include intercarpal and intertarsal joints, zygapophyseal joints in the cervical and thoracic spine, patellofemoral and the costotransverse and costovertebral joints in the lower ribs. The articular surfaces are more or less flat (MacConaill 1953), and, as the name suggests, simple gliding or translational movement can occur.

2. Hinge joints include tibiofemoral, humeroulnar, ankle and interphalangeal joints in the hand and foot. One articular surface is convex and the other concave, allowing rotational flexion and extension movement.

3. Pivot joints include the atlantoaxial and the superior radioulnar joints. One articular surface is round and sits within a ring formed partly by bone and partly by ligament. Rotational movement is

around the longitudinal axis of the bone, producing, for example, in the forearm, pronation and supination.

4. Condyloid or ellipsoidal joints include the radiocarpal joint and the metacarpophalangeal joints. One articular surface is oval and the other elliptical; movement can occur in two planes. For example, at the radiocarpal joint, there is both flexion and extension and radial and ulnar deviation.

5. Saddle joints include the first carpometacarpal joint, pisotriquetral joint and lumbar zygapophyseal joints (MacConaill 1953). The shape of the articular surfaces is like the saddle on a horse: each articular surface is reciprocally concave in one plane and convex in another,

sometimes referred to as sellar (MacConaill 1953). Like the condyloid joints, movement occurs in two planes allowing flexion and extension and abduction and adduction.

6. Ball and socket joints include the glenohumeral and hip joints. One articular surface is shaped like a ball and the other articular surface is shaped as a hand, which holds the ball. Movement occurs in three planes of movement, allowing flexion and extension, abduction and adduction, and medial and lateral rotation.

Joint movement

The study of the movement of joint surfaces is termed arthrokinematics. The type of movement

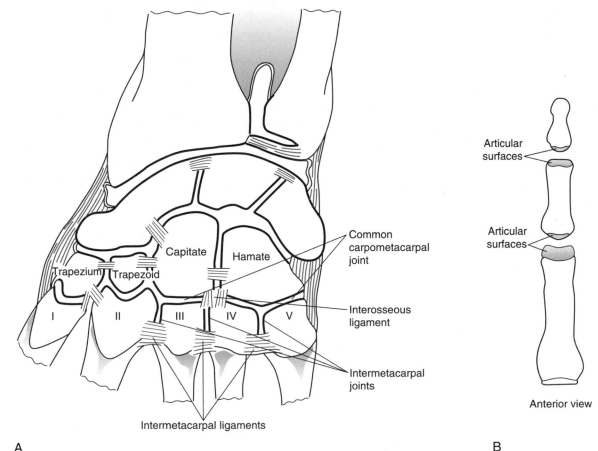

Figure 3.20 Types of synovial joint (after Palastanga et al 2002, with permission). **A** Gliding joints of the intercarpal joints at the wrist. **B** Hinge: interphalangeal joints.

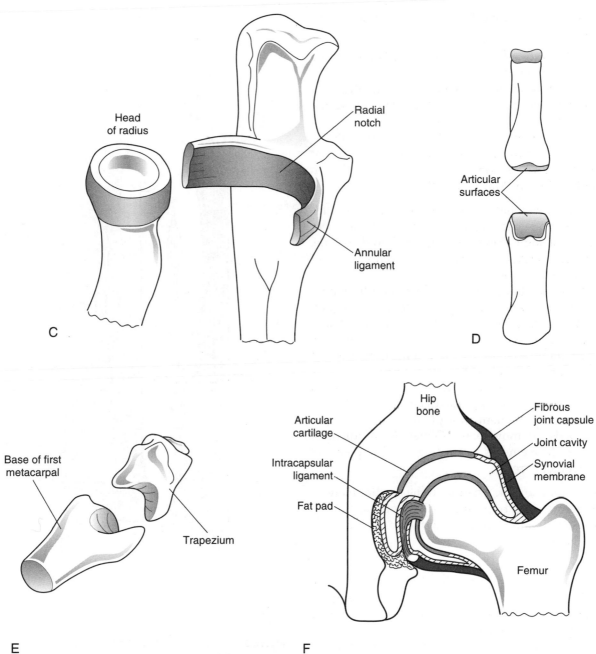

Figure 3.20 **C** Pivot: superior radioulnar joint. **D** Condyloid: metacarpophalangeal joint of the thumb. **E** Saddle: carpometacarpal of the thumb. **F** Ball and socket: hip joint.

at a joint surface can be classified as slide, roll, or spin:

1. Slide or glide is a pure translation of one surface on another.
2. Roll is when the bone rolls or rotates over the articular surface as a wheel rolls along the ground.
3. Spin is pure rotation; it occurs at the humer-oulnar joint during pro- and supination and at the hip and glenohumeral joint during flexion and extension (MaConaill 1966).

The movement that occurs at a plane (or gliding) joint is slide or glide, but at all the other types of joint (hinge, pivot, condyloid, saddle, ball and socket) movement is a combination of slide with roll or spin.

Movement at a joint is further complicated by conjunct rotation, where a secondary rotation occurs during a rotational movement. For example, during flexion of the elbow and the knee joint, there is lateral rotation of the humerus and femur, respectively (MaConaill 1966).

At any joint, there is potentially six degrees of freedom (Fig. 3.21), which can be described in terms of movement in a plane, or according to the axis of movement (Oliver & Middleditch 1991). Movements according to the plane of movement are:

- rotation and translation in the sagittal plane
- rotation and translation in the coronal plane
- rotation and translation in the horizontal plane.

During lumbar spine flexion, for example, there is at each spinal level a combination of anterior sagittal rotation and anterior sagittal translation; during extension there is posterior sagittal rotation and posterior sagittal translation. The amount of sagittal rotation and translation at each segmental level during lumbar spine flexion and extension has been measured using three-dimensional X-ray analysis (Pearcy et al 1984). At each level, there is 8–13° anterior sagittal rotation and 1–3 mm anterior sagittal translation; during extension there is 1–5° posterior sagittal rotation and 1° posterior sagittal translation (Pearcy et al 1984). During lateral flexion,

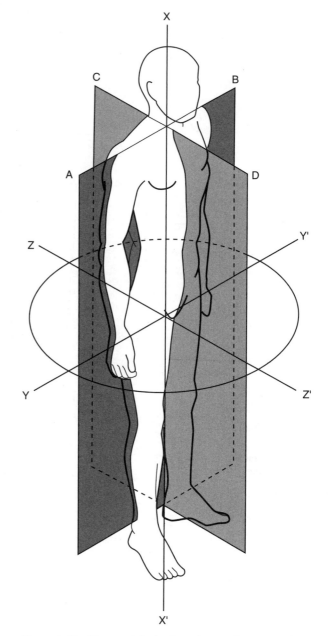

Figure 3.21 Planes of the body and axes of movement. AB is the coronal plane, CD is the sagittal plane and the horizontal circle surrounding the person depicts the horizontal plane; XX′ is the vertical axis, YY′ is the frontal axis and ZZ′ is the sagittal axis (from Oliver & Middleditch 1991, with permission).

there is approximately 3–10° of lateral rotation and 1–2 mm of lateral translation in the frontal plane, and during rotation approximately 2–3°

rotation and 1–2 mm of translation in the horizontal plane (Pearcy & Tibrewal 1984).

Joint glide during physiological movements

Movement at a joint is a combination of roll or spin with a glide; for example, during elbow flexion, the radial head rotates around the capitulum of the humerus and translates (that is, slides) anteriorly. During knee flexion, non-weight-bearing, the tibia rotates posteriorly around the femur and translates posteriorly. Because movement consists of both a roll or spin, and a glide, the axis of movement constantly changes and is referred to as the instantaneous axis of rotation (IAR). Table 3.3 identifies, for each joint movement, the direction of the bone translation.

The direction in which the bone translates (or glides) depends upon the shape of the moving articular surface (Fig. 3.22) (Kaltenborn 1989, MacConaill 1966). When the joint surface of the moving bone is concave, the glide usually occurs in the same direction as the bone is moving so that, with flexion on the knee joint (in non-weight-bearing), posterior glide of the tibial condyles occurs on the femoral condyles. When the joint surface is convex, the glide is usually in the opposite direction to the bone movement so that, with shoulder abduction, there is an inferior glide of the head of the humerus on the glenoid cavity. Exceptions to this general rule occur. For example, at the glenohumeral flexion, where there is movement of a convex humeral head on a concave glenoid, it would be expected that shoulder flexion would involve a posterior glide and extension an anterior glide; however, the opposite occurs, that is, with glenohumeral flexion there is anterior glide and with extension a posterior glide (Harryman et al 1990).

Another consideration is the relative size of the articular surfaces; for example, at the glenohumeral joint the head of the humerus has a much larger surface area than the glenoid cavity. The effect of this is that the head of the humerus, as it rolls, would run out of articular surface on the glenoid. This is overcome by a glide and also by accompanying movement of the scapula, during humeral movements (Norkin & Levangie 1992).

Table 3.3 Direction of bone translation during active physiological movements

Movement	Translation
Glenohumeral	
Flexion	Anterior and superior
Extension	Posterior and inferior
Abduction	Inferior
elbow: humeroulnar	
flexion	anterior
extension	posterior
elbow: radiohumeral	
flexion	anterior
extension	posterior
forearm: superior radioulnar	
pronation	posterior
supination	anterior
forearm: inferior radioulnar	
pronation	anterior
supination	posterior
Wrist: proximal row of carpus on radius and ulnar	
flexion	posterior
extension	anterior
radial deviation	medial
ulnar deviation	lateral
Thumb: base of first metacarpal on trapezium	
flexion	anterior
extension	posterior
abduction	medial
adduction	lateral
Hip	
flexion	posterior
extension	anterior
abduction	medial
adduction	lateral
knee, non-weight-bearing	
flexion	posterior
extension	anterior
Ankle, non-weight-bearing: talus on tibia and fibula	
dorsiflexion	posterior
plantarflexion	anterior

The examples given above refer to peripheral joints. The spinal joints follow the same principles but are worth describing separately here. Each spinal segmental level, between C2 and S1, consists of an interbody joint (two vertebral bodies and the intervening intervertebral disc) and two zygapophyseal joints (Oliver & Middleditch 1991), functionally a triad joint. The shape and direction of the articular surface of the zygapophyseal joints influence the gliding movement available at that segmental level (Table 3.4).

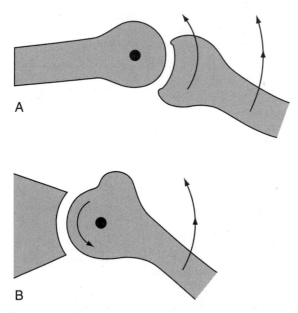

A

B

Figure 3.22 Movement of articular surfaces during physiological movements. The single arrow depicts the direction of movement of the articular surface and the double arrow depicts the physiological movement. **A** With knee extension (non-weight-bearing), the concave articular surface of the tibia slides superiorly on the convex femoral condyles. **B** With shoulder elevation through abduction, the convex articular surface of the humerus slides inferiorly on the concave glenoid cavity. (From Kaltenborn 1989, with permission.)

The shape and direction of the articular surfaces vary throughout the spine (Table 3.5 and Fig. 3.23).

The upper cervical spine, C0/C1 (between the occiput and atlas) and C1/C2 (between C1 and axis) are, anatomically, rather different to the rest of the spine. The superior articular facets of C1 are concave and face upwards and medially; in addition, the lines of the two facets, when viewed superiorly, converge anteriorly (Fig. 3.24A). The occipital condyles are reciprocally shaped. The shape of the facets at C0/C1 facilitates flexion and extension movement. As the head rotates forwards on C1, the occipital condyles slide (or translate) in a posterior direction, following the above principle of a convex surface moving on a concave surface (Fig. 3.24B). With extension of the head on C1, the occipital condyles slide in an anterior direction.

The superior articular facets of C2 are large, oval and convex, and they lie in an anteroposte-

rior direction. They face superiorly and laterally (Fig. 3.25A). The inferior articular facets of C1 are reciprocally shaped. The shape of the facets at C1/C2 facilitates rotation. With rotation to the right, the right inferior facet of C1 glides posteriorly and slightly downwards (Fig. 3.25B). The posterior movement produces the rotation movement, and the downward (inferior) movement produces a right lateral flexion movement. Thus, at this segmental level, rotation to the right is accompanied by ipsilateral (right) lateral flexion. During flexion, the inferior facets of C1 glide backward on the superior facets of C2. During extension, the inferior facets of C1 glide above).

In the cervical spine (C3–C7 levels) the superior articular facets are oval and flat and face upwards and backwards (Fig. 3.23). During cervical spine flexion, the inferior articular facets of each cervical vertebra slide upward and forward on the superior articular facets of the vertebra below. For example, the inferior facets of C5 slide upward and forward on the superior facets of C6. On extension the reverse occurs throughout the cervical spine, so, for example, at C5/6, the inferior facets of C5 slide downward and backward on the superior facets of C6.

On right lateral flexion, the left inferior articular facets of each cervical vertebra slide upward and forward on the vertebra below, and on the right hand side the inferior articular facets slide downward and backward. If we consider the movement of the left inferior articular facets during the movement of right lateral flexion, the upward movement produces the right lateral flexion movement and the forward movement produces a right rotation movement. Thus, in the cervical spine right lateral flexion is accompanied by right (ipsilateral) rotation.

On cervical rotation to the right, the left inferior articular facets at each cervical level glide upward, forward and laterally on the superior facet of the vertebra below (Fig. 3.26). Once again, the opposite movement occurs on the other side: the right inferior articular facets glide downward, backward and medially on the vertebra below. On the left side, the forward movement (of the left inferior articular facet) produces the right rotation movement, and the upward

Table 3.4 Glide of inferior articular facets during physiological movements of the spine. Movement in parenthesis denotes minimal amount of movement

	Flexion	Extension	Left lateral flexion	Right lateral flexion	Left rotation	Right rotation
C2–C7						
Left inferior articular facet	Upward Forward	Downward Backward	Downward Backward	Upward Forward	Downward Backward medial	Upward Forward lateral
Right inferior articular facet	Upward Forward	Downward Backward	Upward Forward	Downward Backward	Upward Forward lateral	Downward Backward medial
T1–T12						
Left inferior articular facet	Upward (Forward)	Downward (Backward)	Downward (Backward)	Upward (Forward)	Medial	Lateral
Right inferior articular facet	Upward (Forward)	Downward (Backward)	Upward (Forward)	Downward (Backward)	Lateral	Medial
L1–S1						
Left inferior articular facet	Upward (Forward)	Downward (Backward)	Downward (Backward)	Upward (Forward)		
Right inferior articular facet	Upward (Forward)	Downward (Backward)	Upward (Forward)	Downward (Backward)		

Table 3.5 Shape and direction of the superior articular surfaces of the zygapophyseal joints in the spine

Spinal level	Shape of superior facets	Direction of superior facets	Movement facilitated by direction of facets
C1	Concave	Upwards and medial	Flexion and extension
C2	Large, oval, convex	Upwards and lateral	Rotation
C2–C7	Oval, flat	Upwards and backwards	All directions
T1–T12	Triangular, flat	Backwards, slightly upwards and lateral	Rotation Lateral flexion
L1–L5	Concave	Backwards and medial	Flexion, extension, lateral flexion

movement produces a right lateral flexion movement. Thus, in the cervical spine, right rotation is accompanied by right (ipsilateral) lateral flexion. In summary, then, cervical lateral flexion is accompanied by ipsilateral rotation, and rotation is accompanied by ipsilateral lateral flexion.

In the thoracic spine the flat, triangular superior articular facets face backward and slightly upward and lateral (Fig. 3.23). During thoracic flexion, the inferior articular facets at each level glide essentially upward, with some forward translation (Fig 3.27). On thoracic extension, the inferior articular facets glide downward with some backward translation. On left lateral flexion, the right inferior articular facets glide upward and slightly forward; the upward movement produces the lateral flexion, the forward movement produces a rotation movement to the left (ipsilateral). The left inferior articular facets glide in a reciprocal manner, that is, they glide downward and slightly backward. On rotation to the left, the right inferior articular facets glide laterally, while the left inferior articular facets glide medially. The combination of rotation and lateral flexion movements in the thoracic spine is not as straightforward as in the cervical spine. The coupled movements vary in different regions of the thoracic spine. At T2, lateral flexion is accompanied by ipsilateral rotation, whereas, at T6 and T11, lateral flexion can be accompanied by ipsilateral rotation or contralateral rotation, the direction varies with individuals (White 1969).

In the lumbar spine, the superior articular facets are concave facing backwards and medially (Fig. 3.23). During lumbar flexion, the inferior articular facets glide upward and forward. On extension, the inferior articular facets glide downward and backward (Fig. 3.28). The movement of the articular facets during lateral flexion is less clear. With lateral flexion, there may be ipsilateral or contralateral rotation (Pearcy & Tibrewal 1984). On lumbar rotation to the left (moving the trunk), the inferior articular facet on the right glides anteriorly and laterally to impact onto the superior articular facet of the vertebra below. The left inferior articular facet glides in a posterior and medial direction, so there is gapping of the joint space. Rotation of the lumbar spine from L1 to L4 is accompanied by contralateral lateral flexion, whereas rotation at L5/S1 is accompanied by ipsilateral lateral flexion (Pearcy & Tibrewal 1984).

Normal function of any synovial joint, then, requires the moving bone to rotate and translate. Each of these movements, rotation and translation, if normal, would be full-range, symptom-free, and with normal through-range and end-range resistance; normal muscle function is assumed. In the examination of a patient, normal rotation and translation is examined during active and passive physiological movements, and normal translation is examined during accessory movements; this is described in detail elsewhere (Maitland et al 2001, Petty & Moore 2001).

A knowledge of the normal rotation and translation of bone during movement of a joint is important when attempting to restore normal joint function. Some examples may highlight this. The examples assume that the patient is lying prone with the spine in a neutral position. To facilitate an increase in cervical flexion at the C4/5 level, a central posteroanterior force with a cephalad inclination could be used on C4 spinous process. This accessory movement will also enhance extension at the C3/4 segmental level. In the same way, to facilitate cervical lateral flexion or rotation to the

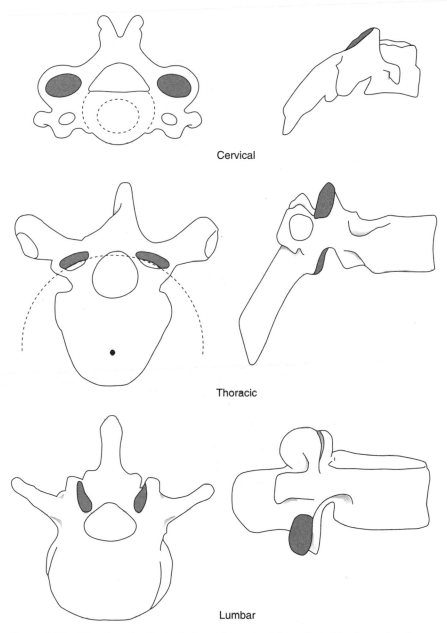

Cervical

Thoracic

Lumbar

Figure 3.23 Direction of articular surfaces in cervical, thoracic and lumbar spine (from Palastanga et al 2002, with permission). The superior articular facets of the cervical face upwards and backwards, the thoracic backwards and laterally and the lumbar backwards and medially.

right at C4/5 level, a unilateral posteroanterior pressure with a cephalad inclination could be applied on the left C4 articular pillar. This accessory movement would also enhance ipsilateral lateral flexion and rotation at the C3/4 level.

In the thoracic spine, similar accessory movements could be used; the major difference is the greater downward obliquity of the middle four spinous processes, which would require the force to be in a more cephalad direction than in the cervical

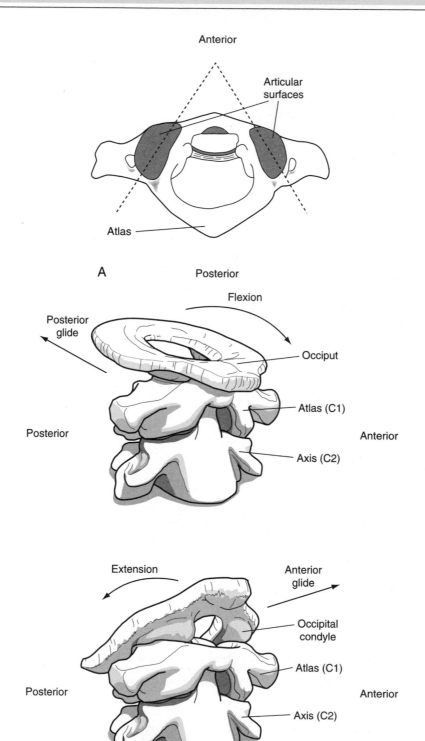

Figure 3.24 **A** Superior surface of atlas (from Palastanga et al 2002, with permission). Superior articular facets of C1 are concave and face upwards and medial. The lines of the two facets, when viewed superiorly, converge anteriorly. **B** Flexion and extension at the C0/C1 joint (after Edwards 1999, with permission). During flexion the occipital condyles glide posteriorly while during extension they glide anteriorly.

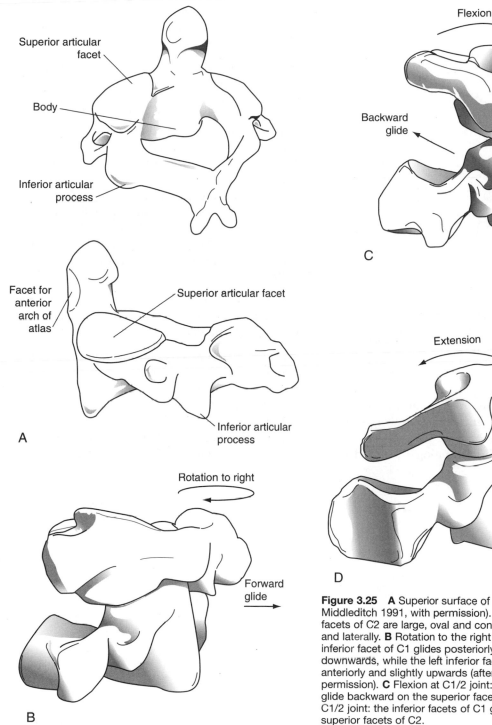

Figure 3.25 **A** Superior surface of C2 (after Oliver & Middleditch 1991, with permission). The superior articular facets of C2 are large, oval and convex and face superiorly and laterally. **B** Rotation to the right at C1/2 joint. The right inferior facet of C1 glides posteriorly and slightly downwards, while the left inferior facet of C1 glides anteriorly and slightly upwards (after Edwards 1999, with permission). **C** Flexion at C1/2 joint: the inferior facets of C1 glide backward on the superior facets of C2. **D** Extension at C1/2 joint: the inferior facets of C1 glide forward on the superior facets of C2.

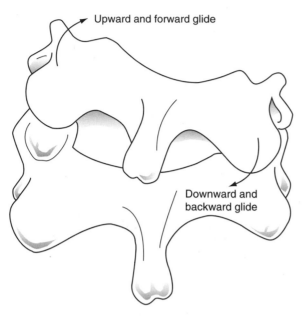

Figure 3.26 Cervical rotation to the right is accompanied by lateral flexion to the right (after Oliver & Middleditch 1991, with permission). The left inferior articular facet glides upward and forward, while the right inferior articular facet glides downward and backward.

spine and possibly also positioning into flexion to achieve an enhancement of thoracic flexion.

In the lumbar spine, there have been quite a number of studies investigating the effect of a central posteroanterior mobilization force to L3 or L4, in terms of stiffness and movement. Stiffness of a PA mobilization has been found to:

- vary widely between asymptomatic subjects (Lee & Svensson 1993)
- increase with increased speed of application of the force (Lee & Evans 1992)
- increase with increased muscle activity (Lee et al 1993, Shirley et al 1999)
- increase in patients with LBP (Latimer et al 1996)
- increase from cephalad to caudad: L5 is stiffest, then L4, then L3 (Edmondston et al 1998)
- vary with the position of the spine: it is increased in flexion (32%) and in extension (12%) compared to neutral (Edmondston et al 1998).

In terms of movement that occurs with a central posteroanterior pressure to L3 or L4, the following have been found:

- a generalized extension movement from T8 to S1 (Lee & Svensson 1993)
- more movement at the caudad level than the cephalad level, apart from L5 (Lee & Evans 1992)
- a sustained central PA results in a greater displacement and more generalized

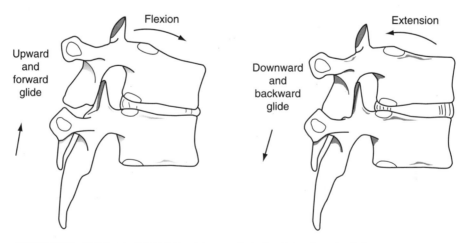

Figure 3.27 Flexion and extension movements in the thoracic spine (after Palastanga et al 2002, with permission). During flexion the inferior articular facets glide upward and slightly forward, and on extension the inferior articular facets glide downward and slightly backward.

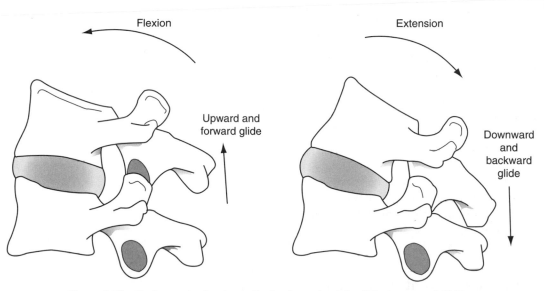

Figure 3.28 Flexion and extension in the lumbar spine (after Palastanga et al 2002, with permission). During lumbar flexion the inferior articular facets glide upward and forward, while on extension they glide downward and backward.

movement throughout the spine than an oscillatory movement (Lee & Svensson 1993)
• an increasing displacement over time with a sustained PA force, with nearly 70% of creep occurring in the first 30 seconds (Lee & Evans 1992).

The biomechanical nature of the PA force means that the composite tissues of the spine, as a whole, behave like viscoelastic tissues. For example, the displacement achieved when applying a PA force depends on the rate of loading and the time of loading. All of this research has focussed on one or two levels of the lumbar spine and so the findings cannot be transferred directly to other types of spinal accessory movement or to different regions of the spine. However, it does provide, in a general sense, the biomechanical effects of spinal accessory movements.

Another concept is that of close pack and loose pack position of a joint. Close pack is where there is maximal congruency of joint surfaces, maximal tension in the joint capsule and ligaments, and least joint play; it is usually found at the extreme of range. Loose pack is any position other than close pack, where the joint capsule and ligaments are relatively slack and there is

some joint play. Joint play is the amount of slack, or give, in the joint.

Summary

A major function of synovial joints is to allow a certain amount of movement, which will often be a combination of glide and rotation. The amount and direction of the glide and rotation movements depend on the shape of the articular surfaces. As a general rule, when the joint surface of the moving bone is concave, the glide occurs in the same direction as the bone is moving; when the joint surface is convex, the glide is in the opposite direction to the bone movement. During physiological movements in the spine there is gliding at the zygapophyseal joints and the direction of the glide can be predicted on the basis of the shape and direction of the articular facets.

The predicted glide and rotation movements in peripheral and spinal joints given in this chapter are based on classic textbook descriptions of joint surface shape and orientation. In the real world, with real people, the shape and orientation of the joint surfaces may vary due to normal anatomical differences and/or congenital anomalies. There are numerous references in the literature to anatomical and biomechanical variation between individuals; some examples here include the shoulder (Maki & Gruen 1976), the spine (Nathan 1962, Penning 1988) and the knee (Frankel et al 1971, Ramsey & Wretenberg 1999). In addition, altered muscle activity (Renstrom et al 1986), altered muscle length (Comerford & Mottram 2001), degenerative changes in the joint (Penning 1988), pathology (Frankel et al 1971) and age (Nathan 1962, Penning 1988) may also affect the quality and range of movement that occurs at a specific joint at any one moment in time. For this reason, the theory of joint movement must be applied cautiously to patients.

Biomechanics of joint movement

The normal function of most joints is to allow full-range movement of the adjacent bones. As the bones move towards the end range of joint movement, resistance to movement increases (Nigg & Herzog 1999, Wright & Johns 1961) as the surrounding joint capsule, ligaments and muscles become taut (Wright & Johns 1961), eventually causing movement to stop. This is a protective mechanism so that the joint does not sublux or dislocate. Force–displacement curves from physiological movements at the knee and at the finger are shown in Figure 3.29, while curves from accessory movements of the lumbar spine, knee and shoulder are shown in Figure 3.30; these curves identify the increasing resistance from the beginning of range to the end of range. Different joints are limited by different structures. For example, elbow extension is limited by bony opposition of the olecranon process of the ulna in the olecranon fossa, knee flexion is limited by soft-tissue opposition between the calf and the thigh, and wrist flexion is limited by the wrist dorsal ligaments as well as the bony configuration of the carpus. Different joints and different movements have different end-feels. The quality of this resistance at the end of range has been categorized by Cyriax (1982) and Kaltenborn (1989), as shown in Table 3.6.

The phenomenon of stress relaxation has been demonstrated in the human wrist (Wright &

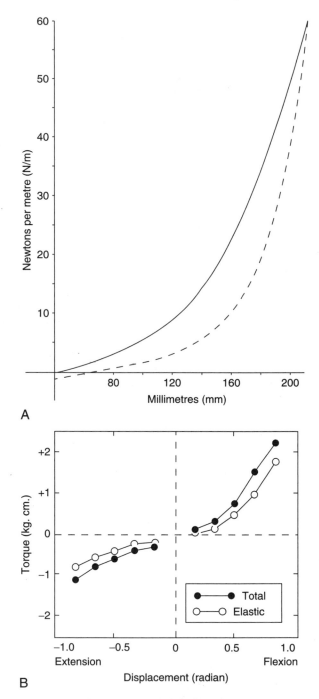

Figure 3.29 Force–displacement curves for physiological movements. **A** The last 20–30 degrees of passive knee extension (from Tindle 1987, with permission). The dotted line depicts the unloading curve and, where it crosses the x axis, demonstrates the increase in length. **B** Finger metacarpophalangeal flexion and extension (after Wright & Johns 1961, with permission).

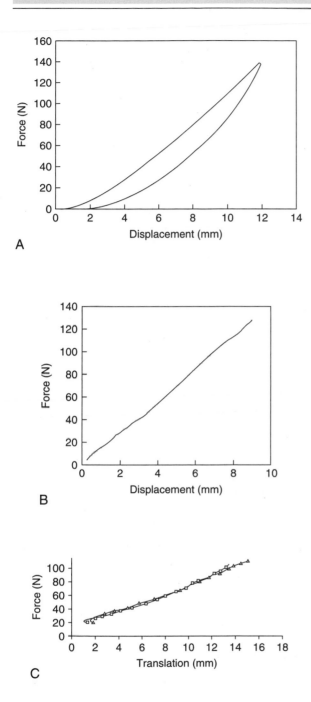

Figure 3.30 Force–displacement curves for accessory movements. **A** Central posteroanterior glide to L3, loading and unloading curves (from Petty et al 2002, with permission). **B** Anteroposterior glide on the tibia with the knee in slight flexion (from Petty et al 2002, with permission). **C** PA to the glenohumeral joint in 90 degrees abduction and in neutral, internal and external rotation (from McQuade et al 1999, with permission).

Johns 1961). When the wrist is held in approximately 38 degrees flexion for 2.5 minutes there is 64% reduction in stress (or force per unit area) within the tissues. The stiffness of the wrist joint flexion and extension differs between males and females, males having significantly greater (P <0.001) stiffness. Stiffness values increases with age (Wright & Johns 1961). Raising skin temperature to 45°C causes a 20% reduction in stiffness on wrist extension, compared to cooling to 33°C (Wright & Johns 1961).

Functional movement

While movement at an individual joint can occur, functional activities often involve movement throughout the limb. For example, in standing, when a person bends at the knees this will be accompanied by hip flexion and ankle dorsiflexion. This predictable movement pattern can be referred to as a closed kinematic chain, a term used in engineering for linkages that make up a system. In contrast, the unpredictable movement patterns that can occur in the upper limb (and the lower limb when not weight-bearing) can be termed an open kinematic chain. The concept of open and closed kinematic chains is useful in that it highlights that movement involves a number of joints, and rarely does a joint move in isolation.

Proprioception

Proprioception is a perception of position and movement gained from skin, joint and muscle receptors (Grigg 1994, McCloskey et al 1987, Strasmann & Halata 1988, Strasmann et al 1990). It seems likely that the brain uses information collectively from joint, muscle and skin afferents, and that isolated information from one of these tissues provides limited information (Macefield et al 1990).

The skin of the hand, for example, contains slowly adapting type II mechanoreceptors that are highly sensitive to static and dynamic skin deformation produced by joint movement (Edin 1992, Edin & Abbs 1991, Hulliger et al 1979). The importance of skin mechanoreceptors in

Table 3.6 Normal end feel (Cyriax 1982, Kaltenborn 1989)

Cyriax	Kaltenborn	Description
Soft tissue approximation	Soft-tissue approximation or soft tissue stretch	Soft end feel, e.g. knee flexion, ankle dorsiflexion
Capsular feel	Firm soft-tissue stretch	Fairly hard halt to movement, e.g. shoulder, elbow or hip rotation due to capsular or ligamentous stretching
Bone to bone	Hard	Abrupt halt to the movement, e.g. elbow extension

proprioception remains unclear (Edin & Abbs 1991, Grigg 1994, Macefield et al 1990, Moberg 1983).

The role of joint afferents in the metacarpophalangeal and interphalangeal joints of the human hand has been investigated (Macefield et al 1990). When joint afferents are electrically stimulated in isolation, the subject has a perception of joint movement, demonstrating their proprioceptive role. Further, when the joints are passively moved, there is increased joint afferent activity, which is greatest at end-of-range positions (Macefield et al 1990). Clearly, joint afferent activity is, in part, responsible for providing proprioceptive information about joint position.

Joint movement does not occur in isolation: there will be movement of skin, muscle, tendon and fascia, as well as intra- and periarticular joint structures. For this reason, it is likely that proprioception is a result of the combined afferent information from all of these structures (Grigg 1994, McCloskey et al 1987, Strasmann & Halata 1988, Strasmann et al 1990).

Normal function of a joint could be summarized from this section as full-range movement, with normal quality of movement and without production of symptoms.

JOINT DYSFUNCTION

Just as the function of joints depends on the function of muscles and nerves, so dysfunction of joints can lead to dysfunction in muscles and nerves. They are dependent on each other in both normal and abnormal conditions, and this relationship is depicted in Figure 3.31. Some examples may help to highlight how joint dysfunction will often be accompanied by muscle and/or nerve dysfunction.

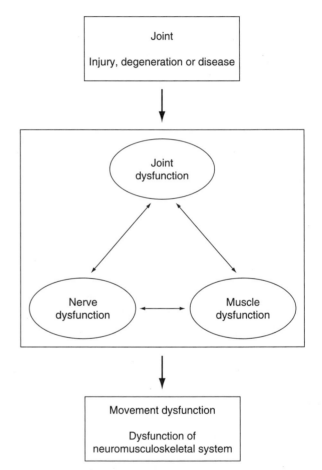

Figure 3.31 Dysfunction of joint can produce muscle and/or nerve dysfunction.

There is overwhelming evidence that pathology in a joint can lead to weakness of the overlying muscle. This has been demonstrated in the knee in the presence of a variety of pathologies: rheumatoid arthritis (deAndrade et al 1965); osteoarthritis (deAndrade et al 1965, Hurley &

Newham 1993); ligamentous knee injuries (DeVita et al 1997, Hurley et al 1992, Hurley et al 1994, Kennedy et al 1982, Newham et al 1989, Snyder-Mackler et al 1994, Urbach & Awiszus 2002) and following meniscectomy (Hurley et al 1994, Shakespeare et al 1985, Stokes & Young 1984, Suter et al 1998); in the elbow in the presence of rheumatoid arthritis (Hurley et al 1991); and in the glenohumeral joint in the presence of anterior dislocation (Keating & Crossan 1992). The inhibition of muscle is thought to be due to inhibitory (Iles et al 1990, Suter & Herzog 2000, Torry et al 2000) or abnormal (Hurley & Newham 1993, Hurley et al 1991) input from joint afferents. Thus, joint pathology leads to altered nervous system activity, which leads to altered muscle activity.

Another example would be the effect of joint immobilization on local muscle and nerve. Three weeks of joint immobilization has been shown to cause a reduced maximal voluntary contraction of the muscles around the joint, and a decrease in the maximal firing rate of motor neurones supplying the muscles (Seki et al 2001). Thus, immobilization of a joint leads to muscle weakness and altered nervous system activity.

Joint instability and ligament insufficiency have been shown to alter nervous system activity, which leads to altered muscle activity. Ligamentous insufficiency at the elbow joint (Glousman et al 1992) and glenohumeral joint (Glousman et al 1988) has been found to alter muscle activity over the elbow and shoulder region respectively, when throwing. In the lower limb, anterior cruciate ligament deficiency has been found to alter electromyographic (EMG) activity of quadriceps and hamstring muscle groups during knee movement (Solomonow et al 1987) and gait (Berchuk et al 1990). A cycle of events leading to dysfunction in ligament, muscle and nerve is shown in Figure 3.32 (Kennedy et al 1982). Thus, ligamentous injury leads to altered nervous system activity, which leads to altered muscle activity.

Reduced activity of joint afferents can lead to joint degeneration. In the dog knee joint, if the joint afferent nerve supply and the anterior cruciate ligament are cut, severe joint degeneration

is evident after just 3 weeks (O'Connor et al 1985, Vilensky et al 1997). Additionally, reduced proprioception may initiate or enhance osteoarthritic change in the knee (Barrett et al 1991) and the proprioceptive loss is thought to be a sensitive measure of degenerative joint disease (Skinner et al 1984), which, if correct, highlights the sensitive relationship of joint and nerve.

Joint nociceptor activity directly affects muscle activity. Pain around the knee causes a nociceptive flexor withdrawal response: hip and knee flexion and ankle dorsiflexion. There is increased alpha motor neurone excitability of the muscles to produce this movement (Stener & Peterson 1963) and reciprocal inhibition of the knee extensors (Stener 1969, Stener & Peterson 1963, Young et al 1987). For example, pressure or tension on a partially ruptured medial collateral ligament results in increased activity of sartorius and semimembranosus (knee flexors), with inhibition of vastus medialis (extensor) (Stener & Peterson 1963). Pain over the lateral femoral epicondyle leads to inhibition of the vastus medialis and lateralis, both knee extensors (Stener 1969), and pain from the lumbar zygapophyseal joint causes increased activity of the hamstring muscle group (Mooney & Robertson 1976). Nociceptor activity is thought to influence muscle activity via the alpha motor neurone (Wyke & Polacek 1975). Interestingly, activation of type I, II and IV receptors in the zygapophyseal joints of the cervical

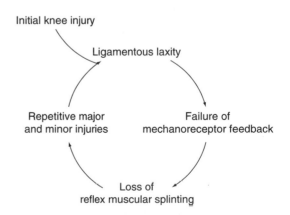

Figure 3.32 A proposed cycle of progressive knee instability following an initial ligament injury (from Kennedy et al 1982, with permission).

spine has more widespread effects than just the muscles around the neck; it also influences the muscles around the eye and mandible (Wyke & Polacek 1975).

Joint nociceptor activity can enhance joint dysfunction. In rats with inflammatory arthritis, joint nociceptors have been found to release substance P, and postganglionic sympathetic neurones to release catecholamines; both of these substances exacerbate joint inflammation (Basbaum & Levine 1991, Levine et al 1985b).

Conversely, dysfunction in muscle is thought to lead to joint dysfunction. For example, abnormal eccentric force of quadriceps muscle is thought to be a contributing factor in anterior knee pain (Hughston et al 1984), and muscle weakness may make a joint more vulnerable to injury (Keating & Crossan 1992, Stokes & Young 1984, Young et al 1982). For example, quadriceps muscle weakness is thought to alter knee joint loading which may, in the long term, lead to osteoarthritis in the joint (Brandt 1997, Felson & Zhang 1998). Thus, joint dysfunction may occur as a result of a muscle dysfunction and this sequence of events is outlined in Figure 3.33.

Summary

This section has sought to highlight that joint dysfunction can lead to muscle and nerve dysfunction, and conversely, that muscle and nerve dysfunction can lead to joint dysfunction. It seems reasonable to suggest that joint dysfunction probably does not occur in isolation – it will always be accompanied, to a greater or lesser extent, by nerve and muscle dysfunction. The term 'joint' in this chapter refers to both intra-articular and periarticular structures.

Classification of joint dysfunction

The description of joint dysfunction flows directly from the description of normal joint function. The function of a joint is to transfer force from one bone to another and to permit limited movement (Nigg & Herzog 1999). Some joints, such as the sacroiliac joint, transmit very high forces and have hardly any movement, whereas other joints, such as the glenohumeral joint, transmit less force and have a large range of movement. The movement available at a joint includes physiological and accessory movements. The signs and symptoms of joint dysfunction are directly related to these functions, that is, there may be one or more of the following: reduced range of joint movement (hypomobility), increased range of joint movement (hypermobility), altered quality of movement, or production of symptoms. A particular mix of these signs and symptoms occurs with a ligamentous sprain, and for clarity this is discussed in a separate section at the end of this chapter. Box 3.1 highlights these characteristics of joint function and dysfunction.

The signs and symptoms of joint dysfunction include reduced range of joint movement (hypomobility), increased range of joint movement (hypermobility), altered quality of movement, and production of symptoms. These signs and symptoms can occur in isolation or in any combination.

Hypomobility

There may be hypomobility of one or more accessory movements and/or hypomobility of

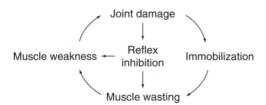

Figure 3.33 Effect of joint damage and/or immobilization on muscle and nerve tissue. (Reproduced, with permission, from Stokes M, Young A 1984 Clinical Science 67:7–14. © The Biochemical Society and the Medical Research Society.)

Box 3.1 Characteristics of joint dysfunction
Hypomobility or hypermobility Altered quality of movement Production of symptoms

one or more physiological movements. It seems reasonable to suggest that if there is a reduced range of translation this will affect, to some degree, the range of rotation of the bone. In the same way, if there is a reduced range of rotation movement, this will affect the range of translation movement.

Limited range of accessory or physiological movement is often associated with an altered quality of movement. This is most commonly increased resistance to movement or production of symptoms; these are depicted in Figure 3.34.

Traumatized or pathological tissues, which may produce a physical resistance to further movement, include intra-articular structures, such as joint capsule, a torn meniscus or a loose body, and peri-articular structures such as ligament, muscle or nerve overlying the joint. Each joint has its own unique range and resistance to movement owing to its particular intra-articular and peri-articular arrangement. In the upper and lower limbs, the clinician compares the left and right side to determine normality for the patient, comparing the range of movement and the through-range and end-range resistance to movement (Petty & Moore 2001). A comparison is made and the clinician judges any difference, while bearing in mind that range of movement

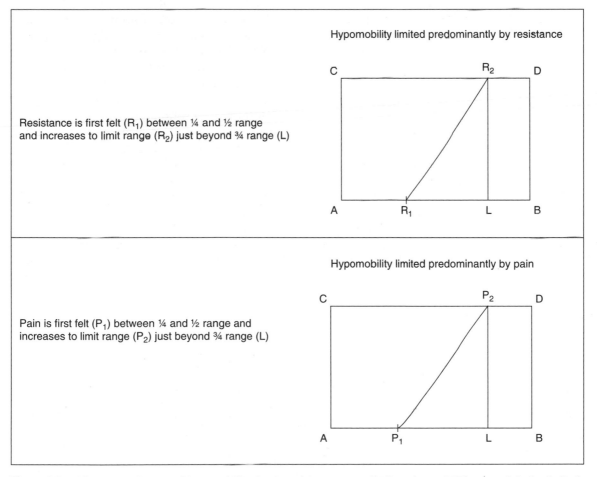

Figure 3.34 Movement diagram of hypomobility due to resistance or production of symptoms, where L is the limit of range, R_1 is the first point of resistance felt by the examiner, R_2 is maximum intensity of resistance which limits further movement, P_1 is point in range where pain is first felt and P_2 is maximum intensity of pain which limits further movement.

varies from side to side in normal asymptomatic subjects. Where there is no other side with which to compare, as with central posteroanterior pressures of the vertebrae, the clinician can compare movement at adjacent levels, but again bearing in mind that there are normal differences in the range of movement at different segmental levels (Oliver & Middleditch 1991).

Limited range of accessory or physiological movements may be caused by the production of symptoms. Symptoms can be any sensation felt by the patient and can include pain, ache, pulling, pins and needles, numbness, a sense of something crawling along the skin, as well as apprehension by the patient to move further into range.

Hypomobility can be more fully appreciated by exploring the effects of immobilization on joint structures, as this produces the most profound joint hypomobility.

Immobilization

Knowledge of the effects of immobilization on joint tissue has come about largely from research on animals, where it is possible to control the environment carefully, immobilize the joint, and then identify the changes that have occurred. Human joints undergo the same effects as the animal joint described below (Enneking & Horowitz 1972), and so this research aids our understanding of the effect of joint immobilization in man.

The time-scales involved with rat knee joint immobilization on the joint space, articular cartilage and subchondral bone are summarized in Table 3.7 (Evans et al 1960). Within 15 days there is connective tissue filling the joint space and the formation of adhesions between the connective tissue and the articular cartilage. At 1 month there is atrophy of the opposing articular cartilage, and at 2 months the formation of dense adhesions, more widespread atrophy and ulceration of the articular cartilage and erosion of subchondral bone. All the knees investigated following immobilization had reduced range of movement and joint stiffness due to the connective tissue and adhesion formation in the joint space (Evans et al 1960).

The detailed effect of immobilization on joint capsule, synovial membrane, ligament and articular cartilage has also been investigated. The fibrils within the joint capsule and synovial membrane have been found to have a reduced ability to glide (Akeson et al 1987). The ligament undergoes alterations in its water and glycosaminoglycans (GAG) content, degradation in collagen synthesis, increase in collagen crosslinks after 9 weeks, bone resorption at the bone–ligament junction, reduced stiffness and increased extensibility of the ligament and a reduction in load to failure (Box 3.2). The substantial change in the load displacement curve of the rabbit femur-medial collateral ligament–tibia complex, after 9 weeks of immobilization, compared to a control group is depicted

Table 3.7 Effect of immobilization on joint

Tissue	Time (Evans et al 1960)	Effect	Study
Joint space	15 days; well established at 1 month	Fibrofatty connective tissue appears within the joint space	Evans et al 1960
Adhesions	15 days; dense at 2 months	Adhesions between the fibrofatty connective tissue and the articular cartilage	Evans et al 1960
Articular cartilage	1 month	Atrophy of opposing articular cartilage	Evans et al 1960
	2 months	Atrophy of unapposing cartilage	
	2 months	Ulceration of articular cartilage	
Subchondral bone	2 months	Under an area of articular cartilage lesion proliferation of very vascular connective tissue	Evans et al 1960
	2 months	Erosion of subchondral bone	
Synovial membrane		Reduced ability of fibres to glide	Akeson et al 1987
Joint capsule		Reduced ability of fibres to glide	Akeson et al 1987

Box 3.2 Effect of immobilization on ligament

Effect on ligament	Author
Decrease in water content and glycoaminoglycan (GAG) level in collagen at 9 weeks	Akeson et al 1973
Initially an increase in collagen synthesis and degradation then a decrease in synthesis and degradation of collagen by 3 months	Amiel et al 1983 Tipton et al 1970
Increase in collagen cross-links at 9 weeks	Akeson et al 1977
Decrease in cross-sectional area	Tipton et al 1970 Woo et al 1987
Increase in osteoclastic activity at the bone–ligament junction, causing an increase in bone resorption in that area	Woo et al 1987
Reduced stiffness	Woo et al 1987
Increased extensibility	Akeson et al 1987
Reduction in load to failure and reduction in energy-absorbing capabilities	Akeson et al 1987 Woo et al 1987

in Figure 3.35 (Woo et al 1988). The structural and mechanical effects of immobilization and remobilization of the bone–ligament–bone complex is depicted in Figure 3.36 (Woo et al 1987).

The detailed changes of articular cartilage following immobilization (Box 3.3) include reduced proteoglycan synthesis, softening of the articular cartilage, softening and reduced thickness, adhesions to the fibrofatty connective tissue in the joint space, and pressure necrosis where adjacent surfaces are in contact with chondrocyte death (Vanwanseele et al 2002).

The position in which the joint is immobilized is important in determining the rate of the tissue changes. If a joint is immobilized in full flexion (Salter & Field 1960) or in a position where there is continuous compression of adjacent articular surfaces (Salter & Field 1960), degeneration of

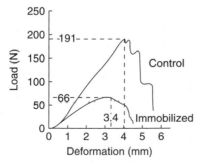

Figure 3.35 The load displacement curve of the rabbit femur-medial collateral ligament–tibia complex after 9 weeks of immobilization compared to a control group (from Woo et al 1988, with permission).

the articular cartilage can occur within 6 days, rather than 30 days (Box 3.3). With prolonged immobilization over 1 year, the ligaments and joint capsule contract, the joint space becomes obliterated with fibrous connective tissue and ossification occurs where the articular surfaces contact each other (Baker et al 1969, Enneking & Horowitz 1972).

Remobilization

The effect of remobilization following 9 weeks of immobilization has been tested in rabbit knee joints (Woo et al 1975). Following immobilization, the knees were repeatedly moved into extension and flexion and the torque necessary to move the knee was measured. With the first cycle, there was a tenfold increase in the resistance to movement but by the 5th cycle, this had reduced to a sevenfold increase, compared to a control group (Woo et al 1975). Cyclic loading thus produced hysteresis and the authors postulated that the underlying mechanism was a physical disruption of adhesions or cross-linkages between collagen fibres in the ligaments developed during the period of immobilization (Woo et al 1975).

The length of time required to gain full recovery following a period of immobilization is much longer than the length of the immobilization (Noyes 1977, Woo et al 1987). Monkey knee joints were immobilized for 8 weeks and it took 12 months for the anterior cruciate ligament to

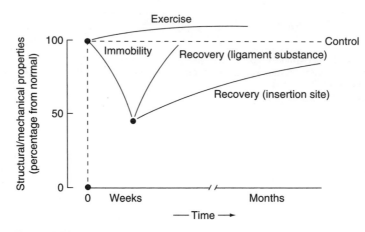

Figure 3.36 The structural and mechanical properties of bone–ligament–bone complex following immobilization and recovery (from Woo et al 1988, with permission of American Academy of Orthopaedic Surgeons).

return to almost full tensile strength (Noyes 1977). In rabbit knees immobilized for 12 weeks, there was a significant reduction ($P = 0.05$) in tensile strength of the medial collateral ligament at 3 months, with full strength at 1 year (Woo et al 1987). If immobilization is not for longer than 30 days, the connective tissue and adhesion formation in the joint space is able to adapt and lengthen with remobilization, although the atrophy of articular cartilage and subchondral bone remains unchanged (Evans et al 1960). Despite the limited reversal of changes, functional movement is restored following a period of remobilization (Evans et al 1960).

Box 3.3 Effect of immobilization on articular cartilage (Vanwanseele et al 2002)

Decrease in proteoglycan synthesis
Softening of articular cartilage
Decrease thickness of articular cartilage
Adherence of fibrofatty connective tissue to cartilage surfaces
Pressure necrosis at points of cartilage–cartilage contact
Chondrocyte death

Summary of hypomobility

A reduced joint range of movement may be due to an increased resistance to movement, or due to the production of symptoms. The movement that is affected may be a physiological and/or accessory movement. Most research into hypomobility has concentrated on the effect of immobilization of a joint where the changes are widespread and profound, and where recovery is limited.

Hypermobility

There may be hypermobility of one or more accessory movements and/or hypermobility of one or more physiological movements. It seems reasonable to suggest that, if there is an increased range of translation, this will affect, to some degree, the range of the rotation of the bone. In the same way, if there is an increased range of rotation this will affect the range of translation. As in hypomobility, the clinician makes a judgement that a joint has more movement than 'normal', which may be based on comparing sides or, in the spine, comparing adjacent levels.

Increased range of accessory or physiological movement is often associated with an altered

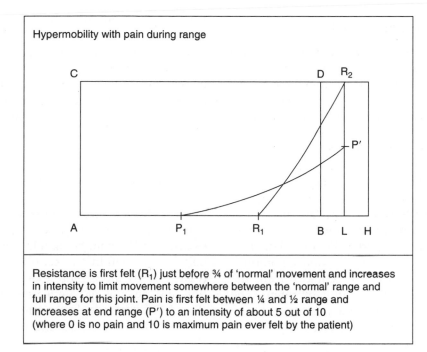

Resistance is first felt (R_1) just before ¾ of 'normal' movement and increases in intensity to limit movement somewhere between the 'normal' range and full range for this joint. Pain is first felt between ¼ and ½ range and increases at end range (P') to an intensity of about 5 out of 10 (where 0 is no pain and 10 is maximum pain ever felt by the patient)

Figure 3.37 Movement diagram of hypermobility with production of symptoms, where ABCD depicts a movement diagram with normal range (AB), L is the limit in range for this movement and H is the 'normal' end of the hypermobile range. R_1 is the first point of resistance felt by the examiner, R_2 is maximum intensity of resistance which limits further movement, P_1 is point in range where pain is first felt and P' is maximum intensity of pain which limits further movement.

quality of movement. This is most commonly associated with the production of symptoms and is depicted in Figure 3.37.

Altered quality of joint movement

Quality of movement includes instability, increased or decreased resistance to movement, poor control of movement, the presence of joint noise such as a clunk or crepitus, excessive effort or reluctance of the patient to move; in short, it is anything considered to be abnormal either by comparison to the other side or from the clinician's experience of what is 'normal'. Altered quality of movement can occur in an otherwise normal joint; for example, muscle weakness will cause active movement to be perceived as greater effort for the patient – there is altered quality of

movement with no dysfunction of the joint. Altered quality of movement can be associated with altered joint range; often hypomobility is associated with increased resistance with or without production of symptoms, and hypermobility with reduced resistance and production of symptoms.

Altered quality of movement has been shown to occur with some pathologies. For example, patients with anterior shoulder instability have been found to have abnormal anterior glide of the humeral head on the glenoid cavity during arm movements (Howell et al 1988). The joint lubricant in synovial fluid, surface-active phospholipid (SAPL), has been found to be deficient in osteoarthritic joints (Hills & Monds 1998) and this reduction causes increased resistance to joint movement (Hills & Thomas 1998).

Production of symptoms

Symptoms from joint dysfunction are most commonly a pain or an ache. Other symptoms include soreness, pulling, and apprehension by the patient to move further into range. Symptoms can come on at any point, or increase through the joint range of movement and/or at the end of the range of joint movement. Sometimes a symptom is felt only during a part of the range, that is, through a particular arc of the movement, and if the symptom is pain it is then commonly referred to as an 'arc or catch of pain'. This would be documented, for example, as 'active shoulder abduction 120 to 140 degrees produces lateral shoulder pain'. More commonly, symptoms are produced sometime during the range and increase to the limit of range. The symptom may be sufficiently intense to be the cause of the limitation in range, depicted as

P_2 on a movement diagram (Figure 3.38), or may reach a particular intensity at the limit of range (P'). Symptoms may be produced in a joint with 'normal', hypomobile or hypermobile range of movement, with or without altered quality of movement. For further information on movement diagrams see Petty & Moore (2001).

Nociception and pain

A distinction needs to be made between nociception and pain. Nociception is the transmission of impulses from nociceptors that occurs with tissue damage. This activation, however, does not necessarily lead to pain being felt. The perception of pain occurs within the central nervous system (Grieve 1994) and is more than simply the sensation and physiological effects of tissue damage (Fig. 3.39). It also includes affective factors such as mood and emotion, cognitive factors such as

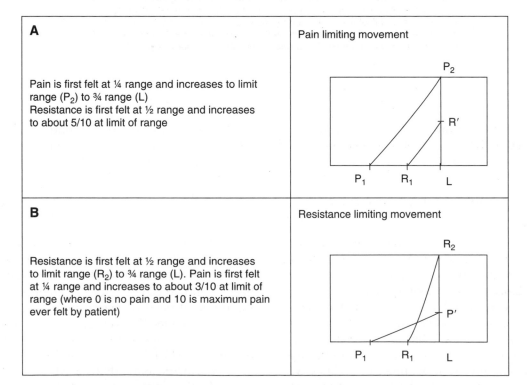

Figure 3.38 Movement diagram depicting **A** P_2 with some resistance and normal range, and **B** P' and resistance limiting movement.

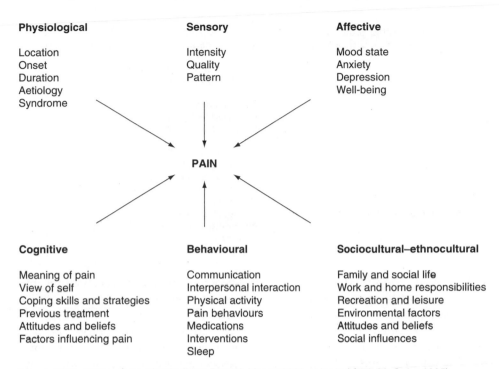

Physiological

Location
Onset
Duration
Aetiology
Syndrome

Sensory

Intensity
Quality
Pattern

Affective

Mood state
Anxiety
Depression
Well-being

PAIN

Cognitive

Meaning of pain
View of self
Coping skills and strategies
Previous treatment
Attitudes and beliefs
Factors influencing pain

Behavioural

Communication
Interpersonal interaction
Physical activity
Pain behaviours
Medications
Interventions
Sleep

Sociocultural–ethnocultural

Family and social life
Work and home responsibilities
Recreation and leisure
Environmental factors
Attitudes and beliefs
Social influences

Figure 3.39 Dimensions of pain (from Petty & Moore 2001, adapted from McGuire 1995).

beliefs and knowledge, behavioural factors such as posture and analgesic intake, and socio-cultural factors such as age, gender and ethnicity (Ahles & Martin 1992, McGuire 1995). Pain has, thus, been defined as 'an unpleasant sensory and emotional experience associated with actual or potential tissue damage, or described in terms of such damage' (Merskey et al 1979). This is not an entirely new idea: Descartes (1985) in the 17th century recognized that pain was accompanied by sadness. He wrote that the body is 'ill-disposed when I feel pain', while unclear of the relationship between 'the thing which causes pain and the sense of sadness to which this feeling gives rise'. In 1940, the classical Christian scholar, C.S Lewis, attempted to unravel the meaning of pain (Lewis 1998), describing it as 'any experience, whether physical or mental, that the patient dislikes and is synonymous with suffering, anguish, tribulation, adversity and trouble'; he clearly associated pain with effects on emotion and thought. Indeed, what person has ever felt indifferent when experiencing pain? Most, if not all,

readers will be able to testify to the sense of suffering and to an emotional response that goes hand in hand with the experience of pain. Pain is an extensive subject and cannot be covered comprehensively in this text. The reader is referred to a number of excellent books on pain, most notably a text by Wall and Melzack (1999). What follows here is an overview of how tissue damage in a joint can cause nociception and potentially cause a person to perceive pain.

The perception of pain affects the sympathetic nervous system (Box 3.4) which has widespread effects on the respiratory, cardiovascular, gastrointestinal and genitourinary systems and on endocrine and metabolic function (Cousins & Power 2002).

Most of the tissues that make up a joint (capsule, ligament, articular disc, meniscus and fat pad) are innervated; in fact, the only structure that is not innervated is the avascular articular cartilage (Messner 1999). The nociceptors in joint are type IV free nerve endings and have been found throughout the joint tissues. In the knee,

Box 3.4 The effect of acute pain on respiratory, cardiovascular, gastrointestinal and genitourinary systems, and endocrine and metabolic function (Cousins & Power 1999)

Respiratory	Splinting of abdominal and thoracic muscles
	Grunting on expiration
	Small tidal volume
	Rapid respiratory rate
Cardiovascular	Increased heart rate
	Increased blood pressure
	Increased cardiac output
	Decreased blood flow in the limbs
Gastrointestinal and genitourinary	Increased intestinal secretions
	Increased smooth-muscle tone
	Reduced intestinal motility
	Urinary retention
Endocrine and metabolic function	Nausea, vomiting
	Altered metabolic rate

for example, they have been found in the collateral ligaments, joint capsule, synovium, cruciate ligaments, infra-patellar fat pad and the outer surface of the menisci (Kennedy et al 1982). All of these tissues are therefore capable of being a source of pain. The type IV fibres that signal pain can be an unmyelinated meshwork, usually associated with blood vessels, or unmyelinated free nerve terminals lying between the collagen and elastic fibres of the connective tissue in which they lie (Messner 1999). These fibres are supplied by myelinated A δ and unmyelinated C fibres.

Nociceptors in joint tissues can be activated by a noxious mechanical force or chemical stimulus (Jessell & Kelly 1991). The effect of nociceptor activity by a mechanical or chemical stimulus alters the physiology of the nociceptor itself; in this way the nociceptor is plastic, that is, it changes. This increased sensitivity of nociceptors leads to a decreased pain threshold and increased pain to supra-threshold stimuli – changes collectively referred to as primary hyperalgesia. If a stimulus is applied which would normally not provoke pain, such as joint movement or light touch, and pain is provoked, this is termed allodynia (Raja et al 1999). In addition, mechanoreceptors in adjacent uninjured tissue develop the ability to evoke pain, a phenomenon known as secondary hyperalgesia (Raja et al 1999). This is thought to be due to an increase in the responsiveness of second-order nociceptor neurones in the spinal cord which

become activated by mechanoreceptor activity, a response known as central sensitization (Raja et al 1999).

Because joint nociceptors are activated by a noxious mechanical force or chemical stimulus (Jessell & Kelly 1991), the pain from joint can be classified as mechanical or chemical nociceptive pain (Gifford 1998).

Mechanical pain occurs where certain movements stress injured tissue, increasing the mechanical deformation and activation of nociceptors; other movements reduce the stress on injured tissue, reducing the mechanical deformation and activation of nociceptors (Box 3.5). Thus, with mechanical pain, there are particular movements which aggravate and ease the pain, sometimes referred to as 'on/off pain'. The magnitude of the mechanical deformation may be directly related to the magnitude of nociceptor activity; this has been found in the skin of the cat where greater forces cause greater nociceptor activity (Garell et al 1996).

Chemical nociceptive pain can be produced by the chemicals released as a result of inflammation, ischaemia or activity of the sympathetic nervous system (Gifford 1998).

Inflammation releases noxious chemicals into the tissues; these chemicals induce or sensitize activity of the nociceptors (Dray 1995, Levine & Reichling 1999), that is, hyperalgesia. It has been proposed that resting pain, pain with movement and pain on local pressure over a joint associated

Box 3.5	Clinical features of mechanical, inflammatory and ischaemic nociceptive pain (Butler 2000)
Mechanical pain	Particular movements that aggravate and ease the pain, sometimes referred to as 'on/off pain'
Inflammatory pain	Redness, oedema and heat
	Acute pain and tissue damage
	Close relationship of stimulus response and pain
	Diurnal pattern with pain and stiffness worst at night and in the morning
	Signs of neurogenic inflammation (redness, swelling or symptoms in neural zone)
	Beneficial effect of anti-inflammatory medication
Ischaemic pain	Symptoms produced after prolonged or unusual activities
	Rapid ease of symptoms after a change in posture
	Symptoms towards the end of the day or after the accumulation of activity
	Poor response to anti-inflammatory medication
	Absence of trauma

with joint inflammation, is caused largely by sensitization of group III and group IV fine articular afferents (Schaible & Schmidt 1985). Prostaglandin E_2 has been identified in inflamed tissue, and this is known to sensitize fine articular afferents (Schaible & Schmidt 1988). Experimentally induced knee joint inflammation of the cat results in a spontaneous discharge from free nerve endings, increased frequency of discharge and reduced threshold for activation by movement (Coggeshall et al 1983, Grigg et al 1986, Schaible & Schmidt 1985). In the rat, some joint afferents and some nociceptors have been found to contain pro-inflammatory chemicals (Levine et al 1985a, 1985b Salo & Theriault 1997); this suggests that mechanoreceptors and nociceptors may contribute to the development of joint inflammation (Holzer 1988, Levine et al 1985a, 1985b).

The effect of joint inflammation on the dorsal horn of the spinal cord has also been investigated. Experimental inflammation in rat and cat ankle and knee joints has been found to cause spontaneous release of substance P, in the dorsal horn of the spinal cord, and this release is increased with passive movements of the inflamed joint (Oku et al 1987, Schaible et al 1990). This may account, at least in part, for the increase in pain when an inflamed joint is passively moved.

Clinical features of inflammatory pain (Box 3.5) are: redness, oedema and heat, acute pain and tissue damage, a close relationship of stimulus response and pain, a diurnal pattern with pain and stiffness worst at night and, in the morning, signs of neurogenic inflammation (redness, swelling or symptoms in neural zone), and a beneficial effect of anti-inflammatory medication (Butler 2000).

In addition, in the cat, it has been demonstrated that knee joint inflammation causes an increased sensitivity of alpha and gamma motor neurones in the hamstring muscles to local pressure and to knee flexion and extension movements (Proske et al 1988). The number of stimulated alpha motor neurones increased, while some gamma motor neurones were stimulated and others were inhibited. The authors consider this to be part of the flexor reflex pattern, with the inhibitory effect on some gamma motor neurones facilitating co-contraction, so that the knee is held in a position of maximum comfort (Proske et al 1988).

Ischaemic nociceptive pain is caused by a lowered pH (acidosis) in tissues, which stimulates nociceptor activity (Steen et al 1995). Lowered pH level is frequently related to both painful ischaemic conditions and painful inflammatory conditions (Steen et al 1995). Clinical features of ischaemic pain (Box 3.5) are thought to be: symptoms produced after prolonged or unusual activities, rapid ease of symptoms after a change in posture, symptoms towards the end of the day or after the accumulation of activity, a poor response to anti-inflammatory medication and sometimes absence of trauma (Butler 2000).

In the presence of tissue injury or inflammation, the sympathetic nervous system activity can maintain the perception of pain or enhance nociception in inflamed tissue. Sympathetically maintained pain can occur with complex regional pain syndromes and may play a part in chronic arthritis and soft-tissue trauma (Raja et al 1999). In rats with inflammatory arthritis, post-ganglionic sympathetic neurones have been found to release catecholamines, a substance that exacerbates joint inflammation (Basbaum & Levine 1991, Levine et al 1985a, 1985b).

It should be noted that the information given here has focused on pain from joint tissue only. Clearly, pain may be felt from a number of tissues, including the skin, muscle and nerve overlying the joint. Discussion of muscle pain is discussed in the chapter on function and dysfunction of muscles, and discussion of pain from skin and nerve is discussed in the chapter on function and dysfunction of nerves.

Summary of symptom production

The commonest symptom from a joint is pain. The perception of pain occurs in the central nervous system and is multidimensional, including sensory, physiological, affective, cognitive, behavioural and socio-cultural factors. Almost all the tissues that make up joint, except for the articular cartilage, contain nociceptors and can therefore be a potential source of pain. Joint nociceptors are sensitive to mechanical deformation and chemical irritation and can thus produce mechanical or chemical nociceptive pain. Chemical irritation may be due to inflammation, ischaemia or sympathetic nervous system activity.

Pain referral areas

Some generalization can be made about the pattern of pain referral from bone, joint, capsule and ligaments. In general, pain does not usually cross the midline of the spine (Cloward 1959, Kellgren 1939), although this has been observed in some individuals (Hockaday & Whitty 1967, Mooney & Robertson 1976). Pain from more superficial tissue, regardless of whether that tissue is bone, joint or ligament, gives rise to more localized pain; deeper tissue gives rise to more diffuse pain that may be referred in a segmental distribution

(Inman & Saunders 1944, Kellgren 1939, Kellgren 1977). Pain from skin is the most localized and accurate (Inman & Saunders 1944), which would seem to make sense because it is the interface between the body and the world around. Because pain from bone, joint, capsule and ligament is diffuse and widespread, the area of a patient's pain will not directly relate to the source of the patient's symptom. For example, pain from the hip joint can produce anterior thigh pain without any pain actually over the joint (Grieve 1994).

The segmental distribution may be related to a dermatome or sclerotome (Fig. 3.40). Dermatomes describe the segmental innervation of the skin, and sclerotomes the segmental innervation of bone (Inman & Saunders 1944). These charts provide a generalized segmental supply of skin and bone and are used clinically to interpret pain referral areas. However, there is such a wide variation of these areas between individuals that they are considered invalid (Hockaday & Whitty 1967, McCall et al 1979). Dermatome and sclerotome charts, therefore, need to be considered as a guideline for clinical practice.

Bone. The sensitivity of the various tissues to producing pain differs, with periosteum having the greatest sensitivity followed by ligaments, joint capsules, tendons, fascia and finally muscle tissues (Inman & Saunders 1944). The sensitivity of the joint capsule and ligamentous tissue varies, and is greatest where it attaches to the periosteum (Inman & Saunders 1944). Superficial irritation of periosteum produces pain over the area, while deep irritation of periosteum causes more of a diffuse pain, which may be referred (Kellgren 1939). Some distributions of pain from the periosteum of the lumbar spine and the scapula are given in Figure 3.41.

Ligaments. The pattern of pain referral from provocative injection of saline into the interspinous ligament has been explored by a number of workers (Hockaday & Whitty 1967, Inman & Saunders 1944, Kellgren 1939). If the interspinous ligament is injected in the midline, pain is felt bilaterally, and if slightly to one side, pain is felt only on that side (Kellgren 1939), although occasionally injection on one side produces

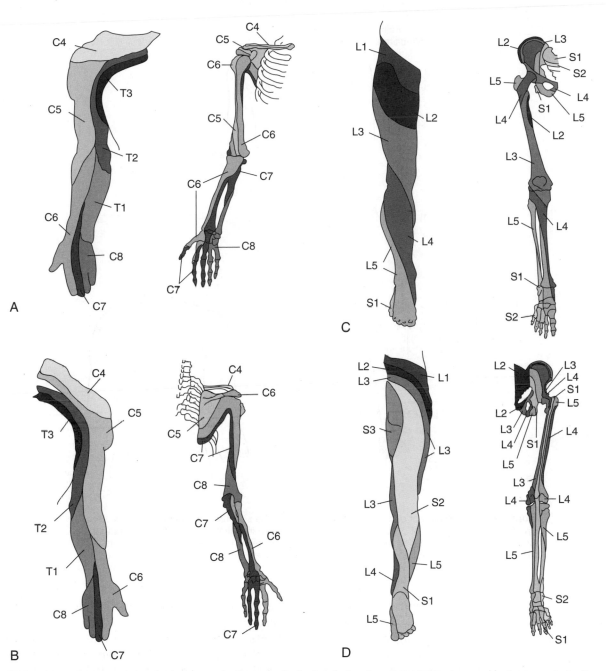

Figure 3.40 Dermatomes and sclerotomes in the upper limb. **A** Anterior view. **B** Posterior view, and in the lower limb. **C** Anterior view. **D** Posterior view. (From Inman & Saunders 1944, Referred pain from skeletal structures. Journal of Nervous and Mental Disease 99:660–667, with permission.)

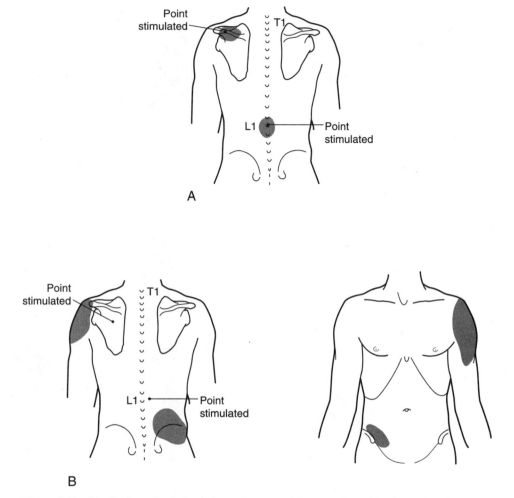

Figure 3.41 Distribution of pain from the periosteum of the scapula and lumbar spine. **A** Superficial irritation of tip of scapula and L1 lamina. **B** Deep irritation of spine and infraspinous fossa of scapula. (Reproduced, with permission, from Kellgren J H 1939 Clinical Science 4:35–46. © The Biochemical Society and the Medical Research Society.)

bilateral pain (Hockaday & Whitty 1967). The pattern of ache and deep tenderness felt by three subjects for each interspinous ligament from C4/5 level to the sacrum is shown in Figure 3.42. In a similar study with 28 subjects, it was found that referral to the arms was rare, with most pain felt around the posterior trunk (Hockaday & Whitty 1967). Two examples from injection of the interspinous ligament at C7/T1 and at T6/7 are shown in Figure 3.43. While there was consistency in the response on different occasions for any one individual, there was a large variation between individuals (Hockaday & Whitty 1967).

Joints. The pattern of pain referral from the cervical interbody joint has been explored with cervical discography (Cloward 1959, Holt 1964, Klafta & Collis 1969). This involves a provocative injection of radio-opaque solution into the outer and middle parts of the intervertebral disc. Stimulation of the disc in the midline produced bilateral pain and stimulation on one side produced unilateral pain (Cloward 1959). While there was variation between individuals, a

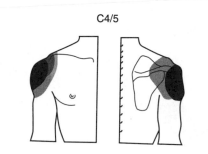

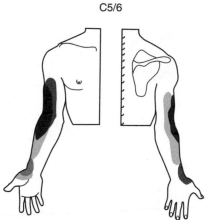
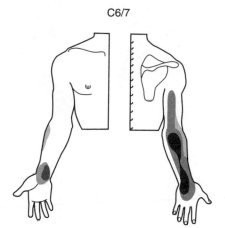

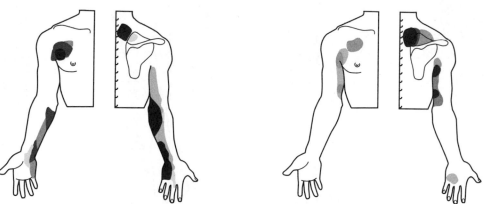

Figure 3.42 Distribution of pain from the interspinous ligament from C4/5 level to sacrum. (Reproduced, with permission, from Kellgren J H 1939 Clinical Science 4:35–46 © The Biochemical Society and the Medical Research Society.)

consistent pattern of more caudad cervical levels producing more caudad thoracic pain was apparent (Cloward 1959). The pattern of pain referral from the anterior aspect of the disc differs from the pain referral from the posterior aspect (Fig. 3.44). When the posterior aspect of the disc was stimulated, the pain was more intense and more widespread (Cloward 1959). Provocation to the left of midline on the posterior aspect of C4/5 produced pain over the base of

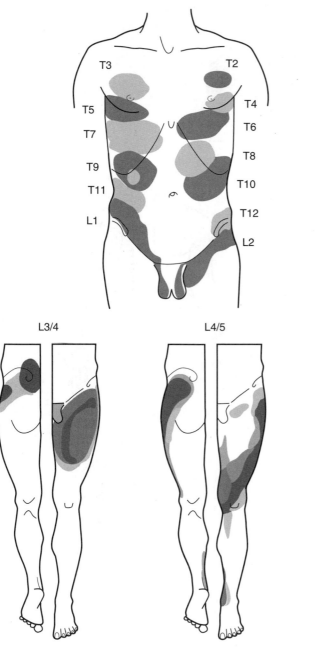
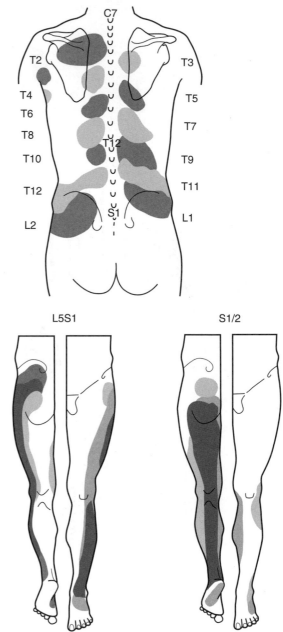

Figure 3.42 *(Cont'd)*

the neck and top of the shoulder (Cloward 1959). These pain referral areas, however, were not substantiated by a similar study a few years later (Holt 1964). In 50 asymptomatic subjects, injection at each level between C3/4 and C7/T1 failed to produce any consistent pattern of pain referral (Holt 1964). The use of discography to identify the intervertebral disc as the source of the patient's symptoms is, however, limited (Holt 1964, Klafta & Collis 1969). For discs with degeneration or protrusion, injection reproduced the patient's symptoms in only 20 or 30% of cases

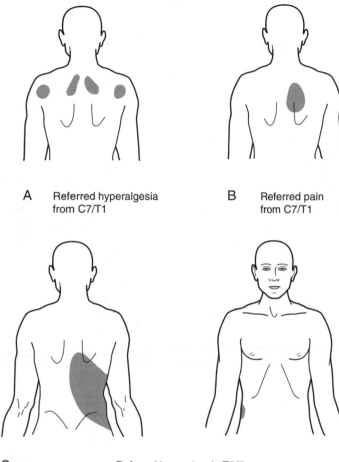

A   Referred hyperalgesia
    from C7/T1

B   Referred pain
    from C7/T1

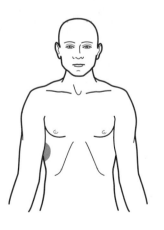

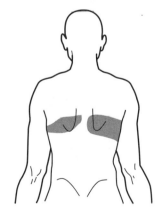

C   Referred hyperalgesia T6/7

D   Referred pain T6/7

Figure 3.43 Distribution of hyperalgesia and pain from the interspinous ligament from C7/T1 and T6/7 (after Hockaday & Whitty 1967, Patterns of referred pain in the normal subject. Brain 90(3):481–495 with permission of Oxford University Press).

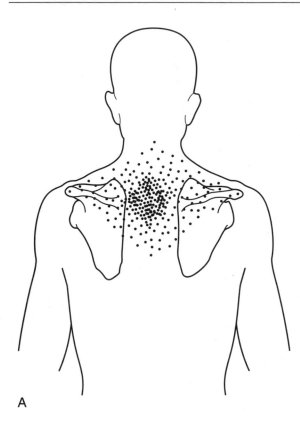

A

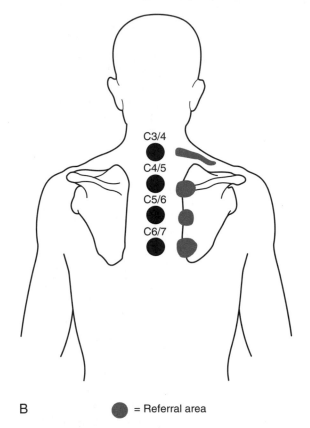

B

⬤ = Referral area

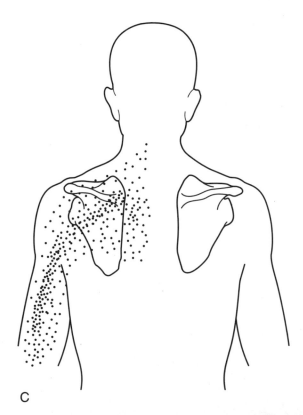

C

Figure 3.44 A Referred pain from the anterior aspect of the cervical intervertebral discs between C3/4, C4/5, C5/6 and C6/7. (After Cloward 1959, Cervical discography: a contribution to the etiology and mechanism of neck, shoulder and arm pain. Annals of Surgery 150:1052–1064, with permission.) **B** Referred pain from the posterior aspect and midline of the cervical intervertebral discs between C3/4, C4/5, C5/6 and C6/7. The midline dots indicate the area of referred pain from provocation of the midline of the disc, while the shaded areas to the right indicate the area of referred pain from provocation to the right of midline. **C** Referred pain from provocation to the left of midline at C5/6 and C6/7.

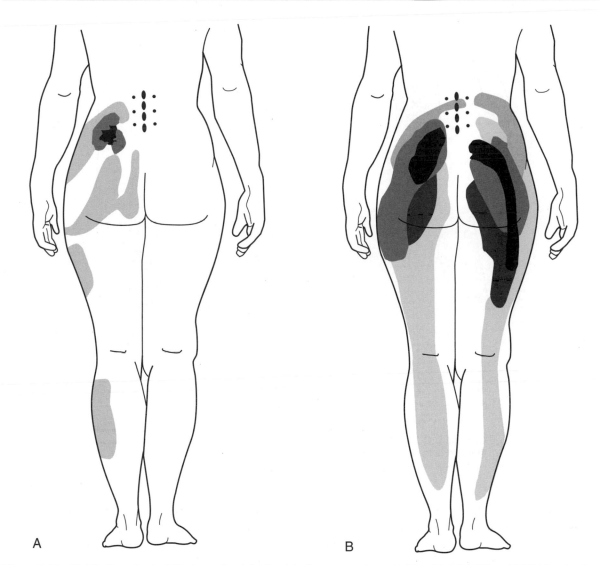

Figure 3.45 Distribution of pain following saline injection into the zygapophyseal joints of **A** left L4/5 and L5/S1 levels of asymptomatic subjects, and **B** all three levels – L3/4, L4/5 and L5/S1 – of chronic LBP patients (after Mooney & Robertson 1976, The facet syndrome. Clinical Orthopaedics and Related Research 115:149–156, with permission).

respectively (Klafta & Collis 1969). Interscapula pain, as well as chest pain, arm pain and occipital headaches, were found to be associated with C4/5, C5/6 and C6/7 disc pain (Brodsky 1985).

Pain arising from the lumbar zygapophyseal joints has been investigated by injection of saline into the joint cavity (McCall et al 1979, Mooney & Robertson 1976). The extent of referral into the leg was dependent on the degree of irritation, greater amounts of saline causing more distal

symptoms (Mooney & Robertson 1976). Saline injection into L4/5 and L5/S1 zygapophyseal joints of five asymptomatic subjects and 15 patients suffering chronic low back pain (LBP) is shown in Figure 3.45. Similar results in asymptomatic subjects were found with injection at L1/2 and L4/5 zygapophyseal joints (McCall et al 1979). Interestingly, the areas of referred pain from L1/2 and L4/5 are close and even overlap (Fig. 3.46) – which makes interpretation of this

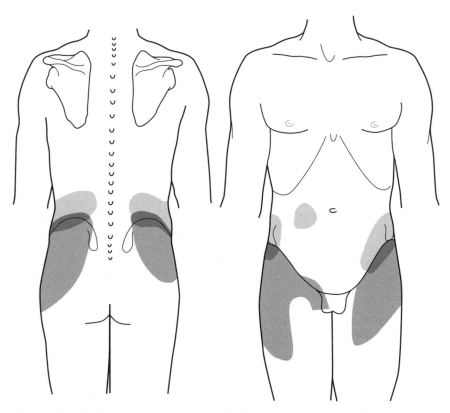

Figure 3.46 Distribution of pain following injection of saline into the L1/2 (lighter shading) and L4/5 (darker shading) zygapophyseal joint (after McCall, Park & O'Brien 1979, Induced pain referral from posterior lumbar elements in normal subjects. Spine 4(5):441–446 with permission).

information in the clinical field difficult. This is compounded by the fact that patients diagnosed with zygapophyseal joint pain with anaesthetic blocks have no clinical features in common (Schwarzer et al 1994). So, while zygapophyseal joints can theoretically be a source of pain, clinicians are unable to identify this joint on the basis of a patient's clinical pain presentation.

Information on pain from the sacroiliac joint has been explored in 10 asymptomatic subjects by radio-opaque injection into the joint (Fortin et al 1994a). Pain was felt fairly locally around the posterior superior iliac spine (Fig. 3.47). In a further study, it was found that this area of referral could not be used accurately to identify patients with sacroiliac joint pain (Fortin et al 1994b).

Pain arising from joints in the upper or lower limb tends to be localized around the joint. This

localization is greatest in the distal joints of the hand and foot, while the hip and shoulder can refer pain in a more segmental distribution (Kellgren 1939). Referral of pain from the tibiofemoral joint by provocation of the medial collateral ligament, lateral and posterior joint capsule is shown in Figure 3.48 (Kellgren 1939).

Joint injury: ligament tear and healing

Ligaments can tear in the middle region by avulsion of bone and, more rarely, at the insertion site (Woo et al 1988). Untreated ligaments have been shown to repair by scar tissue formation that is inferior to the original ligamentous tissue (Frank et al 1983). The natural repair process of ligamentous tissue has been observed in rabbit knees

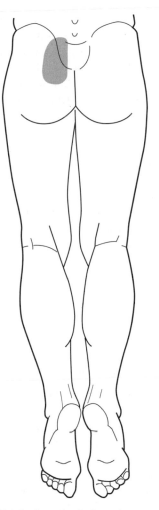

Figure 3.47 Distribution of pain from the sacroiliac joint (after Fortin et al 1994a, Sacroiliac joint: pain referral maps upon applying a new injunction/arthography technique, part I: asymptomatic volunteers. Spine 19(13):1475–1482 with permission).

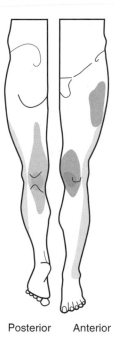

Posterior   Anterior

Figure 3.48 Referred pain from the knee: from medial collateral ligament – horizontal hatching; lateral joint capsule – stippling; posterior joint capsule – vertical hatching. (Reproduced, with permission, from Kellgren J H 1939 Clinical Science 4:35–46 © The Biochemical Society and the Medical Research Society.)

by experimentally transecting the medial collateral ligament (Frank et al 1983). Granulation tissue bridged the gap between the ligament ends within 10 days, with hypertrophy at 3 weeks. Remodelling then occurred so that the ligament looked normal by 14 weeks. Normal ligamentous tissue is made up of type I collagen; ligamentous scar tissue, however, consists of type III collagen, giving the ligament less stiffness and strength than prior to the injury (Woo & Akeson 1987). In the skin, maturation causes a gradual reduction in the type III collagen (Forrest 1983); however, in ligaments even after 40 weeks, there are still significant amounts of type III collagen (Woo & Akeson 1987). Healing can be considered to occur in three stages: an inflammatory response lasting approximately 72 hours, a proliferation phase lasting several weeks and finally the remodelling and maturation phase which can take 1–2 years (Vicenzino et al 2002). The reader is directed to the numerous pathology textbooks for further information on inflammation and healing.

Following a joint sprain, such as a sprained ankle with a tear of the lateral ligament, the dysfunction is more localized to specific movements. Typically, with a lateral ligament sprain, the movements of the foot which cause tension on the lateral ligament are limited in range and may give rise to pain. So the movement dysfunction, in this case, is hypomobility due to resistance and pain produced by plantarflexion, inversion and perhaps anteroposterior and posteroanterior glides of the talus.

Joint effusion may accompany a joint injury and, if excessive, can impair synovial nutrition (Jayson & Dixon 1970a). Knee joint pressure is generally greatest in extension and is reduced at about 30 degrees flexion, which corresponds to the position of ease that a patient often finds in a swollen joint (Jayson & Dixon 1970b).

Summary of joint dysfunction

Common joint dysfunctions seen clinically are hypomobility limited by resistance or pain, hypermobility with pain, altered quality of movement and the production of symptoms.

Joint dysfunction does not exist in isolation. Not only may there be a number of movements affected at any one joint, and a number of joints affected, muscle and nerve tissue will also to some extent be involved. For example, after 3 weeks in plaster of paris following a Colles fracture, there may be hypomobility due to resistance and pain of accessory and physiological movements at the superior and inferior radiocarpal joints, radiocarpal joint, mid-carpal joints, carpometacarpal and metacarpophalangeal joints of the hand, as well as muscle weakness and shortening, nerve shortening and pain and tenderness over the skin.

The next chapter discusses treatment of joint dysfunction.

REFERENCES

Adams M A, Bogduk N, Burton K, Dolan P 2002 The biomechanics of back pain. Churchill Livingstone, Edinburgh

Ahles T A, Martin J B 1992 Cancer pain: a multidimensional perspective. In: Turk D C, Feldman C S (eds) Noninvasive approaches to pain management in the terminally ill. Haworth, New York, p 25–48

Akeson W H, Woo S L-Y, Amiel D et al 1973 The connective tissue response to immobility: biochemical changes in periarticular connective tissue of the immobilized rabbit knee. Clinical Orthopaedics and Related Research 93:356–362

Akeson W H, Amiel D, Mechanic G L et al 1977 Collagen cross-linking alterations in joint contractures: changes in the reducible cross-links in periarticular connective tissue collagen after nine weeks of immobilization. Connective Tissue Research 5:15–19

Akeson W H, Amiel D, Abel M F et al 1987 Effects of immobilization on joints. Clinical Orthopaedics and Related Research 219:28–37

Albright D J, Zimny M L, Dabezies E 1987 Mechanoreceptors in the human medial meniscus. Anatomical Record 218:6A–7A

Amiel D, Akeson W H, Harwood F L, Frank C B 1983 Stress deprivation effect on metabolic turnover of the medial collateral ligament collagen, a comparison between nine- and 12-week immobilization. Clinical Ortho paedics and Related Research 172:265–270

Askew M J, Mow V C 1978 The biomechanical function of the collagen fibril ultrastructure of articular cartilage. Journal of Biomechanical Engineering 100:105–115

Baker W de C, Thomas T G, Kirkaldy-Willis W H 1969 Changes in the cartilage of the posterior intervertebral joints after anterior fusion. Journal of Bone and Joint Surgery 51B(4):736–746

Barrett D S, Cobb A G, Bentley G 1991 Joint proprioception in normal, osteoarthritic and replaced knees. Journal of Bone and Joint Surgery 73B(1):53–56

Basbaum A I, Levine J D 1991 The contribution of the nervous system to inflammation and inflammatory disease. Canadian Journal of Physiology and Pharmacology 69:647–651

Berchuck M, Andriacchi T P, Bach B R, Reider B 1990 Gait adaptations by patients who have a deficient anterior cruciate ligament. Journal of Bone and Joint Surgery 72A(6):871–877

Bogduk N 1997 Clinical anatomy of the lumbar spine and sacrum, 3rd edn. Churchill Livingstone, New York, ch 9, p 105

Brandt K D 1997 Putting some muscle into osteoarthritis. Annals of Internal Medicine 127(2):154–156

Brodsky A E 1985 Cervical angina, a correlative study with emphasis on the use of coronary arteriography. Spine 10(8):699–709

Butler D S 2000 The sensitive nervous system. Noigroup, Adelaide.

Clark F J 1975 Information signaled by sensory fibers in medial articular nerve. Journal of Neurophysiology 38:1464–1472

Clark F J, Burgess P R 1975 Slowly adapting receptors in cat knee joint: can they signal joint angle? Journal of Neurophysiology 38:1448–1463

Cloward R B 1959 Cervical discography: a contribution to the etiology and mechanism of neck, shoulder and arm pain. Annals of Surgery 150:1052–1064

Coggeshall R E, Hong K A H P, Langford L A et al 1983 Discharge characteristics of fine medial articular afferents at rest and during passive movements of inflamed knee joints. Brain Research 272:185–188

Comerford M J, Mottram S L 2001 Functional stability re-training: principles and strategies for managing mechanical dysfunction. Manual Therapy 6(1):3–14

Cooper R R, Misol S 1970 Tendon and ligament insertion: a light and electron microscopic study. Journal of Bone and Joint Surgery 52A(1):1–20

Cousins M, Power I 1999 Acute and postoperative pain. In: Wall P D, Melzack R (eds) Textbook of pain, 4th edn. Churchill Livingstone, Edinburgh, ch 19, p 447–491

Cyriax J 1982 Textbook of orthopaedic medicine-diagnosis of soft tissue lesions, 8th edn. Baillière Tindall, London

deAndrade J R, Grant C, Dixon A St J 1965 Joint distension and reflex muscle inhibition in the knee. Journal of Bone and Joint Surgery 47A(2):313–322

Descartes R 1985 Discourse on method and the meditations. Penguin, Middlesex, 6th meditation p 150–169

DeVita P, Hortobagyi T, Barrier J et al 1997 Gait adaptations before and after anterior cruciate ligament reconstruction surgery. Medicine and Science in Sports and Exercise 29(7):853–859

Dray A 1995 Inflammatory mediators of pain. British Journal of Anaesthetics 75:125–131

Edin B B 1992 Quantitative analysis of static strain sensitivity in human mechanoreceptors from hairy skin. Journal of Neurophysiology 67(5):1105–1113

Edin B B, Abbs J H 1991 Finger movement responses of cutaneous mechanoreceptors in the dorsal skin of the human hand. Journal of Neurophysiology 65(3):657–670

Edmondston S J, Allison G T, Gregg C D et al. 1998 Effect of position on the posteroanterior stiffness of the lumbar spine. Manual Therapy 3(1):21–26

Edwards B C 1999 Manual of combined movements, 2nd edn. Butterworth-Heinemann, Oxford

Enneking W F, Horowitz M 1972 The intra-articular effects of immobilization on the human knee. Journal of Bone and Joint Surgery 54A(5):973–985

Evans E B, Eggers G W N, Butler J K, Blumel J 1960 Experimental immobilization and remobilization of rat knee joints. Journal of Bone and Joint Surgery 42A(5):737–758

Felson D T, Zhang Y 1998 An update on the epidemiology of knee and hip osteoarthritis with a view to prevention. Arthritis and Rheumatism 41(8):1343–1355

Ferrell W R 1980 The adequacy of stretch receptors in the cat knee joint for signalling joint angle throughout a full range of movement. Journal of Physiology 299:85–99

Ferrell W R 1985 The response of slowly adapting mechanoreceptors in the cat knee joint to tetanic contraction of hind limb muscles. Quarterly Journal of Experimental Physiology 70:337–345

Forrest L 1983 Current concepts in soft connective tissue wound healing. British Journal of Surgery 70:133–140

Fortin J D, Dwyer A P, West S, Pier J 1994a Sacroiliac joint: pain referral maps upon applying a new injection/arthrography technique, part I: asymptomatic volunteers. Spine 19(13):1475–1482

Fortin J D, Aprill C N, Ponthieux B, Pier J 1994b Sacroiliac joint: pain referral maps upon applying a new injection/arthrography technique, part II: clinical evaluation. Spine 19(13):1483–1489

Frank C B, Shrive N G 1999 Ligament. In: Nigg B M, Herzog W Biomechanics of the musculo-skeletal system, 2nd edn. John Wiley, Chichester, ch 2.5, p 107–126

Frank C, Woo S L-Y, Amiel D et al 1983 Medial collateral ligament healing a multidisciplinary assessment in rabbits. American Journal of Sports Medicine 11(6):379–389

Frankel V H, Burstein A H, Brooks D B 1971 Biomechanics of internal derangement of the knee. Journal of Bone and Joint Surgery 53A(5):945–962

Freeman M A R, Wyke B 1967a Articular reflexes at the ankle joint: an electromyographic study of normal and abnormal influences of ankle joint mechanoreceptors upon reflex activity in the leg muscles. British Journal of Surgery 54(12):990–1001

Freeman M A R, Wyke B 1967b The innervation of the knee joint. An anatomical and histological study in the cat. Journal of Anatomy 101(3):505–532

Fuller M S, Grigg P, Hoffman A H 1991 Response of joint capsule neurons to axial stress and strain during dynamic loading in cat. Journal of Neurophysiology 65(6):1321–1328

Garell P C, McGillis S L B, Greenspan J D 1996 Mechanical response properties of nociceptors innervating feline hairy skin. Journal of Neurophysiology 75(3):1177–1189

Gifford L 1998 Pain. In: Pitt-Brooke J, Reid H, Lockwood J, Kerr K (eds) Rehabilitation of movement, theoretical basis of clinical practice. W B Saunders, London, ch 5, p 196–232

Glousman R, Jobe F, Tibone J et al 1988 Dynamic electromyographic analysis of the throwing shoulder with glenohumeral instability. Journal of Bone and Joint Surgery 70A(2):220–226

Glousman R E, Barron J, Jobe F W et al 1992 An electromyographic analysis of the elbow in normal and injured pitchers with medial collateral ligament insufficiency. American Journal of Sports Medicine 20(3):311–317

Grieve G P 1994 Referred pain and other clinical features. In Grieve's modern manual therapy, the vertebral column, 2nd edn. Boyling J D, Palastanga N (eds) Churchill Livingstone, Edinburgh, ch 19, p 271–292

Grigg P 1994 Peripheral neural mechanisms in proprioception. Journal of Sport Rehabilitation 3:2–17

Grigg P, Hoffman A H 1982 Properties of Ruffini afferents revealed by stress analysis of isolated sections of cat knee capsule. Journal of Neurophysiology 47(1):41–54

Grigg P, Hoffman A H, Fogarty K E 1982 Properties of Golgi–Mazzoni afferents in cat knee joint capsule, as revealed by mechanical studies of isolated joint capsule. Journal of Neurophysiology 47(1):31–40

Grigg P, Schaible H-G, Schmidt R F 1986 Mechanical sensitivity of group III and IV afferents from posterior articular nerve in normal and inflamed cat knee. Journal of Neurophysiology 55(4):635–643

Harryman D T, Sidles J A, Clark J M et al 1990 Translation of the humeral head on the glenoid with passive glenohumeral motion. Journal of Bone and Joint Surgery 72A(9):1334–1343

Heppelmann B, Messlinger K, Neiss W F, Schmidt R F 1990 Ultrastructural three-dimensional reconstruction of group III and group IV sensory nerve endings ('free nerve endings') in the knee joint capsule of the cat: evidence for multiple receptive sites. Journal of Comparative Neurology 292:103–116

Hills B A 1989 Oligolamellar lubrication of joints by surface active phospholipid. Journal of Rheumatology 16(1):82–91

Hills B A 1995 Remarkable anti-wear properties of joint surfactant. Annals of Biomedical Engineering 23:112–115

Hills B A, Monds M K 1998 Deficiency of lubricating surfactant lining the articular surfaces of replaced hips and knees. British Journal of Rheumatology 37:143–147

Hills B A, Thomas K 1998 Joint stiffness and 'articular gelling': inhibition of the fusion of articular surfaces by surfactant. British Journal of Rheumatology 37:532–538

Hockaday J M, Whitty C W M 1967 Patterns of referred pain in the normal subject. Brain 90(3):481–495

Holt E P 1964 Fallacy of cervical discography: report of 50 cases in normal subjects. Journal of the American Medical Association 188(9):799–801

Holzer P 1988 Local effector functions of capsaicin-sensitive sensory nerve endings: involvement of tachykinins, calcitonin gene-related peptide and other neuropeptides. Neuroscience 24(3):739–768

Hortobagyi T, DeVita P 2000 Muscle pre- and coactivity during downward stepping are associated with leg stiffness in aging. Journal of Electromyography and Kinesiology 10:117–126

Howell S M, Galinat B J, Renzi A J, Marone P J 1988 Normal and abnormal mechanics of the glenohumeral joint in the horizontal plane. Journal of Bone and Joint Surgery 70A(2):227–232

Hughston J C, Walsh W M, Puddu G 1984 Patellar subluxation and dislocation, vol 5. W B Saunders, Philadelphia

Hulliger M, Nordh E, Thelin A-E, Vallbo A B 1979 The responses of afferent fibres from the glabrous skin of the hand during voluntary finger movements in man. Journal of Physiology (Lond) 291:233–249

Hurley M V, Newham D J 1993 The influence of arthrogenous muscle inhibition on quadriceps rehabilitation of patients with early, unilateral osteoarthritic knees. British Journal of Rheumatology 32:127–131

Hurley M V, O'Flanagan S J, Newham D J 1991 Isokinetic and isometric muscle strength and inhibition after elbow arthroplasty. Journal of Orthopaedic Rheumatology 4:83–95

Hurley M V, Jones D W, Wilson D, Newham D J 1992 Rehabilitation of quadriceps inhibited due to isolated rupture of the anterior cruciate ligament. Journal of Orthopaedic Rheumatology 5:145–154

Hurley M V, Jones D W, Newham D J 1994 Arthrogenic quadriceps inhibition and rehabilitation of patients with extensive traumatic knee injuries. Clinical Sciences 86:305–310

Iles J F, Stokes M, Young A 1990 Reflex actions of knee joint afferents during contraction of the human quadriceps. Clinical Physiology 10:489–500

Indahl A, Kaigle A, Reikeras O, Holm S 1995 Electromyographic response of the porcine multifidus musculature after nerve stimulation. Spine 20(24):2652–2658

Indahl A, Kaigle A, Reikeras O, Holm S 1997 Interaction between the porcine lumbar intervertebral disc, zygapophysial joints, and paraspinal muscles. Spine 22(24):2834–2840

Inman V T, Saunders J B DeC M 1944 Referred pain from skeletal structures. Journal of Nervous and Mental Disease 99:660–667

Jayson M I V, Dixon A St J 1970a Intra-articular pressure in rheumatoid arthritis of the knee. II Effect of intra-articular pressure on blood circulation to the synovium. Annals of the Rheumatic Diseases 29:266–268

Jayson M I V, Dixon A St J 1970b Intra-articular pressure in rheumatoid arthritis of the knee. III. pressure changes during joint use. Annals of the Rheumatic Diseases 29:401–408

Jessell T M, Kelly D D 1991 Pain and analgesia. In: Kandel E R, Schwartz J H, Jessell T M (eds) Principles of Neural Science, 3rd edn. Elsevier, New York, ch 27, p 385–399

Johns R J, Wright V 1962 Relative importance of various tissues in joint stiffness. Journal of Applied Physiology 17(5):824–828

Kaltenborn F M 1989 Manual mobilization of the extremity joints: basic examination and treatment, 4th edn. Olaf Norlis Bokhandel, Oslo

Keating J F, Crossan J F 1992 Evaluation of rotator cuff function following anterior dislocation of the shoulder. Journal of Orthopaedic Rheumatology 5:135–140

Kellgren J H 1939 On the distribution of pain arising from deep somatic structures with charts of segmental pain areas. Clinical Science 4:35–46

Kellgren J H 1977 The anatomical source of back pain. Rheumatology and Rehabilitation 16(3):3–12

Kennedy J C, Alexander I J, Hayes K C 1982 Nerve supply of the human knee and its functional importance. American Journal of Sports Medicine 10(6):329–335

Klafta L A, Collis J S 1969 The diagnostic inaccuracy of the pain response in cervical discography. Cleveland Clinical Quarterly 36:35–39

Knatt T, Guanche C, Solomonow M et al 1995 The glenohumeral-biceps reflex in the feline. Clinical Orthopaedics and Related Research 314:247–252

Krauspe R, Schmidt M, Schaible H-G 1992 Sensory innervation of the anterior cruciate ligament. Journal of Bone and Joint Surgery 74A(3):390–397

Latimer J, Lee M, Adams R, Moran C M 1996 An investigation of the relationship between low back pain and lumbar posteroanterior stiffness. Journal of Manipulative and Physiological Therapeutics 19(9):587–591

Lee R, Evans J 1992 Load-displacement-time characteristics of the spine under posteroanterior mobilisation. Australian Journal of Physiotherapy 38:115–123

Lee M, Svensson N L 1993 Effect of loading frequency of the spine to lumbar posteroanterior forces. Journal of Manipulative and Physiological Therapeutics 16(7):439–446

Lee M, Esler M-A, Mildren J, Herbert R 1993 Effect of extensor muscle activation on the response to lumbar posteroanterior forces. Clinical Biomechanics 8:115–119

Levick J R 1983 Joint pressure-volume studies: their importance, design and interpretation. Journal of Rheumatology 10:353–357

Levick J R 1984 Blood flow and mass transport in synovial joints. In: Renkin E M, Michel C C (eds) Handbook of physiology section 2: the cardiovascular system volume IV microcirculation, part 2. American Physiological Society, Bethesda, Maryland, ch 19, p 917–947

Levine J D, Reichling D B 1999 Peripheral mechanisms of inflammatory pain. In: Wall P D, Melzack R (eds) Textbook of pain, 4th edn. Churchill Livingstone, Edinburgh

Levine J D, Dardick S J, Basbaum A I, Scipios E 1985a Reflex neurogenic inflammation 1. Contribution of the peripheral nervous system to spatially remote inflammatory responses that follow injury. Journal of Neuroscience 5(5):1380–1386

Levine J D, Moskowitz M A, Basbaum A I 1985b The contribution of neurogenic inflammation in experimental arthritis. Journal of Immunology 135(2):843s–847s

Lewis C S 1998 The problem of pain. Fount, London

Louie J K, Mote C D 1987 Contribution of the musculature to rotatory laxity and torsional stiffness at the knee. Journal of Biomechanics 20(3):281–300

Louie J K, Kuo C Y, Gutierrez M D, Mote C D 1984 Surface EMG and torsion measurements during snow skiing: laboratory and field tests. Journal of Biomechanics 17(10):713–724

McCall I W, Park W M, O'Brien J P 1979 Induced pain referral from posterior lumbar elements in normal subjects. Spine 4(5):441–446

McCloskey D I, Macefield G, Gandevia S C, Burke D 1987 Sensing position and movements of the fingers. News in Physiological Science 2:226–230

MacConaill M A 1953 The movements of bones and joints, 5. The significance of shape. Journal of Bone and Joint Surgery 35B(2):290–297

MacConaill M A 1966 The geometry and algebra of articular kinematics. Bio-Medical Engineering 32(1):205–211

Macefield G, Gandevia S C, Burke D 1990 Perceptual responses to microstimulation of single afferents innervating joints, muscles and skin of the human hand. Journal of Physiology (Lond) 429:113–129

McGill S M, Norman R W 1986 Partitioning of the L4-L5 dynamic moment into disc, ligamentous, and muscular components during lifting. Spine 11(7):666–678

McGuire D B 1995 The multiple dimensions of cancer pain: a framework for assessment and management. In: McGuire D B, Yarbro C H, Ferrell B R (eds) Cancer pain management, 2nd edn. Jones and Bartlett, Boston

McQuade K J, Shelley I, Cvitkovic J 1999 Patterns of stiffness during clinical examination of the glenohumeral joint. Clinical Biomechanics 14:620–627

Maitland G D, Banks K, English K, Hengeveld E, 2001 Maitland's vertebral manipulation, 6th edn. Butterworth-Heinemann, Oxford

Maki S, Gruen T 1976 Anthropometric study of the gleno humeral joint. 22nd Annual Meeting of the Orthopaedic Research Society 1:173

Merskey R, Albe-Fessard D G, Bonica J J et al 1979 Pain terms: a list with definitions and notes on usage. Pain 6:249–252

Messner K 1999 The innervation of synovial joints. In: Archer C W, Caterson B, Benjamin M, Ralphs J R (eds) Biology of the synovial joint. Harwood, Australia, ch 25, p 405–421

Moberg E 1983 The role of cutaneous afferents in position sense, kinaesthesia, and motor function of the hand. Brain 106:1–19

Mooney V, Robertson J 1976 The facet syndrome. Clinical Orthopaedics and Related Research 115:149–156

Mow V C, Holmes M H, Lai W M 1984 Fluid transport and mechanical properties of articular cartilage: a review. Journal of Biomechanics 17(5):377–394

Mow V C, Proctor C S, Kelly M A 1989 Biomechanics of articular cartilage. In: Nordin M, Frankel V H (eds) Basic biomechanics of the musculoskeletal system, 2nd edn. Lea & Febiger, Philadelphia, ch 2, p 31–58

Nathan H 1962 Osteophytes of the vertebral column, an anatomical study of their development according to age, race, and sex with consideration as to their etiology and significance. Journal of Bone and Joint Surgery 44A(2):243–267

Newham D J, Hurley M V, Jones D W 1989 Ligamentous knee injuries and muscle inhibition. Journal of Orthopaedic Rheumatology 2:163–173

Nigg B M, Herzog W 1999 Biomechanics of the musculo-skeletal system, 2nd edn. John Wiley, Chichester, ch 2.9, p 205

Nordin M, Frankel V H 1989 Basic biomechanics of the musculoskeletal system, 2nd edn. Lea & Febiger, Philadelphia

Norkin C C, Levangie P K 1992 Joint structure and function, a comprehensive analysis, 2nd edn. F A Davis, Philadelphia

Noyes F R 1977 Functional properties of knee ligaments and alterations induced by immobilization: a correlative biomechanical and histological study in primates. Clinical Orthopaedics and Related Research 123:210–242

Noyes F R, Grood E S 1976 The strength of the anterior cruciate ligament in humans and rhesus monkeys, age-related and species-related changes. Journal of Bone and Joint Surgery 58A(8):1074–1082

Noyes F R, DeLucas J L, Torvik P J 1974 Biomechanics of anterior cruciate ligament failure: an analysis of strain-rate sensitivity and mechanisms of failure in primates. Journal of Bone and Joint Surgery 56A(2):236–253

Noyes F R, Butler D L, Paulos L E, Grood E S 1983 Intra-articular cruciate reconstruction, 1: perspectives on graft strength, vascularization, and immediate motion after replacement. Clinical Orthopaedics and Related Research 172:71–77

O'Connor B L, Palmoski M J, Brandt K D 1985 Neurogenic acceleration of degenerative joint lesions. Journal of Bone and Joint Surgery 67A(4):562–572

O'Hara B P, Urban J P G, Maroudas A 1990 Influence of cyclic loading on the nutrition of articular cartilage. Annals of the Rheumatic Diseases 49:536–539

Oku R, Satoh M, Takagi H 1987 Release of substance P from the spinal dorsal horn is enhanced in polyarthritic rats. Neuroscience Letters 74:315–319

Oliver J, Middleditch A 1991 Functional anatomy of the spine. Butterworth-Heinemann, Oxford

Palastanga N, Field D, Soames R 2002 Anatomy and human movement – structure and function, 4th edn. Butterworth-Heinemann, Oxford

Panjabi M M 1992a The stabilizing system of the spine. Part 1. Function, dysfunction, adaptation, and enhancement. Journal of Spinal Disorders 5(4):383–389

Panjabi M M 1992b The stabilizing system of the spine. Part II. Neutral zone and instability hypothesis. Journal of Spinal Disorders 5(4):390–396

Panjabi M M, White A A 2001 Biomechanics in the musculoskeletal system. Churchill Livingstone, New York

Panjabi M, Abumi K, Duranceau J, Oxland T 1989 Spinal stability and intersegmental muscle forces: a biomechanical model. Spine 14(2):194–200

Pearcy M J, Tibrewal S B 1984 Axial rotation and lateral bending in the normal lumbar spine measured by three-dimensional radiography. Spine 9(6):582–587

Pearcy M, Portek I, Shepherd J 1984 Three-dimensional X-ray analysis of normal movement in the lumbar spine. Spine 9(3):294–297

Penning L 1988 Differences in anatomy, motion, development and aging of the upper and lower cervical disk segments. Clinical Biomechanics 3:37–47

Perry J, Antonelli D, Ford W 1975 Analysis of knee-joint forces during flexed-knee stance. Journal of Bone and Joint Surgery 57A(7):961–967

Petty N J, Moore A P 2001 Neuromusculoskeletal examination and assessment, a handbook for therapists, 2nd edn. Churchill Livingstone, Edinburgh

Petty N J, Maher C, Latimer J, Lee M 2002 Manual examination of accessory movements-seeking R1. Manual Therapy 7(1):39–43

Phillips D, Petrie S, Solomonow M et al 1997 Ligamentomuscular protective reflex in the elbow. Journal of Hand Surgery 22A(3):473–478

Pope M H, Johnson R J, Brown D W, Tighe C 1979 The role of musculature in injuries to the medial collateral ligament. Journal of Bone and Joint Surgery 61A(3):398–402

Proske X HE U, Schaible H-G, Schmidt R F 1988 Acute inflammation of the knee joint in the cat alters responses of flexor motoneurons to leg movements. Journal of Neurophysiology 59(2):326–340

Raja S N, Meyer R A, Ringkamp M, Campbell J N 1999 Peripheral neural mechanisms of nociception. In: Wall P D, Melzack R (eds) Textbook of pain, 4th edn. Churchill Livingstone, Edinburgh

Ramsey D K, Wretenberg P F 1999 Biomechanics of the knee: methodological considerations in the in vivo kinematic analysis of the tibiofemoral and patellofemoral joint. Clinical Biomechanics 14:595–611

Renstrom P, Arms S W, Stanwyck T S 1986 Strain within the anterior cruciate ligament during hamstring and quadriceps activity. American Journal of Sports Medicine 14(1):83–87

Salo P T, Theriault E 1997 Number, distribution and neuropeptide content of rat knee joint afferents. Journal of Anatomy 190:515–522

Salter R B, Field P 1960 The effects of continuous compression on living articular cartilage: an experimental investigation. Journal of Bone and Joint Surgery 42A(1):31–49

Schaible H-G, Schmidt R F 1983 Responses of fine medial articular nerve afferents to passive movements of knee joint. Journal of Neurophysiology 49(5):1118–1126

Schaible H-G, Schmidt R F 1985 Effects of an experimental arthritis on the sensory properties of fine articular afferent units. Journal of Neurophysiology 54(5):1109–1122

Schaible H-G, Schmidt R F 1988 Excitation and sensitization of fine articular afferents from cat's knee joint by prostaglandin E2. Journal of Physiology 403:91–104

Schaible H-G, Jarrott B, Hope P J, Duggan A W 1990 Acute arthritis in cat's knee joint leads to release of immunoreactive substance P (ir SP) in the spinal cord. Pain (suppl 5) S230 (abstract 447)

Schwarzer A C, Aprill C N, Derby R et al 1994 Clinical features of patients with pain stemming from the lumbar zygapophyseal joints: is the lumbar facet syndrome a clinical entity? Spine 19(10):1132–1137

Seki K, Taniguchi Y, Narusawa M 2001 Effects of joint immobilization on firing rate modulation of human motor units. Journal of Physiology 530(3):507–519

Shakespeare D T, Stokes M, Sherman K P, Young A 1985 Reflex inhibition of the quadriceps after meniscectomy: lack of association with pain. Clinical Physiology 5:137–144

Shirley D, Lee M, Ellis E 1999 The relationship between submaximal activity of the lumbar extensor muscles and lumbar posteroanterior stiffness. Physical Therapy 79(3):278–285

Shoemaker S C, Markolf K L 1982 In vivo rotary knee stability: ligamentous and muscular contributions. Journal of Bone and Joint Surgery 64A(2):208–216

Shrive N G, Frank C B 1999 Articular cartilage. In: Nigg B M, Herzog W Biomechanics of the musculo-skeletal system, 2nd edn. John Wiley, Chichester, ch 2.4 p 86–106

Skinner H B, Barrack R L, Cook S D 1984 Age-related decline in proprioception. Clinical Orthopaedics and Related Research 184:208–211

Skoglund S 1956 Anatomical and physiological studies of knee joint innervation in the cat. Acta Physiologica Scandinavica 36 (suppl):124

Snyder-Mackler L, De Luca P F, Williams P R et al 1994 Reflex inhibition of the quadriceps femoris muscle after injury or reconstruction of the anterior cruciate ligament. Journal of Bone and Joint Surgery 76–A(4):555–560

Solomonow M, Guzzi A, Baratta R et al 1986 EMG-force model of the elbows antagonistic muscle pair: the effect of joint position, gravity and recruitment. American Journal Physical Medicine 65(5):223–244

Solomonow M, Baratta R, Zhou B H et al 1987 The synergistic action of the anterior cruciate ligament and thigh muscles in maintaining joint stability. American Journal of Sports Medicine 15(3):207–213

Solomonow M, Zhou B-H, Harris M et al 1998 The ligamento-muscular stabilizing system of the spine. Spine 23(23):2552–2562

Steen K H, Issberner U, Reeh P H 1995 Pain due to experimental acidosis in human skin: evidence for non-adapting nociceptor excitation. Neuroscience Letters 199:29–32

Stener B 1969 Reflex inhibition of the quadriceps elicited from a subperiosteal tumour of the femur. Acta Orthopaedica Scandinavica 40:86–91

Stener B, Petersen I 1963 Excitatory and inhibitory reflex motor effects from the partially ruptured medial collateral ligament of the knee joint. Acta Orthopaedica Scandinavica 33:359

Stokes M, Young A 1984 The contribution of reflex inhibition to arthrogenous muscle weakness. Clinical Science 67:7–14

Strasmann T, Halata Z 1988 Applications for 3-D image processing in functional anatomy: reconstruction of the cubital joint region and spatial distribution of mechanoreceptors surrounding this joint in mondelphius domestica, a laboratory marsupial. European Journal of Cell Biology 48 (25) (suppl):107–110

Strasmann T, van der Wal J C, Halata Z, Drukker J 1990 Functional topography and ultrastructure of periarticular mechanoreceptors in the lateral elbow region of the rat. Acta Anatomica 138:1–14

Suter E, Herzog W 2000 Muscle inhibition and functional deficiencies associated with knee pathologies. In: Herzog W (ed) Skeletal Muscle Mechanics, from Mechanisms to Function. Wiley, Chichester, ch 21, p 365

Suter E, Herzog W, Bray R C 1998 Quadriceps inhibition following arthroscopy in patients with anterior knee pain. Clinical Biomechanics 13:314–319

Threlkeld A J 1992 The effects of manual therapy on connective tissue. Physical Therapy 72(12):893–902

Tindle P 1987 Force/displacement curves of the knee. In Dalziel B A & Snowsill J C (eds) Manipulative Therapists' Association of Australia 5th biennial conference proceedings, Melbourne, 271–296

Tipton C M, James S L, Mergner W, Tcheng T-K 1970 Influence of exercise on strength of medial collateral knee ligaments of dogs. American Journal of Physiology 218(3):894–902

Torry M R, Decker M J, Viola R W et al 2000 Intra-articular knee joint effusion induces quadriceps avoidance gait patterns. Clinical Biomechanics 15:147–159

Urbach D, Awiszus F 2002 Impaired ability of voluntary quadriceps activation bilaterally interferes with function testing after knee injuries. A twitch interpolation study. International Journal of Sports Medicine 23(4):231–236

Vanwanseele B, Lucchinetti E, Stussi E 2002 The effects of immobilization on the characteristics of articular cartilage: current concepts and future directions. Osteoarthritis and Cartilage 10:408–419

Vicenzino B, Souvlis T, Wright A 2002 Musculoskeletal pain. In: Strong J, Unruh A M, Wright A, Baxter G D (eds) Pain a textbook for therapists. Churchill Livingstone, Edinburgh, ch 17, p 327–349

Vilensky J A, O'Connor B L, Brandt K D et al 1997 Serial kinematic analysis of the canine hindlimb joints after deafferentation and anterior cruciate ligament transection. Osteoarthritis and Cartilage 5:173–182

Wall P D, Melzack R 1999 Textbook of pain, 4th edn. Churchill Livingstone, Edinburgh

Walla D J, Albright J P, McAuley E et al 1985 Hamstring control and the unstable anterior cruciate ligament-deficient knee. American Journal of Sports Medicine 13(1):34–39

White A A 1969 Analysis of the mechanics of the thoracic spine in man an experimental study of autopsy specimens. Acta Orthopaedica Scandinavica 127 (suppl):1–105

Wilke H-J, Wolf S, Claes L E et al 1995 Stability increase of the lumbar spine with different muscle groups: a biomechanical in vitro study. Spine 20(2):192–198

Williams P L, Bannister L H, Berry M M et al 1995 Gray's anatomy, 38th edn. Churchill Livingstone, New York

Woo S L-Y, Akeson W H 1987 Response of tendons and ligaments to joint loading and movements. In: Helminen H J, Kiviranta I, Saamanen A-M et al (eds) Joint loading, biology and health of articular structures. Wright, Bristol

Woo S L-Y, Matthews J V, Akeson W H et al 1975 Connective tissue response to immobility: correlative study of biomechanical and biochemical measurements of normal and immobilized rabbit knees. Arthritis and Rheumatism 18(3):257–264

Woo S L-Y, Gomez M A, Sites T J et al 1987 The biomechanical and morphological changes in the medial collateral ligament of the rabbit after immobilization and remobilization. Journal of Bone and Joint Surgery 69A(8):1200–1211

Woo S, Maynard J, Butler D et al 1988 Ligament, tendon, and joint capsule insertions to bone. In: Woo S L-Y, Buckwalter J (eds) Injury and repair of the musculoskeletal soft tissues. American Academy of Orthopaedic Surgeons, Park Ridge, Illinois ch 4, p 133–166

Wright V, Johns R J 1961 Quantitative and qualitative analysis of joint stiffness in normal subjects and in patients with connective tissue diseases. Annals of the Rheumatic Diseases 20:36–46

Wyke B D 1970 The neurological basis of thoracic spinal pain. Rheumatology and Physical Medicine 10(7):356–367

Wyke B D, Polacek P 1975 Articular neurology: the present position. Journal of Bone and Joint Surgery 57B(3):401

Yamashita T, Minaki Y, Ozaktay A C et al 1996 A morphological study of the fibrous capsule of the human lumbar facet joint. Spine 21(5):538–543

Young A, Hughes I, Round J M, Edwards R H T 1982 The effect of knee injury on the number of muscle fibres in the human quadriceps femoris. Clinical Science 62:227–234

Young A, Stokes M, Iles J F 1987 Effects of joint pathology on muscle. Clinical Orthopaedics and Related Research 219:21–27

Zimny M L 1988 Mechanoreceptors in articular tissue. American Journal of Anatomy 182:16–32

Zimny M L, St Onge M 1987 Mechanoreceptors in the temporomandibular articular disk. Journal of Dental Research 66:237

4

Principles of joint treatment

There is no pure treatment for joint, that is, treatment cannot be isolated to joint alone, it will always, to a greater or lesser extent, affect muscle and/or nerve tissues. However, some sort of classification system for treatment is needed in order to have meaningful communication between clinicians, and this text follows the traditional classification of joint, muscle and nerve treatment. In this text, a 'joint treatment' is defined as a 'treatment to effect a change in joint'; that is, the intention of the clinician is to produce a change in joint, and therefore it is described as a joint treatment. Similarly, where a technique is used to effect a change in a muscle, it will be referred to as a 'muscle treatment' and where a technique is used to effect a change in nerve, it will be referred to as a 'nerve treatment'. Thus, techniques are classified according to which tissue the clinician is predominantly attempting to affect. This relationship of joint, nerve and muscle treatment is depicted in Figure 4.1.

An example may help to illustrate the impurity of a joint technique. A posteroanterior glide on the head of the fibula will move the superior tibiofibular joint, the lateral collateral ligament of the tibiofemoral joint and also the common peroneal nerve, soleus and biceps femoris. A posteroanterior glide to the head of the fibula can therefore be applied to affect any of these structures. It may be used to affect the superior tibiofibular joint, in which case it would be described as a joint treatment, or, for example, it may be used to affect the common peroneal nerve, in which case it is referred to as a nerve treatment. Similarly, physiological joint movements will

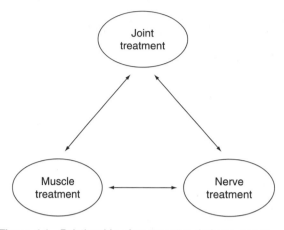

Figure 4.1 Relationship of treatment techniques one to another, joint, nerve and muscle.

move local joint, nerve and muscle tissues. For example, passive physiological hip flexion will move the hip joint, pelvis and lumbar spine, as well as lengthen the hip extensor muscles and the sciatic nerve. If the movement is carried out actively, there will be, in addition, isotonic contraction of the hip flexor muscles. Passive physiological hip flexion may be given to effect a change in the hip joint – in which case it would be classified as a joint treatment, but could equally be used to effect a change in the sciatic nerve, in which case it would be classified as a nerve treatment. The possible desired effects of joint mobilization on joint, nerve and muscle tissue are summarized in Box 4.1. Further information on treatment of muscle and nerve tissue using joint mobilization can be found in Chapters 6 and 8. In this chapter it is assumed that joint mobilization treatment is being applied to affect joint tissues.

Box 4.1 Desired effect of joint mobilization
Glide joint surface parallel to plane of joint Move joint surface to lengthen periarticular tissues Move joint to rotate joint surfaces Move joint in such a way as to reproduce the patient's symptoms Move joint to affect nerve tissue (including pain relief) Move joint to affect muscle tissue Don't know, but it improves the patient's signs and symptoms!

There is a variety of joint treatments. Treatments are categorized in this text from the dysfunctions identified in the previous chapter, namely, reduced range of movement due to increased resistance and/or pain, hypermobility with pain, altered quality of movement and symptom production (Table 4.1). From this a classification of joint treatment can be identified:

- treatment of hypomobility due to increased resistance and/or pain
- treatment of hypermobility with pain through the range
- treatment of altered quality of movement
- treatment to reduce symptoms.

The reader is reminded that there are a number of precautions and contraindications to joint mobilization treatment; these are given in Chapter 2. Various techniques to address each of these treatments are shown in Table 4.1.

TREATMENT OF HYPOMOBILITY DUE TO INCREASED RESISTANCE AND/OR PAIN

Range of movement may be limited by resistance or by the production of symptoms, most commonly pain. With resistance limiting movement, there may, or may not, be production of symptoms during the range of movement. With pain limiting movement, there may, or may not, be increased resistance during the movement. The most common presentation is a reduced range of movement, due to resistance, with production of symptoms during the range. However, other presentations seen include (i) resistance limiting a movement without production of symptoms – in this case the joint is essentially stiff; and (ii) pain limiting a movement with no resistance – in this case the joint is very painful. All of the above presentations could involve accessory movements and/or physiological movements. A joint may display limitation of one accessory movement, or one physiological movement, or a number of accessory and/or physiological movements. The method of treatment for each of these possible presentations is much the same – the only differ-

Table 4.1   Joint dysfunction, aims of joint treatment and treatment techniques

Dysfunction	Aims of joint treatment	Treatment techniques
Hypomobility limited by resistance or pain	Increase range of movement and reduce resistance or pain	Accessory movements Physiological movements (active or passive) Accessory with physiological movements (active or passive) Soft-tissue mobilizations Frictions PNF Electrotherapy
Hypermobility with pain	Reduce pain	Accessory movements Physiological movements (active or passive) Accessory with physiological movements (active or passive) Soft-tissue mobilizations PNF Electrotherapy
Altered quality of movement	Normalize quality of movement e.g. instability Increased or decreased resistance to movement	Exercises to enhance motor control and coordination (see chapter on muscle treatment) As for hypomobility/hypermobility above
Symptom production with hypomobility, hypermobility or instability	Reduce symptoms	Accessory movements Physiological movements (active or passive) Accessory with physiological movements (active or passive) Soft-tissue mobilizations Frictions Electrotherapy

ence lies in the choice of the treatment dose, which is discussed below.

Joint treatments for increasing the range of movement include: joint mobilizations (accessory and physiological movements), specific soft-tissue mobilizations, frictions, proprioceptive neuromuscular facilitation (PNF) and electrotherapy (Table 4.2). Having identified a dysfunction, treatment aims to restore normal function, whether this be restoration of the rotation movement, the translation movement or a combination of the two. The method of treating joints can therefore be broadly divided into physiological movements (which emphasize rotation of the bone) and accessory movements (which emphasize translation of the bone), or a combination of the two (Figure 4.2). The physiological movements can be further subdivided into passive or active physiological movements; accessory movements, by definition, will always be passive. Combinations of accessory and physiological movements are then possible, and include accessory movements with passive or active physiological movements. Details of these acces-

sory and physiological movements are provided in the companion text (Petty & Moore 2001).

Accessory movements

Every accessory movement available at a joint can be used as a treatment technique. Having examined and identified a dysfunction of an accessory movement, the clinician can draw a movement diagram and then choose a suitable treatment dose, described in the next section. The accessory movement can be carried out in any part of the physiological range of that joint; for example, an anteroposterior glide to the tibiofemoral joint can be applied with the knee in flexion, extension or tibial rotation. The chosen position depends on the desired effects of the treatment, discussed later in this chapter.

Physiological movements

Every physiological movement available at a joint can be converted to a treatment technique and can be carried out actively by the patient or

Table 4.2 Aspects of treatment dose for joint mobilization

Factors	Variables
Patient position	e.g. prone, side lie, sitting
Movement	This may be a physiological movement, e.g. flexion, lateral rotation, or an accessory movement or a mixture of the two
Direction of force applied	e.g. anteroposterior, posteroanterior, medial, lateral, caudad, cephalad
Magnitude of force applied	Related to therapist's perception of resistance: grades I to V
Amplitude of oscillation	None: sustained (quasistatic) Small: grades I and IV Large: grades II and III
Speed	Slow or fast
Rhythm	Smooth or staccato
Time	Of repetition and number of repetitions
Symptom response	Short of symptom production Point of onset or increase in resting symptom Partial reproduction of symptom Full reproduction of symptom

passively by the clinician. Active repetitive movements of the spine have, for example, been advocated by McKenzie (1981, 1983, 1985). Having examined the passive physiological movement, and drawn a movement diagram, the clinician can then choose a suitable treatment dose, described in the next section.

The principles of applying passive physiological movement are:

- the body part is fully supported
- the movement is fully controlled by the clinician, in terms of: where in range the movement begins and ends, the amplitude of oscillation, the smoothness of the movement, and the speed of the movement
- the clinician constantly monitors symptoms during the application of the technique.

Passive physiological movement combined with accessory movements

A physiological movement can be applied while also applying an accessory movement. Thus, the physiological movement and the accessory movement can both be oscillated at the same time; the physiological movement can be oscillated while the accessory movement is sustained; or the physiological movement can be sustained while the accessory movement is oscillated. For example, a longitudinal caudad and shoulder abduction can each be oscillated at the same time, the shoulder abduction can be oscillated while the longitudinal caudad is sustained, or the shoulder abduction can be sustained while the longitudinal caudad is oscillated. Other

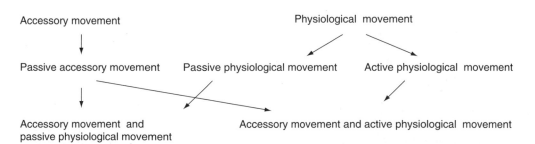

Figure 4.2 Classification of joint mobilizations.

examples of using physiological movement with accessory movements include:

- knee flexion with a posteroanterior glide on the tibia
- ankle dorsiflexion with an anteroposterior glide to the talus
- cervical lateral flexion with a transverse glide to a spinous process.

The reader should note that these techniques can be applied in a variety of positions. Knee flexion with a posteroanterior glide can be applied with the patient in crook lie, sitting, standing, prone etc. Similarly, shoulder abduction with a longitudinal glide can be applied in sitting, lying or standing, and cervical lateral flexion with a transverse glide can be applied in supine or sitting. These are aspects of the treatment dose.

Active physiological movement with accessory movement

As the patient performs an active physiological movement the clinician can apply an accessory movement. For example, the clinician can apply an anteroposterior glide to the talus and ask the patient to dorsiflex the foot actively. For the cervical spine, the clinician can apply the transverse glide to a spinous process and then ask the patient to flex the head laterally. When the physiological movement is performed actively by the patient, as opposed to passively by the clinician, this can sometimes enable the technique to be carried out in a more functional position. For example, it would be extremely difficult, if not impossible, to dorsiflex the foot passively while the patient is weight-bearing. For further information on accessory movement with active physiological movements see Mulligan (1995).

Joint treatment dose

The term 'treatment dose' is often used by the medical profession when prescribing the quantity of a drug. The term is used here to describe the nature of the movement applied by the clinician or by the patient. The treatment dose incorporates quite a large number of factors, most of

which have a number of variables; these variables are outlined in Table 4.2.

Some examples of treatment dose, which might be used and documented in the patient's notes, are given below:

1. 'In left side lie with arm back and pelvis rotated, did left rotation grade II in line of femur, slowly and smoothly, for 30 seconds, to partial reproduction of patient's back pain'. This clinical note describes the patient in left side lie, with arm resting on trunk and right hip and knee flexed so that the knee rests on the couch, in front of the underlying leg. The clinician applies a slow and smooth passive physiological movement (grade II) to the pelvis, in the direction of the line of the femur, for 30 seconds, such that the patient feels only partial reproduction of the back pain.

2. 'In right lateral flexion did Γ with cephalad inclination, on left C3, Grade IV, fast and smoothly, for 1 minute, to total reproduction of patient's cervical & left trapezius pain'.

3. 'In prone with knee flexion 130 degrees, did ↓ tibiofemoral joint, IV+, fast and staccato, for 1 minute, to full reproduction of the patient's knee pain'.

4. 'In standing with foot on a stool, did ↑ talus, sustained Grade IV, with patient moving over foot, for 10 repetitions, to full reproduction of patient's posterior ankle and calf pain'.

The clinician, when choosing a treatment dose, has to make a decision about each variable. The choice of each variable depends on the desired effect of treatment.

The patient's position

This includes the general position of the patient, such as lying, sitting or standing, and the specific position of the body part, for example, the knee may be flexed or extended during the application of an anteroposterior glide on the tibia. The choice of general and specific positioning will depend on a number of factors, including:

- the comfort and support of the patient
- the comfort of the clinician applying the technique

- the desired effect of the treatment
- whether the joints are to be weight-bearing or non-weight-bearing
- to what extent the movement is to be functional
- to what extent symptoms are to be produced.

So, for example, a patient with limitation of knee flexion due to resistance may be positioned in long sitting with the knee flexed to the end of the available range, while the clinician applies an anteroposterior (AP) glide to the tibia. This technique is comfortable for the patient and the clinician and allows the clinician to apply a strong AP force. An alternative position could be to apply the AP force with the patient in prone, and the knee flexed to the end of available range. The clinician may find this an easier position in which to apply a strong force; however, in this position there may be passive insufficiency of the rectus femoris muscle. The clinician must, therefore, consider carefully the best general, and specific, position of the patient when deciding how to apply a technique.

It should be noted that the resistance to passive accessory movements will depend on the position of the joint; for example, the resistance to a posteroanterior force to the humeral head is greatest with the glenohumeral joint in full lateral rotation, while the resistance to an anteroposterior force is greatest in medial rotation (McQuade et al 1999).

Direction of movement

Where a physiological movement is used a description of the physiological movement and naming the joint will describe this aspect of the treatment dose. For example, knee flexion, hip lateral rotation or lumbar rotation to the left, each identifies the direction of the movement and the joint complex. Where an accessory movement is used, the direction of the force and the joint will describe the movement. Examples include an AP to the tibiofemoral joint, a lateral glide of the glenohumeral joint or an AP to the talocrural joint. Again, each identifies the direction of the force and the joint complex. The general conven-

tion would assume that the force was applied to the distal bone of the joint – in the above examples, to the tibia, humerus and talus, respectively. Techniques, of course, can be applied to the proximal bone; when this occurs the bone needs to be identified in the written description. For example, the description may read 'AP to tibiofemoral joint, on femur'.

In the spine, where each spinal level consists of a number of joints, an additional descriptor is added for accessory movements. The point of application of the force needs to be identified. For example, a central PA on L3, a transverse glide to left on T5, a unilateral PA on C5. In these examples, the word 'central' means that the force is applied over the spinous process, 'transverse' to the lateral aspect of the spinous process, and 'unilateral' to the articular pillar.

Magnitude of the force

Whenever a clinician passively moves a joint, with either a physiological or accessory movement, the clinician is applying a force. Clearly, this has a certain magnitude and it is commonly described using a grade of movement (Magarey 1985, Magarey 1986, Maitland et al 2001). Grades of movement in this text are defined according to where the movement occurs, within joint resistance. The resistance to movement perceived by the clinician is depicted on a movement diagram (described in Petty & Moore 2001). Grades of movement (I to IV+) are then defined according to the resistance curve. The grades of movement defined in this text (Fig. 4.3 and Table 4.3) are a modification of Magarey (1985, 1986). The modification allows every possible position in range to be described (cf. Magarey 1985, 1986), and each grade to be distinct from one another (cf. Maitland et al 2001). A grade V technique is a manipulative thrust.

With most physiological joint movements there is minimal resistance within the range of movement. For example, elbow flexion or knee extension will have little resistance in the early part of the range, and the clinician may mark the onset of resistance (R_1) somewhere towards the end of the movement (Fig. 4.3A). Grades of

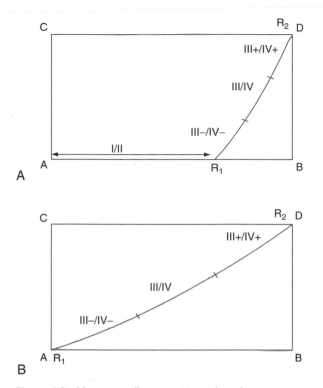

Figure 4.3 Movement diagram with grades of movement for **A** a typical asymptomatic physiological movement, and **B** a typical asymptomatic accessory movement. The resistance is divided into thirds, so that a large-amplitude movement within the middle third will be a grade III.

and IV+ (Fig. 4.3B); that is, a grade I and II may not be possible as these grades are defined as movements within a resistance-free range (Table 4.3). The grade of movement is defined according to where the maximum force is applied in resistance, and whether the clinician considers the movement to be large or small. For example, a grade III– is to the first third of resistance; the fact that the amplitude may be sufficiently large that the return movement may be earlier than the first onset of resistance (in a resistance-free range) is not relevant.

Amplitude of oscillation

A movement can be a sustained or an oscillatory force. It is impossible for a truly sustained force to be applied – there will always be some variation in the force, albeit very small. For this reason, it is sometimes referred to as a quasistatic force. If the force is oscillated it is described as having a small or large amplitude. The amplitude is relative to the available range of any particular movement so it will vary quite dramatically between physiological and accessory movements. For example, small-amplitude accessory movements may be a few millimetres of movement, compared to a 40-degree arc of movement for a physiological movement. The amplitude of oscillatory movement is described within the definition of grades of movement: grades I and IV are small-amplitude movements and grades II and III are large-amplitude movements. Where a clinician applies a sustained force it is suggested that the description would use grades I and IV, with the word 'sustained'

movement available for physiological movements include I, II, III–, IV–, III, IV, III+, IV+ (Fig. 4.3A). With accessory movements, however, resistance occurs at the beginning of range (Petty et al 2002), that is, R_1 is at A on the movement diagram (Fig. 4.3B). Grades of movement available will be limited to grades III–, IV–, III, IV, III+

Table 4.3 Grades of movement

Grade	Definition
I	Small-amplitude movement short of resistance
II	Large-amplitude movement short of resistance
III–	Large-amplitude movement in the first third of resistance
IV–	Small-amplitude movement in the first third of resistance
III	Large-amplitude movement in the middle third of resistance
IV	Small-amplitude movement in the middle third of resistance
III+	Large-amplitude movement in the last third of resistance
IV+	Small-amplitude movement in the last third of resistance
V	Manipulative thrust

written prior to the grade; for example, treatment notes would read 'sustained grade IV'. In this way, the grade is used to describe where in resistance the movement is carried out.

It can be seen that grades of movement describe both the magnitude of force applied and the amplitude of oscillation. The choice of grade of movement is determined by the relationship of pain (or other symptom) and resistance through the range of movement; this is depicted on a movement diagram (Maitland et al 2001). Where resistance limits the range of movement (Fig. 4.4A), and there is minimal pain, a grade III+ or IV+, provoking only a small amount of pain, may be appropriate. Where pain limits the range of movement (Fig. 4.4B), and there is minimal resistance, a grade I or II that does not produce any pain may be appropriate. A grade III− or IV− may be chosen if the pain is not severe and not irritable and there is no caution related to the nature of the disorder. Where resistance limits the movement, and there is a significant amount of pain, or where pain limits the movement and there is significant resistance, the choice of grade will depend on the degree to which symptoms can be provoked (Fig. 4.4C and D). For example, in Figure 4.4C, if a grade IV is chosen at about 50% of resistance, the patient may report an intensity of pain about 2 out of 10 (where A is 0 and C is 10). If a grade IV is chosen for Figure 4.4D, this may provoke about 6 out of 10, which may, or may not, be acceptable to the patient or clinician.

Speed and rhythm of movement

The speed of the movement can be described as slow or fast, and the rhythm as smooth or staccato (jerky); of course, these descriptors will apply only to oscillatory forces. Speed and rhythm go hand in hand; movements will tend to be either slow and smooth, fast and smooth, or

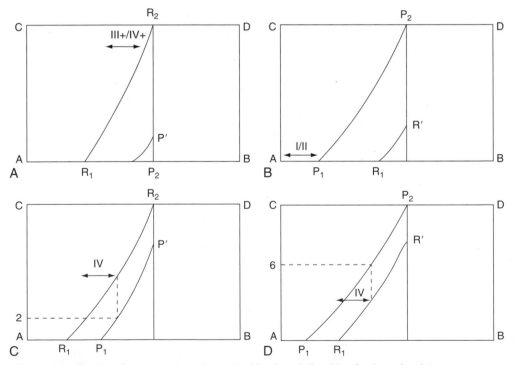

Figure 4.4 Grades of movement are determined by the relationship of pain and resistance through the range of movement; this is depicted on a movement diagram. **A** Resistance limiting movement. **B** Pain limiting movement. **C** Resistance limiting movement with a significant amount of resistance. **D** Pain limiting movement with a significant amount of pain.

fast and staccato – it would be difficult to apply a slow staccato movement. Using the descriptors of speed as slow or fast, a grade V manipulative thrust may be described as a very fast speed! Grade V techniques to the spine can be referred to as high-velocity, low-amplitude thrust techniques, shortened to HVLAT (Evans 2002, Gibbons & Tehan 2001).

The tissues around a joint are viscoelastic and, as such, are sensitive to the speed of the applied force. A force applied quickly will produce less movement, provoking a greater stiffness in the tissues; a force applied more slowly, on the other hand, will cause more movement as the stiffness is relatively less (Noyes et al 1974).

Time

In terms of treatment dose, this relates to the duration for which a movement is carried out in a treatment session, the number of times this is repeated within a treatment session, and the frequency of appointments.

Typical clinical practice involves about three repetitions of a treatment technique, each lasting between 30 seconds and 1 minute. These times are given as a guideline only, however, for inexperienced clinicians. The frequency of appointments is decided by the clinician and the patient and will depend on a number of factors. These factors include: the nature of the patient's condition, the severity and irritability of symptoms, the area of the symptoms, the functional limitations of the patient, the stage of the patient's condition, the prognosis, the available time the patient has to attend for treatment and the workload of the clinician.

Temperature

Temperature influences the mechanical behaviour of connective tissue under tensile load. As temperature rises to about 40–45° C, stiffness decreases and extensibility increases (LaBan 1962, Rigby 1964). At about 40° C, a change in the microstructure of collagen occurs; this significantly enhances the extensibility and potential for a permanent (plastic) change in length (Rigby 1964, Rigby et al 1959). A higher temperature will induce less weakening than a lower temperature (Sapega et al 1981, Warren et al 1971). Once the heat is removed it has been found that maintaining the tension as the tissue cools enhances the plastic deformation (Sapega et al 1981). Increasing the temperature of a tissue depends on its depth; it will obviously be easier to heat more superficial joints.

The ability of short-wave diathermy to increase the temperature of joint tissue has been investigated. Twenty minutes of continuous short-wave diathermy has been shown to increase knee intra-articular temperature by 4.5° C (Millard 1961). If normal joint temperature is assumed to be the same as normal body temperature (37° C), then this would raise the temperature of joint tissues to 41.5° C, sufficient to enhance the effect of stretching. Ultrasound is also thought to raise the temperature of joint tissues (Lehmann et al 1966) and thus enhance the ability to lengthen collagenous tissue.

It appears, then, that raising the joint temperature prior to stretching to increase range of movement, and maintaining the stretch as the temperature lowers, may enhance the effects of stretching (Sapega et al 1981).

Symptom response

The clinician decides which, and to what extent, each symptom is to be provoked during treatment. Choices include:

- no provocation
- provocation to the point of onset, or increase, in resting symptoms
- partial reproduction
- total reproduction.

The decision as to what extent each symptom is provoked during treatment depends on the severity and irritability of the symptom(s) and the nature of the condition. If the symptoms are severe, that is, the patient is unable to tolerate the symptom being reproduced, the clinician would choose to apply treatment that did not provoke the symptoms. The clinician may also choose not to provoke symptoms if they are irritable, that is, once symptoms are provoked, they take some time to ease. If, however, the symptoms are not severe and not irritable, then the clinician is able to reproduce the patient's symptoms during treatment, and the extent to which the symptoms are provoked will depend on the tolerance of the patient. The nature of the condition may also limit the extent to which symptoms are produced, such as a recent traumatic injury.

Choice of treatment dose

Where a joint (which includes both intra- and peri-articular tissues) is considered to be the source of the symptoms, the clinician may be able to link the findings of the active and passive physiological movements with the findings of the accessory movements. For example, limited range of wrist extension may be accompanied by limited PA glide of the radiocarpal joint; this would make sense because wrist extension at the radiocarpal joint involves a PA glide of the scaphoid and lunate on the radius. The clinician could choose a physiological wrist extension movement, a PA glide of the proximal carpal bones, or could choose to combine physiological wrist extension with a PA glide to the proximal carpal bones. In the same way, limited dorsiflexion of the ankle may be accompanied by limited AP glide of the talus because these two movements occur together. In this case the clinician could choose to apply a physiological ankle dorsiflexion movement, an AP glide to the talus, or combine physiological ankle dorsiflexion with an AP to the talus. In both examples, the choice would depend on the relative dysfunction of the physiological movement and the accessory movement.

Let us consider treatment to the wrist. If the movements (physiological and accessory) are limited in range by resistance, then the treatment dose will tend to be with the wrist in extension. In this position, the clinician might then apply an end-range sustained or oscillatory grade IV+ PA, to the radiocarpal joint, fast with a staccato rhythm, and continuing for three repetitions of 1 minute each, producing some ache in the wrist. These treatment doses are given in Table 4.4.

At the other end of the spectrum, if the movements are limited in range by pain, then the treatment dose will tend to be applied with the wrist in a pain-free position, such as wrist flexion. In this position, the clinician might apply a sustained or oscillatory PA to the radiocarpal joint, grade I or II technique, slowly and smoothly, continuing for three repetitions of 1 minute each, with no production of symptoms. This example highlights how the treatment dose can be varied in terms of grade of movement, speed and rhythm.

Where the clinical presentation is such that there is no clear link between the active/passive physiological movements and the accessory movements, the clinician has to choose a movement(s) to treat. The decision will be based on a number of factors, including the:

- number of abnormal joint movement tests
- type of abnormality found
- degree of abnormality
- aim of treatment, in terms of the patient's functional goals
- desired therapeutic effect
- severity and irritability of the symptoms
- nature of the condition.

The underlying mechanisms by which joint mobilizations can increase range of movement and reduce pain can be broadly divided into mechanical effects and neurophysiological effects. The neurophysiological effects are discussed later in the chapter.

Table 4.4 Variation in treatment dose depending on whether the joint movement is limited by resistance or by pain

	Resistance limiting movement	Pain limiting movement
Limited radiocarpal extension and limited PA glide of radiocarpal joint	In wrist extension, did sustained IV+ PA radiocarpal joint fast and staccato ×3 (1 min) with some ache	In wrist flexion did II PA radiocarpal joint slowly and smoothly ×3 (1 min) with no pain provoked

Mechanical effects of joint mobilizations

The mechanism by which joint mobilizations increase range of movement remains unclear. If the underlying cause of hypomobility is shortening of the periarticular tissues, then the underlying mechanism of treatment would aim to elongate these collagenous tissues permanently. This would require the application of a force of sufficient magnitude to produce micro-trauma (Threlkeld 1992). The force needs to lie within the plastic zone of the force displacement curve (Fig. 3.6). A force of lesser magnitude, within the elastic zone, will result in only a temporary increase in length owing to creep and hysteresis (Panjabi & White 2001). A rough guide to the amount of force needed to cause a permanent change in length has been estimated to be between 224 N and 1136 N (Threlkeld 1992), with micro-failure of connective tissue beginning at approximately 3% elongation, and macro-failure at approximately 8% (Noyes et al 1983). Forces used by clinicians during mobilization of the lumbar spine have been measured up to about 350 N (Harms & Bader 1997) which, in asymptomatic subjects, failed to produce a significant increase in range of movement (Petty 1995, Petty 2000). Whether these forces would produce a mechanical effect on patients with low back pain, with perhaps some pathological process, has not been determined.

It is, as yet, unknown whether clinically applied forces are able to cause a permanent increase in length. There has been some suggestion that manual forces applied are insufficient to produce micro-trauma and that the clinically applied forces lie within the elastic range of the tissues (McQuade et al 1999).

There is some evidence to suggest that force applied to the tissues has a therapeutic effect. Ligament strength is enhanced with longitudinal tension applied to the ligament (Gomez et al 1991) and by exercise (Tipton et al 1970, Woo et al 1987). In rabbits, a continuous tension applied to a transected ligament enhanced joint stability, strength and stiffness, with longitudinally aligned collagen fibres (Gomez et al 1991). Exercise has been demonstrated to increase the strength of ligament (Tipton et al 1970, Woo et al 1987), although excessive exercise of unstable joints has been found to increase ligament laxity (Burroughs & Dahners 1990). The application of force, whether manually or by movement, would therefore seem beneficial during ligament healing.

Repetitive active joint movements (Giovanelli-Blacker et al 1985) and passive joint movements (Giovanelli-Blacker et al 1985, Nade & Newbold 1983) have been found to cause a reduction in intra-articular pressure, while another study found a rhythmical increase and decrease in pressure, with active and passive movements (Levick 1979). Intra-articular pressure depends on fluid volume and joint angle (Levick et al 1999), as well as pressure on the joint capsule by overlying muscles and ligaments (Levick 1979). When synovial fluid volume is greater than normal, in the presence of a joint effusion, for example, the joint angle affects the pressure within the joint (Levick 1979, Levick et al 1999). In the knee joint, for example, it has been found that flexion increases intra-articular joint pressure (Levick et al 1999), particularly at end range (Levick 1979, Nade & Newbold 1983). However, moving a joint to a fully flexed position, and holding this position for a period of time, will cause a reduction in intra-articular pressure at all joint angles. This is thought to be due to absorption of the fluid through the synovial membrane (Levick 1979, Nade & Newbold 1983). This suggests that, where an increased joint pressure is contributing to a patient's symptoms, treatment with positioning and movement may be beneficial.

Soft-tissue mobilization

Hunter (1998) has coined the phrase 'specific soft tissue mobilization' (SSTM) and has described the following types of treatment technique: physiological SSTM, accessory SSTM and combined SSTM (physiological and accessory).

1. Physiological SSTM involves full exploration of all anatomical regions of the ligamentous tissue by a combination of physiological movements. For example, to explore the anterior

talofibular ligament fully, various degrees of plantarflexion need to be used in combination with inversion (Hunter 1998).

2. Accessory SSTM involves applying manual force to the ligament. It is recommended that the force be applied in the plane of the ligament and at right angles to the site of dysfunction (Hunter 1998). In this regard, it differs from transverse frictions (Fig. 4.5). Manual force can be applied with the ligament relaxed, or on stretch; for example, a horizontal force to the anterior talofibular ligament can be applied with the foot in neutral or in plantarflexion and inversion.

3. Combined accessory and physiological SSTM involves the ligament in a lengthened position while an accessory force is applied to the soft tissue.

Treatment dose

Soft-tissue mobilization is essentially the application of manual force to soft tissues – which can be considered to include ligament as well as skin, fascia, muscle, tendon and nerve. The decision to be made by the clinician, in terms of treatment dose, includes: the patient's position, movement, direction and magnitude of force applied, amplitude of oscillation, speed and rhythm of movement, time and symptom response. Table 4.5 provides a summary of the treatment options.

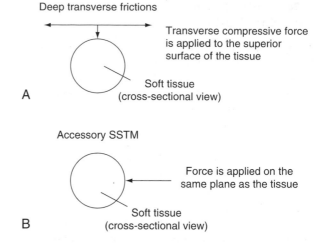

Figure 4.5 Direction of force and position of force for **A** deep transverse frictions, and **B** accessory specific soft-tissue mobilization (from Hunter 1998, with permission).

The underlying effect of soft-tissue mobilization is not yet known. Soft-tissue mobilization is considered to be appropriate following soft-tissue injury during the regeneration and remodelling phase of healing (Hunter 1998), described at the end of Chapter 3. During the regeneration and remodelling phases, soft-tissue mobilization is thought to enhance collagen synthesis and cross-linkage development, promote the orientation of collagen fibres along functional lines of stress, and promote 'normal' viscoelastic behaviour (Hunter

Table 4.5 Treatment dose for specific soft-tissue mobilization

Factors	Variables
Patient's position	e.g. prone, side lie, sitting
Movement	Physiological movement
	Accessory movement or a mixture of accessory and physiological
Direction of force applied	e.g. medial transverse, lateral transverse, AP, PA, caudad, cephalad
Magnitude of force applied	Related to therapist's perception of resistance: grades I to V
Amplitude of oscillation	None: sustained (quasistatic)
	Small: grades I and IV
	Large: grades II and III
Speed	Slow or fast
Rhythm	Smooth or staccato
Time	Of repetition and number of repetitions
Symptom response	Short of symptom production
	Point of onset or increase in resting symptom
	Partial reproduction of symptom
	Full reproduction of symptom

1998). SSTM is also proposed to be beneficial for degenerative lesions by stimulating an inflammatory response that initiates healing (Hunter 1998).

Frictions

Frictions are small-amplitude, deep-pressure movements, which can be applied to ligamentous tissue. A finger or thumb moves with the patient's skin across the tissue. Frictions are usually applied with the tissue in a lengthened position.

It has been proposed that frictions cause hyperaemia, breakdown of adhesions and stimulation of mechanoreceptors (Cyriax 1984). This has not been supported in a study on rabbit ligament in which 3–10 minutes of frictions on alternate days over a period of 10 days produced no change in the tissues (Walker 1984). There was a significant time period before the tissues were analysed, and it may be that healing had already taken place. Certainly in muscle, frictions have been found to have a profound effect (Gregory et al 2003).

Proprioceptive neuromuscular facilitation (PNF)

While PNF essentially affects muscle tissue by causing muscle relaxation, it can also be used to increase joint range of movement (Knott & Voss 1968, Waddington 1999). The techniques include rotational movement patterns through full range of movement, hold–relax, contract–relax and agonist–contract.

Rotational movement patterns

These patterns of movement take muscles from full outer range where they are fully lengthened to a fully shortened position. Specific patterns of movement for the head and neck, trunk and limbs have been described elsewhere (Knott & Voss 1968, Waddington 1999).

Hold–relax

The muscle is positioned in its stretched position, either actively or passively. A strong isometric contraction of the muscle is achieved by the cli-nician providing manual resistance. The muscle contraction needs to be carefully controlled by the clinician. This is achieved by saying to the patient 'don't let me move you', or 'hold', and by slowly and smoothly increasing the manual resistance to contraction. Following maximum contraction, the patient is asked to relax, the clinician gradually reduces the resistance, and time is allowed for muscle relaxation to occur. The clinician then moves the joint further into range to increase the length of the muscle. The procedure of contraction followed by relaxation is then repeated until no further increase in muscle length can be achieved.

Contract–relax

This is the same as hold–relax except that, following the isometric contraction, the patient actively contracts to further lengthen the antagonistic muscle – rather than the clinician passively lengthening the muscle. For example, to lengthen quadriceps, the patient isometrically contracts the quadriceps at, for example, 60 degrees flexion for 3–6 seconds. The patient is then asked to relax and to contract the hamstrings actively in an attempt to increase knee flexion and stretch the quadriceps muscle group. As in hold–relax, the procedure is repeated in the new range of movement and repeated until no further increase in muscle length is achieved.

Agonist–contract

The muscle is put in a position of stretch, and a contraction of the agonist attempts to increase movement, and thus increase stretch of the muscle. The clinician facilitates this movement by carefully applying a passive force. For example, to lengthen quadriceps, the knee is positioned 60 degrees flexion. The patient actively contracts the hamstrings in an attempt to increase knee flexion and stretch the quadriceps muscle group. The clinician applies a force to the lower leg to enhance this movement.

TREATMENT OF HYPERMOBILITY WITH PAIN THROUGH THE RANGE

Treating a hypermobile joint with pain through the range of movement follows the same principles as a hypomobile joint with pain through the range. Hypermobility is an increase in the range of movement beyond the average range of movement in the population and is thus, in itself, not a cause for treatment. If, however, the movement is also associated with pain, then this is abnormal and may require treatment. The treatment choice will follow exactly the same principles as discussed earlier for a joint with limited range of movement and pain through the range. The aim of treatment, however, will not be to increase range; rather, it will be to reduce pain.

TREATMENT OF ALTERED QUALITY OF MOVEMENT

Altered quality of movement includes: increased or decreased resistance to movement, instability, poor control of movement, the presence of joint noise such as a clunk or crepitus, excessive effort or reluctance of the patient to move; in short, it is anything considered to be abnormal, either by comparison to the other side or from the clinician's experience of what is 'normal'.

Increased resistance is most commonly associated with reduced range of movement and has been discussed earlier with hypomobility. Poor control of movement, joint noises, excessive effort or reluctance of the patient to move are signs of a movement dysfunction and need to be assessed, along with the full subjective and physical examination findings, to determine their relevance to the patient's symptoms, and if relevant, to identify suitable treatment.

Instability

Joint instability is due to a deficit in the ligamentous, muscular and/or neural functioning around a joint. For example, ligament insufficiency and joint instability have been found to be associated with altered muscle activity during functional movements at the elbow (Glousman et al 1992), shoulder (Glousman et al 1988) and knee (Solomonow et al 1987).

Instability has been defined as 'a significant decrease in the capacity of the stabilizing system of the spine to maintain the intervertebral neutral zones within the physiological limits so that there is no neurological dysfunction, no major deformity, and no incapacitating pain' (Panjabi 1992). This definition was put forward to describe instability of the vertebral column; however, it can be extended to include any joint. The neutral zone is equivalent to the toe region of a force displacement curve and is discussed more fully in Chapter 3.

Treatment of joint instability will depend on the degree and underlying cause of instability. For example, gross joint subluxation or dislocation that ruptures the ligamentous support system may require surgery to provide the necessary stability to the joint. This is frequently required at the glenohumeral joint, for example (Gerber & Ganz 1984).

Treatment of less severe cases of instability, due to a soft-tissue traumatic injury around the joint, will focus on optimizing the natural healing process and preventing complications; this has been outlined under ligamentous injuries at the end of Chapter 3. Ligamentous injuries are commonly seen, for instance, in the knee joint.

Minor joint instability may be suspected in patients without a traumatic injury. For example, spondylolisthesis, a slip of one vertebra anteriorly on the vertebra below, is an example of a joint instability with subluxation. Minor shoulder instability occurs and has been associated with muscle impingement around the shoulder (Fu et al 1991, Glousman 1993). Treatment in these cases will aim to improve muscle activation and muscle control of the joint to improve joint stability and reduce symptoms. In patients with spondylolysis and spondylolisthesis, for example, specific exercises for the muscles around the lumbar spine have been found to improve the patient's functional status and reduce pain (O'Sullivan et al 1997).

TREATMENT TO REDUCE SYMPTOMS

The assumption here is that the cause of the joint pain is from the joint tissues. In this situation, the pain will be a result of mechanical and/or chemical irritation of the joint nociceptors. The subjective information from the patient, particularly the behaviour of symptoms and the mechanism of injury, may enable the clinician to identify what structure(s) have been injured. For example, medial knee pain and a history of a traumatic abduction force to the knee may suggest a torn medial ligament. Anterior knee pain, on the other hand, aggravated by walking down stairs, may be suggestive of a patellofemoral dysfunction.

Various palpatory techniques can be used to reduce symptoms emanating from joint, including: massage, connective-tissue massage, specific soft-tissue mobilization, taping, frictions and joint mobilizations (accessory and physiological movements). Joint mobilizations and specific soft-tissue mobilization have been discussed above. Electrotherapy is beyond the scope of this text – the reader is referred to Low & Reed (1990) as well as an excellent review by Watson (2000).

Massage can be applied to reduce pain, using: stroking, effleurage, kneading, picking up, wringing and skin rolling (Thomson et al 1991). Additional effects are thought to include: an increase in the flow of the circulation, muscle relaxation, lengthening of tissues, an increase in tissue drainage, and pain relief (Thomson et al 1991). For further details, see Thomson et al (1991).

Connective-tissue massage (CTM) involves applying specific strokes to the skin and subcutaneous tissues, from the lumbar spine to the upper limbs, or from the lumbar spine to the lower limbs. It has been suggested that it affects the autonomic nervous system and, via this system, increases circulation, which aids healing and eases pain (Thomson et al 1991). For further details see Thomson et al (1991).

The mechanism by which pain is relieved with each of these manual techniques is still unclear. This is based on the finding that type I mechanoreceptors in joints have been found to have an inhibitory effect at the spinal cord, on type IV nociceptor afferent activity (Wyke & Polacek 1975). Clearly, large-diameter afferents in the skin and any overlying muscle may also contribute to this inhibition of pain. One of the factors involved in primary hyperalgesia is thought to be a reduction in the activation of low-threshold mechanoreceptors in the area of

injury (Raja et al 1999); treatment may increase this activation, which may reduce pain. Certainly, in normal circumstances, mechanoreceptors in the skin have been shown to inhibit pain (Bini et al 1984, Van Hees & Gybels 1981). The pain may also be reduced via a descending inhibitory system, discussed later.

Taping may be used to relieve joint pain. A useful principle is to apply the tape in such a way that it replicates the direction of the pain-relieving force applied by the clinician during treatment. For details of methods of taping the reader is referred to other texts such as Macdonald (1994).

Joint mobilizations

A greater knowledge and understanding of the underlying neurophysiological effects of joint mobilization have begun to emerge over the last few years.

It has been proposed that passive joint movement stimulates large-diameter joint afferents which, at the level of the spinal cord, cause inhibition of joint nociceptor activity (Wyke & Polacek 1975), in accordance with the pain gate theory (Melzack & Wall 1965). This is based on the finding that type I mechanoreceptors in joints have been found to have an inhibitory effect, at the spinal cord, on type IV nociceptor afferent activity (Wyke & Polacek 1975). In normal joints, the large-diameter joint afferents are stimulated mainly at the end of joint range (Burgess & Clark 1969, Clark 1975, Grigg 1975, Grigg & Greenspan 1977, Guilbaud et al 1984a, Millar 1975, Schaible & Schmidt 1983, Tracey 1979). This response is increased with muscle contraction and by movement (Ferrell 1985). This suggests that movements need to be carried out at the end of range to induce pain relief.

However, end-of-range passive movements also cause stimulation of the small-diameter afferents (Clark 1975, Grigg & Greenspan 1977, Guilbaud et al 1984a, Schaible & Schmidt 1983), and mid-range passive movements of inflamed joints stimulate small-diameter joint nociceptors (Coggeshall et al 1983, Guilbaud et al 1984b, 1985, Schaible & Schmidt 1985). This suggests that both mid- and end-range movements would provoke pain, not relieve pain.

In addition, experimentally induced joint arthritis in rats has been found to cause a discharge of previously silent small-diameter joint afferents and a reduction in the mechanical threshold of neurones in the dorsal horn of the spinal cord (Menetrey & Besson 1982) and thalamic nuclei (Gautron & Guilbaud 1982, Kayser & Guilbaud 1984). This has been associated with altered sensory motor cortex activity (Lamour et al 1983). In addition, with joint inflammation, static and oscillatory joint movements have been found to cause an increase in activity of the sympathetic nervous system, with associated increase in blood pressure and heart rate (Sato et al 1986).

Another consideration is that passive joint movements will always involve touching the skin, which may affect nociceptor activity. In normal skin, it is known that stimulation of the large-diameter afferents causes inhibition of the skin nociceptors in the spinal cord (Woolf 1983, Woolf & Wall 1982). There is a possibility that, in a painful joint, the increase in skin afferent activity by the clinician may reduce the perception of pain.

Overall, these studies would seem to suggest that the pain gate mechanism does not completely block the transmission of pain from the spinal cord to the brain, and does not fully explain the relief of pain with passive joint movement (Zusman 1986, Zusman 1994).

Zusman (1986) proposed a theory for the relief of pain with passive end-range joint movement. It was suggested that end-of-range passive movements reduce pain by inhibiting reflex muscle contraction, reducing intra-articular pressure and reducing the level of joint afferent activity (Fig. 4.6). A number of studies have demonstrated that end-of-range passive joint movements cause a reduction in the local and distant reflex muscle contraction (Baxendale & Ferrell 1981a, 1981b, Freeman & Wyke 1967, Taylor et al 1994) and reduction in muscle tension at the limits of joint movement (Lundberg et al 1978). This reduction in muscle contraction is thought to reduce ischaemic muscle pain (Freeman & Wyke 1967) and to reduce muscle tension on periartic-

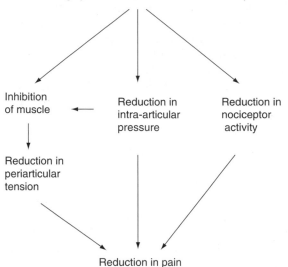

Figure 4.6 Proposed mechanism for pain relief following end-of-range joint mobilization treatment (Zusman 1986).

ular and aponeurotic structures, with subsequent reduction in the peripheral afferent activity (Grigg 1976, Millar 1973). However, activation of joint afferents does not always induce a reduction in muscle activity; stimulation of spinal articular nerves has been found to cause a bilateral increase in EMG activity in the paraspinal, thigh and abdominal muscles (Nade et al 1978). It seems reasonably clear, though, that movement of a joint will, somehow or other, alter local and probably distant muscle groups. Exactly what effect, and whether there is a therapeutic effect, remains uncertain.

Active and passive flexion of a joint has been shown initially to increase, and then reduce, intra-articular pressure (Levick 1979, Nade & Newbold 1983). When intra-articular pressure is experimentally induced it is accompanied by an increase in joint afferent activity (Ferrell et al 1986) owing to the increase in tension in the joint capsule (Wood & Ferrell 1985). Stimulation of joint afferents with joint movement may additionally cause a reduction in the reflex muscle contraction (Spencer et al 1984). This reduction in reflex muscle contraction may reduce pain, as suggested earlier. After 2 minutes of maintained end-of-range movement there is a decrease in intra-articular pressure (Levick 1979, Nade & Newbold 1983). High intra-articular pressure can be caused by high levels of intra-articular fluid or increased muscle tension on the joint capsule (Levick 1979) and is considered to be partly responsible for the pain and limitation of movement in injured or arthritic joints (Ferrell et al 1986). If this is so, then end-range passive movement may help to reduce intra-articular pressure, reduce pain and increase range of movement.

The final mechanism put forward by Zusman (1986) to explain the reduction in pain following end-range passive joint movement involves a reduction in the overall joint afferent activity. Oscillatory end-range passive movement have been shown to cause an increase in range of movement (Gibson et al 1993, Grigg & Greenspan 1977, McCollam & Benson 1993, Twomey & Taylor 1982). When the joint is passively maintained at the end of the range, there is a linear correlation between the stretching of the joint capsule and a reduction in the joint afferent activity (Grigg & Greenspan 1977). If the joint is then moved away from this end-range position, and then re-positioned, the level of joint afferent activity is substantially reduced or absent (Grigg & Greenspan 1977, Millar 1975), and this can last up to 10 minutes (McCall et al 1974). This delay is known as hysteresis. McCall et al (1974) found that this hysteresis effect could be produced with both static and oscillatory passive end-range movements. In arthritic joints, repetitive (Guilbaud et al 1985) and maintained (Iggo et al 1984) mechanical stimulation of small-diameter joint afferents produces an increased response, followed by a greater reduced response lasting a few minutes, compared to normal joints. Thus, end-range mobilizations may cause a reduction in joint afferent activity, and hence reduced pain.

In summary, then, there is some evidence to support the proposal that end-of-range passive movements reduce pain by inhibiting reflex muscle contraction, reducing intra-articular pressure and reducing the level of joint afferent activity (Zusman 1986).

Descending inhibition of pain

The periaqueductal grey (PAG) area has been found to be important in the control of nociception. PAG projects to the dorsal horn and has a descending control of nociception (Fig. 4.7). It also projects upwards to the medial thalamus,

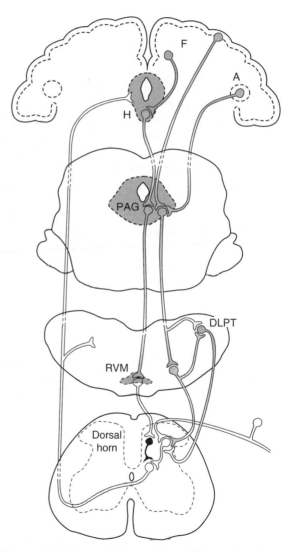

Figure 4.7 Pain-modulating pathway. PAG receives input from the frontal lobe (F), the amygdala (A) and the hypothalamus (H). Afferents from PAG travel to the rostral ventromedial medulla (RVM) and the dorsolateral pontomesencephalic tegmentum (DLPT) and on to the dorsal horn. The RVM has bi-directional control of nociceptive transmission. There are inhibitory (filled) and excitatory (unfilled) interneurones. (From Fields & Basbaum 1999, with permission.)

orbital frontal cortex, and so may have an ascending control of nociception (Fields & Basbaum 1999). The PAG has two distinct regions: the dorsolateral PAG (dPAG) and the ventrolateral PAG (vPAG).

dPAG

The dorsolateral PAG (dPAG) runs to the dorsolateral pons and ventrolateral medulla, which is involved in autonomic control (Fields & Basbaum 1999). In the rat, stimulation of the dPAG causes analgesia, increased blood pressure, increased heart rate, vasodilation of the hind limb muscles, increased rate and depth of respiration, and coordinated hind limb, jaw and tail movements, suggesting increased activity of the sympathetic nervous system (SNS), and alpha motor neurones (Lovick 1991). The neurotransmitter from dPAG is noradrenaline (norepinephrine), and the analgesic effect appears to mediate morphine analgesia of mechanical nociceptor stimuli (Kuraishi et al 1983). At the spinal cord level, dPAG causes inhibition of substance P from peripheral noxious mechanical stimulation (Kuraishi 1990).

vPAG

The ventrolateral PAG (vPAG) runs mainly to the nucleus raphe magnus. In the rat, stimulation of vPAG causes analgesia with decreased blood pressure, decreased heart rate, vasodilation of the hind limb muscles and reduced hind limb, jaw and tail movements, suggesting inhibition of the SNS and inhibition of alpha motor neurones (Lovick 1991). The neurotransmitter used in vPAG is serotonin, and the analgesic effect appears to mediate morphine analgesia of thermal nociceptive stimuli (Kuraishi et al 1983). At the dorsal horn vPAG inhibits the release of somatostatin, produced by peripheral noxious thermal stimulation (Kuraishi 1990). These mechanisms have been linked to the behaviour of an animal under threat, which initially acts with a defensive flight-or-fight response, followed by recuperation (Fanselow 1991, Lovick 1991); this is summarized in Figure 4.8.

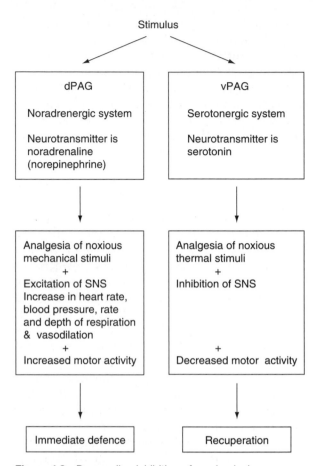

Figure 4.8 Descending inhibition of mechanical nociception from dPAG (noradrenergic system), and thermal nociception from vPAG (serotonergic system).

Noxious stimuli can cause activation of the descending control system (Fields & Basbaum 1999, Yaksh & Elde 1981), which may reduce nociceptive transmission. Noxious stimulation has been found to cause release of enkephalins at the supraspinal and spinal levels (Yaksh & Elde 1981). It has also been found that stimulation of the spinothalamic tract transmitting nociceptive information from one foot can be inhibited by noxious input from the contralateral foot, hand, face or trunk (Gerhart et al 1981). It has been suggested that this may explain the relief of pain with acupuncture, and pain behaviours such as 'biting your lip and banging your head against a wall'(!) (Melzack 1975). Painful joint mobilizations may also activate the descending control system.

The proposed mechanism by which joint mobilizations relieve pain is outlined in Figure 4.9 (Wright 1995). It is suggested that joint mobilizations almost immediately stimulate the dPAG, to cause hypoalgesia. Using research from acupuncture, it is suggested that vPAG may be stimulated 20–45 minutes later (Takeshige et al 1992).

A number of research studies that support the proposal by Wright (1995) have investigated the immediate effects of joint mobilization on noxious mechanical and thermal thresholds, and sympathetic nervous system activity. In a number of the studies, noxious mechanical thresholds have been measured using a digital pressure algometer, and noxious thermal thresholds have used a contact thermode system (Wright 1995). Increased activity of the sympathetic nervous system (SNS) has been measured indirectly by measuring a decrease in skin temperature and an increase in skin conductance (due to a decrease in skin resistance). Skin temperature has been measured using an AT42 skin temperature monitor (Autogenic Advanced Technology, Chicago), and skin conductance has been measured using an AT64 skin conductance monitor (Autogenic Advanced Technology, Chicago).

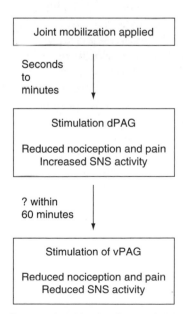

Figure 4.9 Proposed mechanism by which joint mobilizations may reduce pain (Wright 1995).

In a number of studies joint mobilizations have been found to have an immediate hypoalgesic effect on mechanical nociceptor activity and/or to produce increased activity of the sympathetic nervous system (SNS) (Chiu & Wright 1996, Petersen et al 1993, Sterling et al 2001, Vicenzino 1995, Vicenzino et al 1994, 1996, 1998, Wright & Vicenzino 1995). This has been found following a:

• grade III central posteroanterior (PA) pressure to C5 for three repetitions of 1 minute, on asymptomatic subjects (Petersen et al 1993).

• grade III central posteroanterior (PA) pressure to C5 for three repetitions of 1 minute, on asymptomatic subjects (Chiu & Wright 1996). An oscillation frequency of 2 Hz (two cycles per second) caused a greater increase in sympathetic nervous system activity than a slower frequency of 0.5 Hz (one cycle every 2 seconds).

• grade III lateral glide to C5/6 for 30 seconds with the arm in upper limb tension test positions, on asymptomatic subjects (Vicenzino et al 1994).

• grade III lateral glide to C5/6 for three repetitions of 30 seconds, on asymptomatic subjects (Vicenzino 1995). This study found an increase in mechanical pain threshold with no increase in noxious thermal threshold.

• grade III lateral glide to C5/6 for three repetitions of 30 seconds on patients with chronic lateral epicondylalgia (Vicenzino et al 1996, 1998).

• grade III unilateral posteroanterior (PA) pressure to C5/6 articular pillar for three repetitions of 1 minute (Sterling et al 2001). This study additionally found that the EMG activity of the superficial neck muscles was reduced during controlled active upper cervical flexion.

• grade III unilateral posteroanterior pressure on C5 articular pillar, on asymptomatic subjects (Wright & Vicenzino 1995). This study found an increase in mechanical pain threshold and no increase in noxious thermal threshold.

A correlation between the increased sympathetic activity and the reduction in mechanical pain thresholds has been identified (Vicenzino

1995, Vicenzino et al 1996, 1998). This supports the hypothesis that joint mobilizations initiate the descending pain inhibitory system because an increase in sympathetic activity and hypoalgesia have been found to occur together (Lovick 1991).

Summary of reduction of symptoms with joint mobilization

An understanding of the mechanism by which joint mobilizations cause a reduction in a patient's pain is beginning to emerge but is far from complete. Initially, theories that joint mobilization affected the peripheral painful tissue were put forward and may still partly explain the mechanism of pain relief. More recently, greater emphasis has been placed on the role of the descending inhibitory pathways, with evidence suggesting that joint mobilization activates this system, causing a reduction in nociceptor activity and thus pain perception.

Effect of grade V manipulations (HVLAT)

The effect of a grade V manipulative thrust technique on the spine is somewhat unclear. The audible 'crack' is due to a mechanism known as cavitation, and is the result of bubbles within the joint being collapsed (Unsworth et al 1971). The set up position for a grade V causes the pressure within one part of the joint to be lowered such that carbon dioxide bubbles are formed. Within 0.01 seconds, synovial fluid moves into the area of low pressure and bursts the bubbles, creating the audible sound (Unsworth et al 1971). The after-effects of cavitation are thought to be therapeutic; there is an increase in the joint space for approximately 15 minutes (Unsworth et al 1971), increased range of movement (Surkitt et al 2000), and muscle inhibition (Brodeur 1995). These immediate effects of manipulation would seem to enhance joint movement, and so active or passive movements may be helpful after carrying out a manipulation. The reader is referred to two useful articles for further information on manip-

ulation: Evans (2002) and Gibbons & Tehan (2001).

Addressing the biopsychosocial aspects of symptoms

Injury, or the perception of injury, produces anxiety and fear (Craig 1999). Who has ever injured themselves, however minimally, and not experienced an emotional reaction? The psychological aspects of pain sometimes focus on 'emotional individuals', or on chronic pain patients. However, all of us will have a cognitive and emotional response to injury because injury interrupts our lives. There is never a right time for an injury: it will always be, to a greater or lesser degree, a nuisance to us. That 'nuisance' will drive our emotional reactions. It seems reasonable to suggest, therefore, that all patients with neuromusculoskeletal dysfunction will have thoughts and feelings about their problem, and it would be an oversight on the part of the clinician not to enquire about these. This enquiry involves the clinician understanding the patient's thoughts and feelings. This is no easy task, and to do it well requires a high level of skill in active listening. Active listening involves putting our own thoughts, beliefs and feelings to one side and choosing instead to hear what the patient has to say. It involves trying to understand the patient and their world, through their eyes, and avoiding the all-too-easy error of re-interpreting through our own eyes. It requires the clinician to listen with compassion, patience and without judgement. It involves the clinician using words carefully and meaningfully and using open-ended questions to search for information until understanding is reached. It involves sensitive verbal and non-verbal communication, encouraging safe and open communication. This is a tall order, but the benefits of truly being able to come alongside the patient will far outweigh the effort of developing these skills.

The use of 'yellow flags' was devised specifically for acute low back pain to identify beliefs, emotions and behaviours that may contribute to long-term disability (Watson & Kendall 2000). Screening questionnaires (e.g. Main & Waddell

1999) have been devised which, like all questionnaires, have major limitations. Questions provide a superficial and sometimes false understanding of the problem, as anyone who has filled in a questionnaire knows only too well. For example, while a question may ask 'how much have you been bothered by feeling depressed in the last week' and the recipient answers on a 0 to 10 scale from 'not at all' to 'extremely', little information is gleamed from this: there may be a wide variety of factors underlying the given score. For this reason, if a questionnaire is used, a discussion with the patient will also be necessary to understand the problems the patient faces (Watson & Kendall 2000). The questionnaire can be useful in providing the clinician with aspects to discuss with the patient; however, there is a danger that it becomes a mechanistic form-filling exercise. It is worth remembering that the clinical management of patients is fundamentally based on a human relationship, which is not normally enriched by form filling!

Following the enquiry of the patient, as to their thoughts and feelings, two further steps are recommended: education and exposure (Vlaeyen & Crombez 1999). Education involves the clinician carefully facilitating the patient's understanding of their problem. The way this is carried out with patients will vary depending on a number of factors, including the patient's prior knowledge, thoughts and beliefs, and how they feel about the problem. All the listening skills discussed above will be imperative in this process. The ability of the clinician to be honest is important. The clinician needs to be careful about the way the problem is explained to a patient. There is a world of difference between 'the pain in your back is from the disc' and 'I think that the pain in your back could be coming from the disc'. The former explanation suggests that you know that the pain is coming from the disc, and yet there is overwhelming evidence that you cannot make such claims. It has been estimated that a definite diagnosis of the pathology can be made in only about 15% of cases (Waddell 1999). Furthermore, there is a long-term problem with being so confident as the patient may in the future have a recurrence of the same pain and may see another clinician

who may say 'the pain in your back is from your sacroiliac joint'. The patient is aware that this is a repeat episode, and now, quite rightly, begins to have doubts about the ability of these two clinicians. This will be a familiar story to experienced clinicians who will have come across patients who have received perhaps three, four or even more confident 'diagnoses' of the same problem and have come to you depressed, cynical and disillusioned with the medical profession.

The final aspect is exposure, which involves careful and graded exposure to the movements or postures that provoke pain (Vlaeyen & Crombez 1999). While this is designed for chronic pain patients who learn to avoid movements and posture through fear (Waddell & Main 1999), it may also be an important part of the treatment of acute tissue damage. Using movements and postures in a careful, controlled and graded way may help to avoid long-term movement dysfunctions.

MODIFICATION, PROGRESSION AND REGRESSION OF TREATMENT

The best treatment is the one that improves the patient's signs and symptoms in the shortest period of time. Any physical test that reproduces or eases the patient's symptoms can be converted to a treatment technique by applying components of a treatment dose. Converting positive physical testing procedures to treatment techniques would seem the most logical approach to choosing treatment, as the clinician can be confident that the treatment is, somehow or other, affecting the structure at fault. Reproduction of the patient's symptoms is a vital anchor from which to decide aspects of the treatment dose. Only when symptoms are produced can the clinician be sure that they are affecting, somehow or other, the structure(s) at fault. This may require some careful and time-consuming examination procedures, taking an attitude of the explorer, the researcher or the detective who must explore all possible avenues of investigation. For example, testing elbow flexion overpressure is fully explored only if variations of forearm pronation and supination and variations in direction of flexion medially and laterally are carried out. Similarly, when applying accessory movements, a wide variation in the direction of the force needs to be used before deciding that the accessory movement is not symptomatic.

The clinician monitors the patient's signs and symptoms within and between treatment sessions in order to identify the effectiveness of the treatment choice. Any change in signs and symptoms is considered in the light of the prognosis and treatment goals, following the examination and assessment on day one. In this way, the clinician can be creative and imaginative in considering all the possible treatment choices, while constantly monitoring the effectiveness of treatment. If the treatment is proved to be ineffective, then the clinician can alter the treatment; if it proves to be effective, and the patient is improving at the expected rate, then the treatment can be continued or progressed. The nature of this alteration can be to modify the technique in some way, to progress the treatment or regress the treatment. Regardless of which alteration is made, the clinician makes every effort to determine what effect this alteration has on the patient's subjective and physical asterisks. In order to do this, the clinician alters one aspect of treatment at a time and reassesses immediately to determine the value of the alteration.

Modification of treatment

The clinician may modify the treatment given to a patient by altering an existing treatment, adding a new treatment or stopping a treatment. At all times the treatment should have the functional goals of the patient in mind. Altering an existing treatment involves altering some aspect of the treatment dose, discussed earlier. The immediate and more long-term effect of the alteration is then evaluated by reassessment of the subjective and physical asterisks; this process is outlined in Figure 4.10. The clinician then decides whether, overall, the patient is better, the same or worse, relating this to the prognosis. For instance, if a quick improvement was expected

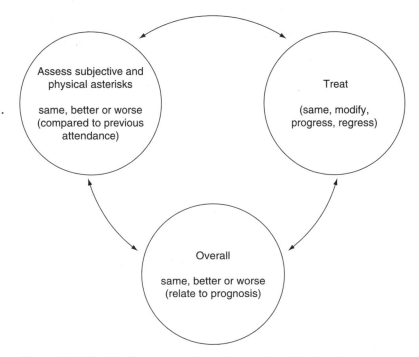

Figure 4.10 Modification, progression and regression of treatment.

but only some improvement occurred, the clinician may progress treatment. If the patient is worse after treatment the dose may be regressed in some way, and if the treatment made no difference at all then a more substantial modification may be made. Before discarding a treatment, it is worth making sure that it has been fully utilized as it may be that a much stronger or much weaker treatment dose may be effective.

Progression and regression of treatment

A treatment is progressed or regressed by altering appropriate aspects of the treatment dose in such a way that more or less treatment is applied to the tissues. The aspects of treatment dose that can be altered are outlined in Table 4.6.

The immediate and more long-term effect of the alteration can then be evaluated by reassess-

ment of the subjective and physical asterisks. Table 4.7 provides an example of how a treatment dose may be progressed and regressed. It can be seen that, for the first treatment for the cervical spine, regression is accomplished by reducing the intensity of the patient's pain, from full reproduction to partial reproduction, and progession is achieved by increasing the time from 30 seconds to 1 minute.

Prognosis

A full discussion on joint injuries and their prognosis is beyond the scope of this text. The rehabilitation, following an anterior cruciate ligament tear, is briefly outlined to highlight the difficulties in obtaining a restoration of function. Six months of intensive rehabilitation, following ACL reconstruction, has been found to result in a normal gait pattern, but altered joint

Table 4.6   Progression and regression of treatment dose

Treatment dose	Progression	Regression
Position	Joint towards end of available range	Joint towards beginning of available range
Direction of force	More provocative	Less provocative
Magnitude of force	Increase	Decrease
Amplitude of oscillation	Decreased	Increased
Rhythm	Staccato	Smoother
Time	Longer	Shorter
Speed	Slower or faster	Slower
Symptom response	Allowing more symptoms to be provoked	Allowing fewer symptoms to be provoked

Table 4.7   Examples of how a treatment dose can be progressed and regressed

Regression	Dose	Progression	Explanation
In cervical extension: did central PA C4 IV ×3 (1 min) slowly & smoothly to partial reproduction of patient's neck pain	In cervical neutral did: central PA C4 IV ×3 (1 min) slowly & smoothly to partial reproduction of patient's neck pain	In cervical flexion did: central PA C4 IV ×3 (1 min) slowly & smoothly to partial reproduction of patient's neck pain	The starting position has been altered. It might be assumed that extension is a position of ease and flexion a more provocative position
In 90 degrees knee flexion did: medial glide tibiofemoral joint I ×3 (1 min) slowly & smoothly short of P1	In 90 degrees knee flexion did: medial glide tibiofemoral joint II slowly & smoothly ×3 (1 min) short of P1	In 90 degrees knee flexion did: medial glide tibiofemoral joint III– ×3 (1 min) slowly & smoothly short of P1	The grade of movement has been altered
Physiological plantarflexion III ×3 (1 min) slowly & smoothly to full reproduction of ankle pain	Physiological plantarflexion III+ ×3 (1 min) slowly & smoothly to full reproduction of ankle pain	Physiological plantarflexion III+ ×3 (1 min) fast & staccato to full reproduction of ankle pain	Grade has been altered as a regression. Speed and rhythm have been altered as a progression

torque and power patterns (DeVita et al 1998). A deficit in joint proprioception (Gillquist & Messner 1999), motor performance (Pfeifer & Banzer 1999) and quadriceps strength (Hurley et al 1994) has been found during the first year following an injury or reconstruction of the anterior cruciate ligament of the knee. Patients who had greater muscle inhibition at the beginning of treatment had a poorer outcome by the end of the year (Hurley et al 1994). A deficit in strength of up to 20% may continue for 4 to 9 years (Arangio et al 1997, Natri et al 1996, Seto et al 1988) owing to muscle atrophy (Arangio et al 1997) and incomplete muscle activation (Suter & Herzog 2000). The consequences of these deficits are unclear; it has been suggested that alterations in muscle activity may alter joint loading and this may, in the long term, lead to osteoarthritis in the joint (Brandt 1997). This is partly supported by the prediction that 50–70% of patients with a rupture of the anterior cruciate ligament will develop radiographic signs of osteoarthritis 15 to 20 years post-injury (Gillquist & Messner 1999). This evidence suggests that joint injury will have profound effects on muscles, and restoration of full function may take a considerable length of time, and even then, may be incomplete.

Summary

This chapter has outlined the principles of joint treatment. Treatment is only a part of the overall management of a patient; the reader is therefore encouraged to go now to Chapter 9, where the principles of management are discussed.

REFERENCES

Arangio G A, Chen C, Kalady M, Reed J F 1997 Thigh muscle size and strength after anterior cruciate ligament reconstruction and rehabilitation. Journal of Orthopaedics and Sports Physiotherapy 26(5):238–243

Baxendale R H, Ferrell W R 1981a The effect of knee joint afferent discharge on transmission in flexion reflex pathways in decerebrate cats. Journal of Physiology 315:231–242

Baxendale R H, Ferrell W R 1981b Modulation of transmission in forelimb flexion reflex pathways by elbow joint afferent discharge in decerebrate cats. Brain Research 221:393–396

Bini G, Cruccu G, Hagbarth K-E et al 1984 Analgesic effect of vibration and cooling on pain induced by intraneural electrical stimulation. Pain 18:239–248

Brandt K D 1997 Putting some muscle into osteoarthritis. Annals of Internal Medicine 127(2):154–156

Brodeur R 1995 The audible release associated with joint manipulation. Journal of Manipulative and Physiological Therapeutics 18(3):155–164

Burgess P R, Clark F J 1969 Characteristics of knee joint receptors in the cat. Journal of Physiology 203:317–335

Burroughs P, Dahners L E 1990 The effect of enforced exercise on the healing of ligament injuries. American Journal of Sports Medicine 18(4):376–378

Chiu T W, Wright A 1996 To compare the effects of different rates of application of a cervical mobilisation technique on sympathetic outflow to the upper limb in normal subjects. Manual Therapy 1(4):198–203

Clark F J 1975 Information signaled by sensory fibers in medial articular nerve. Journal of Neurophysiology 38:1464–1472

Coggeshall R E, Hong K AH P, Langford L A et al 1983 Discharge characteristics of fine medial articular afferents at rest and during passive movements of inflamed knee joints. Brain Research 272:185–188

Craig K D 1999 Emotions and psychobiology. In: Wall P D, Melzack R (eds) Textbook of pain, 4th edn. Churchill Livingstone, Edinburgh, ch 12, p 331–343

Cyriax J 1984 Textbook of orthopaedic medicine, vol 2 Treatment by manipulation, massage and injection. Baillière Tindall, London

DeVita P, Hortobagyi T, Barrier J 1998 Gait biomechanics are not normal after anterior cruciate ligament reconstruction and accelerated rehabilitation. Medicine and Science in Sports and Exercise 30(10):1481–1488

Evans D W 2002 Mechanisms and effects of spinal high-velocity, low-amplitude thrust manipulation: previous theories. Journal of Manipulative and Physiological Therapeutics 25(4):251–262

Fanselow M S 1991 The midbrain periaqueductal gray as a coordinator of action in response to fear and anxiety. In: Depaulis A, Bandler R (eds) The midbrain periaqueductal gray matter. Plenum Press, New York, p 151–173

Ferrell W R 1985 The response of slowly adapting mechanoreceptors in the cat knee joint to tetanic contraction of hind limb muscles. Quarterly Journal of Experimental Physiology 70:337–345

Ferrell W R, Nade S, Newbold P J 1986 The interrelation of neural discharge, intra-articular pressure, and joint angle in the knee of the dog. Journal of Physiology 373:353–365

Fields H L, Basbaum A I 1999 Central nervous system mechanisms of pain modulation. In: Wall P D, Melzack R (eds) Textbook of pain, 4th edn. Churchill Livingstone, Edinburgh, ch 11, p 309–329

Freeman M A R, Wyke B D 1967 Articular reflexes at the ankle joint: an electromyographic study of normal and abnormal influences of ankle-joint mechanoreceptors upon reflex activity in the leg muscles. British Journal of Surgery 54(12):990–1001

Fu F H, Harner C D, Klein A H 1991 Shoulder impingement syndrome, a critical review. Clinical Orthopaedics and Related Research 269:162–173

Gautron M, Guilbaud G 1982 Somatic responses of ventrobasal thalamic neurones in polyarthritic rats. Brain Research 237:459–471

Gerber C, Ganz R 1984 Clinical assessment of instability of the shoulder with special reference to anterior and posterior drawer tests. Journal of Bone and Joint Surgery 66B(4):551–556

Gerhart K D, Yezierski R P, Giesler G J, Willis W D 1981 Inhibitory receptive fields of primate spinothalamic tract cells. Journal of Neurophysiology 46(6):1309–1325

Gibbons P, Tehan P 2001 Patient positioning and spinal locking for lumbar spine rotation manipulation. Manual Therapy 6(3):130–138

Gibson H, Ross J, Allen J et al 1993 The effect of mobilization on forward bending range. Journal of Manual and Manipulative Therapy 1(4):142–147

Gillquist J, Messner K 1999 Anterior cruciate ligament reconstruction and the long term incidence of gonarthrosis. Sports Medicine 27(3):143–156

Giovanelli-Blacker B, Elvey R, Thompson E 1985 The clinical significance of measured lumbar zygapophyseal intracapsular pressure variation. Proceedings Manipulative Therapists Association of Australia 4th Biennial Conference, Brisbane Queensland, p 127–139

Glousman R E 1993 Instability versus impingement syndrome in the throwing athlete. Orthopaedic Clinics of North America 24(1):89–99

Glousman R, Jobe F, Tibone J et al 1988 Dynamic electromyographic analysis of the throwing shoulder with glenohumeral instability. Journal of Bone and Joint Surgery 70A(2):220–226

Glousman R E, Barron J, Jobe F W et al 1992 An electromyographic analysis of the elbow in normal and injured pitchers with medial collateral ligament insufficiency. American Journal of Sports Medicine 20(3):311–317

Gomez M A, Woo S L-Y, Amiel D et al 1991 The effects of increased tension on healing medial collateral ligaments. American Journal of Sports Medicine 19(4):347–354

Gregory M A, Deane M N, Mars M 2003 Ultrastructural changes in untraumatised rabbit skeletal muscle treated with deep transverse friction. Physiotherapy 89(7):408–416

Grigg P 1975 Mechanical factors influencing response of joint afferent neurons from cat knee. Journal of Neurophysiology 38:1473–1484

Grigg P 1976 Response of joint afferent neurons in cat medial articular nerve to active and passive movements of the knee. Brain Research 118:482–485

Grigg P, Greenspan B J 1977 Response of primate joint afferent neurons to mechanical stimulation of knee joint. Journal of Neurophysiology 40(1):1–8

Guilbaud G, Iggo A, Tegner R 1984a Sensory receptors in the joints of rats with adjuvant-induced arthritis. Journal of Physiology 346: 58P

Guilbaud G, Iggo A, Tegner R 1984b Sensory changes in joints of arthritic rats. Pain (suppl 2):S7(7)

Guilbaud G, Iggo A, Tegner R 1985 Sensory receptors in ankle joint capsules of normal and arthritic rats. Experimental Brain Research 58:29–40

Harms M C, Bader D L 1997 Variability of forces applied by experienced therapists during spinal mobilization. Clinical Biomechanics 12(6):393–399

Hunter G 1998 Specific soft tissue mobilization in the management of soft tissue dysfunction. Manual Therapy 3(1):2–11

Hurley M V, Jones D W, Newham D J 1994 Arthrogenic quadriceps inhibition and rehabilitation of patients with extensive traumatic knee injuries. Clinical Sciences 86:305–310

Iggo A, Guilbaud G, Tegner R 1984 Sensory mechanisms in arthritic rat joints. In: Kruger L & Liebeskind J C (eds) Advances in pain research and therapy, vol 6 Neural mechanisms of pain. Raven, New York, p 83–93

Kuraishi Y 1990 Neuropeptide-mediated transmission of nociceptive information and its regulation. Novel mechanisms of analgesics. Yakugaku Zasshi 110(10):711–726

Kuraishi Y, Harada Y, Aratani S et al 1983 Separate involvement of the spinal noradrenergic and serotonergic systems in morphine analgesia: the differences in mechanical and thermal algesic tests. Brain Research 273:245–252

Kayser V, Guilbaud G 1984 Further evidence for changes in the responsiveness of somatosensory neurons in arthritic rats: a study of the posterior intralaminar region of the thalamus. Brain Research 323:144–147

Knott M, Voss D E 1968 Proprioceptive neuromuscular facilitation. Harper Row, New York

LaBan M M 1962 Collagen tissue: implications of its response to stress in vitro. Archives of Physical Medicine and Rehabilitation 43(9):461–466

Lamour Y, Guilbaud G, Willer J C 1983 Altered properties and laminar distribution of neuronal responses to peripheral stimulation in the Sml cortex of the arthritic rat. Brain Research 273:183–187

Lehmann J F, DeLateur B J, Silverman D R 1966 Selective heating effects of ultrasound in human beings. Archives of Physical Medicine and Rehabilitation 47:331–339

Levick J R 1979 An investigation into the validity of subatmospheric pressure recordings from synovial fluid and their dependence on joint angle. Journal of Physiology 289:55–67

Levick J R, Mason R M, Coleman P J, Scott D 1999 Physiology of synovial fluid and trans-synovial flow. In: Archer C W, Caterson B, Benjamin M, Ralphs J R (eds) Biology of the synovial joint. Harwood, Australia, ch 15, p 235–252

Lovick T A 1991 Interactions between descending pathways from the dorsal and ventrolateral periaqueductal gray matter in the rat. In: Depaulis A, Bandler R (eds) The midbrain periaqueductal gray matter. Plenum Press, New York, p 101–120

Low J, Reed A 1990 Electrotherapy explained, principles and practice. Butterworth-Heinemann, London

Lundberg A, Malmgren K, Schomburg E D 1978 Role of joint afferents in motor control exemplified by effects on reflex pathways from 1b afferents. Journal of Physiology 284:327–343

McCaffery M 1979 Nursing the patient in pain. Harper & Row, London

McCall W D, Farias M C, Williams W J, BeMent S L 1974 Static and dynamic responses of slowly adapting joint receptors. Brain Research 70:221–243

McCollam R L, Benson C J 1993 Effects of postero-anterior mobilization on lumbar extension and flexion. Journal of Manual and Manipulative Therapy 1(4):134–141

Macdonald R 1994 Taping techniques. Butterworth-Heinemann, Oxford

McKenzie R 1981 The lumbar spine, mechanical diagnosis and therapy. Spinal Publications, New Zealand

McKenzie R 1983 Treat your own neck. Spinal Publications, New Zealand

McKenzie R 1985 Treat your own back. Spinal Publications, New Zealand

McQuade K J, Shelley I, Cvitkovic J 1999 Patterns of stiffness during clinical examination of the glenohumeral joint. Clinical Biomechanics 14:620–627

Magarey M E 1985 Selection of passive treatment techniques. In: Proceedings of 4th Biennial Conference of the Manipulative Therapists' Association of Australia, Brisbane, p 298–320

Magarey M E 1986 Examination and assessment in spinal joint dysfunction. In: Grieve G P (ed) Modern manual therapy of the vertebral column. Churchill Livingstone, Edinburgh, ch 44, p 481–497

Main C J, Waddell G 1999 Psychological distress. In: Waddell G (ed) The back pain revolution. Churchill Livingstone, Edinburgh, ch 11 p 173–186

Maitland G D, Banks K, English K, Hengeveld E 2001 Maitland's vertebral manipulation, 6th edn. Butterworth-Heinemann, Oxford

Melzack R 1975 Prolonged relief of pain by brief, intense transcutaneous somatic stimulation. Pain 1:357–373

Melzack R, Wall P D 1965 Pain mechanisms: a new theory. Science 150:971–979

Menetrey D, Besson J M 1982 Electrophysiological characteristics of dorsal horn cells in rats with cutaneous inflammation resulting from chronic arthritis. Pain 13:343–364

Millar J 1973 Joint afferent fibres responding to muscle stretch, vibration and contraction. Brain Research 63:380–383

Millar J 1975 Flexion–extension sensitivity of elbow joint afferents in cat. Experimental Brain Research 24:209–214

Millard J B 1961 Effect of high-frequency currents and infrared rays on the circulation of the lower limb in man. Annals of Physical Medicine 6(2):45–66

Mulligan B R 1995 Manual Therapy 'Nags', 'Snags', 'MWMS' etc, 3rd edn. Plane View Series, Wellington

Nade S, Newbold P J 1983 Factors determining the level and changes in intra-articular pressure in the knee joint of the dog. Journal of Physiology 338:21–36

Nade S, Bell E, Wyke B 1978 Articular neurology of the feline lumbar spine. Journal of Bone and Joint Surgery 60B:292 (abstract)

Natri A, Jarvinen M, Latvala K, Kannus P 1996 Isokinetic muscle performance after anterior cruciate ligament surgery. International Journal of Sports Medicine 17:223–228

Noyes F R, DeLucas J L, Torvik P J 1974 Biomechanics of anterior cruciate ligament failure: an analysis of strain-rate sensitivity and mechanisms of failure in primates. Journal of Bone and Joint Surgery 56A(2):236–253

Noyes F R, Butler D L, Paulos L E, Grood E S 1983 Intraarticular cruciate reconstruction, 1: perspectives on graft strength, vascularization, and immediate motion after replacement. Clinical Orthopaedics and Related Research 172:71–77

O'Sullivan P B, Twomey L T, Allison G T 1997 Evaluation of specific stabilising exercise in the treatment of chronic low back pain with radiologic diagnosis of spondylolysis and spondylolisthesis. Spine 22(24):2959–2967

Panjabi M M 1992 The stabilizing system of the spine. Part II. Neutral zone and instability hypothesis. Journal of Spinal Disorders 5(4):390–397

Panjabi M M, White A A 2001 Biomechanics in the musculoskeletal system. Churchill Livingstone, New York

Petersen N, Vicenzino B, Wright A 1993 The effects of a cervical mobilisation technique on sympathetic outflow to the upper limb in normal subjects. Physiotherapy Theory and Practice 9:149–156

Petty N J 1995 The effect of posteroanterior mobilisation on sagittal mobility of the lumbar spine. Manual Therapy 1:25–29

Petty N J 2000 Spinal mobilisation-the effect of treatment dose on lumbar extension. International Federation of Orthopaedic Manipulative Therapists Conference Proceedings p 365

Petty N J, Moore A P 2001 Neuromusculoskeletal examination and assessment, a handbook for therapists, 2nd edn. Churchill Livingstone, Edinburgh

Petty N J, Maher C, Latimer J, Lee M 2002 Manual examination of accessory movements-seeking R1. Manual Therapy 7(1):39–43

Pfeifer K, Banzer W 1999 Motor performance in different dynamic tests in knee rehabilitation. Scandinavian Journal of Medicine and Science in Sports 9:19–27

Raja S N, Meyer R A, Ringkamp M, Campbell J N 1999 Peripheral neural mechanisms of nociception. In: Wall P D, Melzack R (eds) Textbook of pain, 4th edn. Churchill Livingstone, Edinburgh, ch 1, p 11–84

Rigby B J 1964 The effect of mechanical extension upon the thermal stability of collagen. Biochimica et Biophysica Acta 79(SC 43008):634–636

Rigby B J, Hirai N, Spikes J D, Eyring H 1959 The mechanical properties of rat tail tendon. Journal of General Physiology 43:265–283

Sapega A A, Quedenfield T C, Moyer R A, Butler R A 1981 Biophysical factors in range-of-motion exercise. The Physician and Sportsmedicine 9(12):57–65

Sato A, Sato Y & Schmidt R F 1986 Catecholamine secretion and adrenal nerve activity in response to movements of normal and inflamed knee joints in cats. Journal of Physiology 375:611–624

Schaible H-G, Schmidt R F 1983 Responses of fine medial articular nerve afferents to passive movements of knee joint. Journal of Neurophysiology 49(5):1118–1126

Schaible H-G, Schmidt R F 1985 Effects of an experimental arthritis on the sensory properties of fine articular afferent units. Journal of Neurophysiology 54(5):1109–1122

Seto J L, Orofino A S, Morrissey M C et al 1988 Assessment of quadriceps/hamstring strength, knee ligament stability, functional and sports activity levels five years after anterior cruciate ligament reconstruction. American Journal of Sports Medicine 16(2):170–180

Solomonow M, Baratta R, Zhou B H et al 1987 The synergistic action of the anterior cruciate ligament and thigh muscles in maintaining joint stability. American Journal of Sports Medicine 15(3):207–213

Spencer J D, Hayes K C, Alexander I J 1984 Knee joint effusion and quadriceps reflex inhibition in man. Archives of Physical Medicine and Rehabilitation 65:171–177

Sterling M, Jull G, Wright A 2001 Cervical mobilisation: concurrent effects on pain, sympathetic nervous system activity and motor activity. Manual Therapy 6(2):72–81

Surkitt D, Gibbons P, McLaughlin P 2000 High velocity low amplitude manipulation of the atlanto-axial joint: effect on atlanto-axial and cervical spine rotation asymmetry in asymptomatic subjects. Journal of Osteopathic Medicine 3(1):13–19

Suter E, Herzog W 2000 Muscle inhibition and functional deficiencies associated with knee pathologies. In: Herzog W (ed) Skeletal muscle mechanics, from mechanisms to function. John Wiley, Chichester, ch 21, p 365–376

Takeshige C, Sato T, Mera T et al 1992 Descending pain inhibitory system involved in acupuncture analgesia. Brain Research Bulletin 29:617–634

Taylor M, Suvinen T, Reade P 1994 The effect of Grade IV distraction mobilisation on patients with temporomandibular pain-dysfunction disorder. Physiotherapy Theory and Practice 10:129–136

Thomson A, Skinner A, Piercy J 1991 Tidy's physiotherapy, 12th edn. Butterworth-Heinemann, Oxford

Threlkeld A J 1992 The effects of manual therapy on connective tissue. Physical Therapy 72(12):893–902

Tipton C M, James S L, Mergner W, Tcheng T-K 1970 Influence of exercise on strength of medial collateral knee ligaments of dogs. American Journal of Physiology 218(3):894–902

Tracey D J 1979 Characteristics of wrist joint receptors in the cat. Experimental Brain Research 34:165–176

Twomey L, Taylor J 1982 Flexion creep deformation and hysteresis in the lumbar vertebral column. Spine 7(2):116–122

Unsworth A, Dowson D, Wright V 1971 'Cracking joints' a bioengineering study of cavitation in the metacarpophalangeal joint. Annals of the Rheumatic Diseases 30:348–358

Van Hees J, Gybels J 1981 C nociceptor activity in human nerve during painful and non painful skin stimulation. Journal of Neurology, Neurosurgery and Psychiatry 44:600–607

Vicenzino B 1995 An investigation of the effects of spinal manual therapy on forequarter pressure and thermal pain thresholds and sympathetic nervous system activity in asymptomatic subjects: a preliminary report. In: Shacklock M O (ed) Moving in on pain. Butterworth-Heinemann, Australia, p 185–193

Vicenzino B, Collins D, Wright T 1994 Sudomotor changes induced by neural mobilization techniques in asymptomatic subjects. Journal of Manual and Manipulative Therapy 2(2):66–74

Vicenzino B, Collins D, Wright A 1996 The initial effects of a cervical spine manipulative physiotherapy treatment on the pain and dysfunction of lateral epicondylalgia. Pain 68:69–74

Vicenzino B, Collins D, Benson H, Wright A 1998 An investigation of the interrelationship between manipulative therapy-induced hypoalgesia and sympathoexcitation. Journal of Manipulative and Physiological Therapeutics 21(7):448–453

Vlaeyen J W S, Crombez G 1999 Fear of movement/(re)injury, avoidance and pain disability in chronic low back pain patients. Manual Therapy 4(4):187–195

Waddell G 1999 Diagnostic triage. In: Waddell G (ed) The back pain revolution. Churchill Livingstone, Edinburgh, ch 2 p 9

Waddell G, Main C J 1999 Beliefs about back pain. In: Waddell G (ed) The back pain revolution. Churchill Livingstone, Edinburgh, ch 12 p 187–202

Waddington P J 1999 Proprioceptive neuromuscular facilitation (PNF). In: Hollis M & Fletcher-Cook P (ed) Practical exercise therapy. Blackwell Scientific, Oxford, ch 19, p 202–205

Walker J M 1984 Deep transverse frictions in ligament healing. Journal of Orthopaedic and Sports Physical Therapy 6(2):89–94

Warren C G, Lehmann J F, Koblanski J N 1971 Elongation of rat tail tendon: effect of load and temperature. Archives of Physical Medicine and Rehabilitation 52:465–474

Watson T 2000 The role of electrotherapy in contemporary physiotherapy practice. Manual Therapy 5(3):132–141

Watson P, Kendall N 2000 Assessing psychological yellow flags. In: Gifford L (ed) Topical issues in pain 2, biopsychosocial assessment and management relationships and pain. CNS, Kestral, ch 3 p 111–129

Woo S L-Y, Gomez M A, Sites T J et al 1987 The biomechanical and morphological changes in the medial collateral ligament of the rabbit after immobilization and remobilization. Journal of Bone and Joint Surgery 69A(8):1200–1211

Wood L, Ferrell W R 1985 Fluid compartmentation and articular mechanoreceptor discharge in the cat knee joint. Quarterly Journal of Experimental Physiology 70:329–335

Woolf C J 1983 C-primary afferent mediated inhibitions in the dorsal horn of the decerebrate-spinal rat. Experimental Brain Research 51:283–290

Woolf C J, Wall P D 1982 Chronic peripheral nerve section diminishes the primary afferent A-fibre mediated inhibition of rat dorsal horn neurones. Brain Research 242:77–85

Wright A 1995 Hypoalgesia post-manipulative therapy: a review of a potential neurophysiological mechanism. Manual Therapy 1(1):11–16

Wright A, Vicenzino B 1995 Cervical mobilization techniques, sympathetic nervous system effects and their relationship to analgesia. In: Shacklock M O (ed) Moving in on pain. Butterworth-Heinemann, Australia, p 164–173

Wyke B D, Polacek P 1975 Articular neurology: the present position. Journal of Joint and Bone Surgery 57B(3):401

Yaksh T L, Elde R P 1981 Factors governing release of methionine enkephalin-like immunoreactivity from mesencephalon and spinal cord of the cat in vivo. Journal of Neurophysiology 46(5):1056–1075

Zusman M 1986 Spinal manipulative therapy: review of some proposed mechanisms, and a new hypothesis. Australian Journal of Physiotherapy 32(2):89–99

Zusman M 1994 What does manipulation do? The need for basic research. In: Boyling J D, Palastanga N (eds) Grieve's modern manual therapy, the vertebral column, 2nd edn. Churchill Livingstone, Edinburgh, ch 47 p 651–659

5

Function and dysfunction of muscle

In this text the word 'muscle' is used to denote both the muscle and its tendinous attachments.

The function of the neuromusculoskeletal system is to produce movement and this is dependent on optimal functioning of each component, that is, muscles, joints and nerves. This interrelationship is depicted in Figure 5.1, which was originally devised to describe the stability of the spine (Panjabi 1992) but is applicable to the function of the whole neuromusculoskeletal system. This interrelationship has been described in relation to the knee as 'a complex systematic sensory-motor synergy, which includes the ligaments, antagonistic muscle pair (flexors and extensors), bones, and sensory mechanoreceptors in the ligaments, joint capsule, and associated muscles' (Solomonow et al 1987). Once again, this description could be applied equally to the entire neuromusculoskeletal system. Therefore, while this chapter is concerned with the function of muscle it is important to stress that muscles do not function in isolation but in a highly interdependent way with joints and nerves. For a muscle to function normally there must be normal functioning of the relevant joints and nerves.

Some examples of how muscle, joint and nerve function together may help to highlight this close relationship. Anatomically, muscle often blends with ligaments to form one stability system (Strasmann et al 1990). For example, the supraspinous ligament and the superficial part of the interspinous ligament is actually the attachment of longissimus thoracis pars thoracis (Adams et al 2002). In the lumbar spine, multifidus blends with the zygapophyseal joint

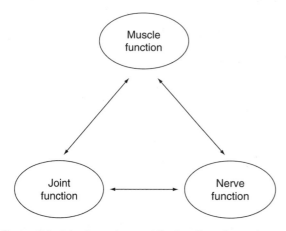

Figure 5.1 Interdependence of the function of muscle, joint and nerve for normal movement (after Panjabi 1992, with permission). Normal function of the neuromusculoskeletal system requires normal function of muscle, joint and nerve.

capsules (Yamashita et al 1996), in the shoulder, supraspinatus and teres minor blend with the glenohumeral joint capsule, and at the knee joint, biceps femoris fuses with the lateral collateral ligament (Williams et al 1995). These examples provide evidence that muscle is not an entirely separate tissue – it blends with the periarticular tissue of joint. As a consequence of this there will be a very close functional relationship between these tissues.

There are numerous examples of the close functional relationship between muscle, joint and nerve. When a muscle contracts and produces movement, the movement that occurs will depend on the shape of the articular surface, the ligaments of the joint, other local muscles, intrinsic and extrinsic forces opposing the movement, as well as the cortical control of movement. Thus, the effect of muscle contraction is dependent on joint and nerve function.

The level of activity of a muscle is dependent on the position of its associated joints. For example, in standing with the knee flexed 15 degrees, the quadriceps force required to support body weight is about 20% of maximum quadriceps strength; when the knee joint angle is increased to 30 degrees the quadriceps force is increased to about 50% (Perry et al 1975).

Muscles contribute to the stability of a joint by contributing to joint stiffness. In the cat wrist joint, muscle contributes 41% and tendon 10% to the joint stiffness (Johns & Wright 1962). In the human knee, contraction of the quadriceps and contraction of the hamstring muscles can substantially increase joint stiffness (Louie & Mote 1987, Zhang et al 1998), with increases of between 200 and 300% for quadriceps and between 100 and 250% for hamstrings (Louie & Mote 1987). Additionally, it has been estimated that co-contraction of the quadriceps and hamstring muscle groups can reduce knee joint laxity by about 70% (Louie & Mote 1987). Contraction of quadriceps and contraction of hamstring muscle groups can each reduce the strain on the anterior cruciate ligament (ACL) (Renstrom et al 1986). Quadriceps and hamstring contraction thus contributes to joint stiffness and therefore enhances joint stability. At the glenohumeral joint with the arm elevated (Fig. 5.2) it can readily be seen that the position and direction of the deltoid muscle produces a force that will compress the humerus against the glenoid cavity, and therefore stabilize the joint (Elftman 1966). It is clear from these studies that muscle contraction directly affects joint stiffness and thus joint stability.

Muscle also enhances joint stability during joint movement (Hortobagyi & DeVita 2000, Louie et al 1984, Louie & Mote 1987, Knatt et al

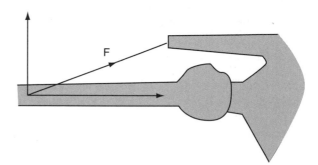

Figure 5.2 Contribution of deltoid muscle to stability of the glenohumeral joint. The force of contraction F can be resolved into two lines of force: vertically, away from the bone producing the rotation of the humerus, and along the shaft of the humerus to the glenohumeral joint, thus aiding stability. (After Elftman 1966, with permission.)

1995, McGill & Norman 1986, Panjabi et al 1989, Perry et al 1975, Phillips et al 1997, Pope et al 1979, Shoemaker & Markolf 1982, Solomonow et al 1986, Solomonow et al 1987, Walla et al 1985, Wilke et al 1995). For example, in the upper limb, isometric contraction of the elbow flexors or extensors at 45, 90 and 135 degrees elbow flexion is coupled with activity in the antagonistic triceps or biceps muscle, which varies with joint angle (Solomonow et al 1986). The pattern of activity of the antagonistic muscle suggests that it regulates the joint torque, thus enhancing elbow joint stability (Solomonow et al 1986). In the lumbar spine, during flexion and extension movements, muscles have been shown to affect segmental stability (Panjabi et al 1989, Wilke et al 1995). The posterior layer of thoracolumbar fascia is considered to act as an accessory ligament, helping to stabilize the lumbar spine during movement (Bogduk & MacIntosh 1984). It can be concluded that, during movement, muscle directly affects joint stability.

In all of the above examples, where muscle enhances joint stability, a normal functioning nervous system is a prerequisite. A number of studies have identified that muscle activity is directly affected by joint afferent activity. In the cat, for example, stimulation of the articular nerve in the glenohumeral joint produces a reflex activation of the biceps muscle (Knatt et al 1995). Similarly, the activity of the muscles overlying the medial ligament of the elbow (flexor carpi radialis and ulnaris, flexor digitorum profundus and superficialis, and pronator teres) is increased with stimulation of afferents in the ulnar collateral ligament; this is thought to be a protective reflex to avoid excessive ligamentous tension (Phillips et al 1997). In the lower limb, in the anaesthetized cat, reflex facilitation of gastrocnemius and inhibition of tibialis anterior is brought about by stimulation of mechanoreceptors in the posterior joint capsule; similarly, facilitation of tibialis anterior and inhibition of gastrocnemius occurs with stimulation of mechanoreceptors in the anterior joint capsule (Freeman & Wyke 1967). In the human lumbar spine, reflex contraction of multifidus muscle occurs with stimulation of mechanoreceptors in the supraspinous

ligament (Solomonow et al 1998). In the pig, this also occurs with stimulation of the mechanoreceptors in the facet joint capsule and intervertebral disc (Indahl et al 1995, 1997) and is thought to be a reflex response for enhancement of spinal stability (Indahl et al 1995, 1997, Solomonow et al 1998). Conversely, contraction of muscle around the cat knee joint has been shown to enhance joint mechanoreceptor activity (Ferrell 1985). It has been postulated that the small muscles, such as the intertransversarii and interspinales in the lumbar spine, are thought to be too weak to have a significant role in producing torque; they have been considered to have a sensory feedback role and have thus been regarded primarily as proprioceptive transducers (Bogduk 1997). Afferents in muscle, as well as in joint and skin, are considered to provide the brain with proprioceptive information necessary for movement (Gandevia et al 1983, McCloskey et al 1987, Macefield et al 1990). Collectively, this research clearly links the interdependent relationship of muscle, joint and nerve function during movement.

Summary

This section has sought to highlight the complex interrelationship of muscle with joint and nerve. It seems clear from the research findings that normal joint and nerve function are prerequisites for normal muscle function.

MUSCLE FUNCTION

This text is limited to the skeletal muscle, as opposed to smooth muscle (in the walls of organs, blood vessels and respiratory passages), and cardiac muscle (in the atria and ventricles of the heart).

The following aspects of joint function will be considered:

- anatomy, biomechanics and physiology of muscle
- nerve supply of muscle
- muscle contraction (strength), power, endurance and motor control and muscle length
- classification of muscle function.

Anatomy, biomechanics and physiology of muscle

Muscle constitutes approximately 40% of the total body weight (Panjabi & White 2001). Muscle is essentially a machine that converts chemical energy into mechanical work, and has been regarded as 'the most efficient and adaptable machine known to man' (Williams et al 1995). A muscle (that is, muscle and its tendons) can be divided grossly into contractile tissue and non-contractile tissue. The non-contractile tissue includes the connective tissue layers within muscle and the tendons.

Contractile tissue of muscle

The smallest unit of muscle is the myofibril, made up of thin actin and thick myosin filaments, giving a striated appearance under the light microscope (Fig. 5.3). The myosin filaments produce the dark A band, and the actin filaments produce the light I band. In addition, elastic titin filaments lie between the myosin filaments (Williams et al 1995). The titin filaments act like a spring, with increased tension when the sarcomere is lengthened, thus enabling it to return to its resting length when the tension is removed; this is also thought to keep the myosin in the centre of the sarcomere when there is an asymmetrical pull (Horowits et al 1989). The Z line demarcates the sarcomere, which is the basic contractile unit of muscle.

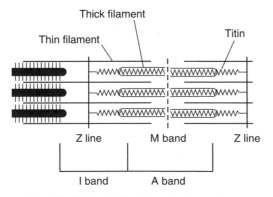

Figure 5.3 The basic contractile unit of muscle, the sarcomere, formed by the thin actin and thick myosin filaments (from Herzog 1999, with permission).

Individual muscle fibres (or cells) are covered in a membrane called the sarcolemma and by a connective tissue sheath called the endomysium (Fig. 5.4). The individual muscle fibres are collected into bundles (or fascicles) by a connective tissue sheath called the perimysium. Numbers of muscle bundles constitute the muscle and are surrounded by a connective tissue sheath called the epimysium and by an outer layer of fascia. These muscle fibres are known as extrafusal fibres, compared to intrafusal fibres, which lie within the muscle spindle (discussed later under nerve supply).

Non-contractile tissue of muscle

Connective tissue is found in layers within the muscle and in the tendons. Connective tissue makes up 30% of muscle mass (Alter 1996) and is vital for normal muscle function. The connective tissue of muscle consists of collagen fibres, and some elastin fibres, held together in a ground substance. The elastin fibres enable muscle to regain its shape, following shortening with a concentric muscle contraction, or after being in a lengthened position.

Connective tissue forms a sheath around each muscle fibre (endomysium), around bundles of muscle fibres (perimysium) and around the whole muscle (epimysium), as shown in Fig. 5.4. The connective tissue, along with the nerves and blood vessels, forms the non-contractile element of the muscle belly. The outer layer of connective tissue enables identification of particular muscles, for example, semitendinosus muscle in the thigh, and allows sliding of muscle on adjacent tissues, for example, movement of semitendinosus on the biceps femoris and the sciatic nerve. The perimysium around a bundle of muscle fibres provides a channel for blood vessels and nerves. The endomysium, perimysium and epimysium join to form the tendon or aponeurosis that attaches the muscle to bone.

The function of connective tissue in muscle can be summarized as follows:

1. It is the architectural structure of the muscle.

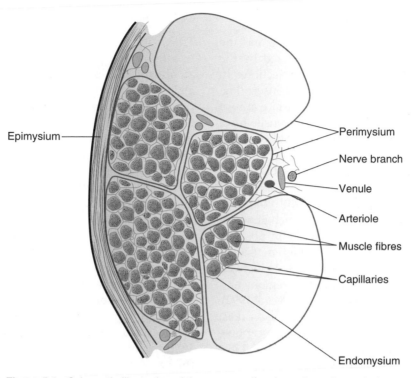

Figure 5.4 Schematic illustration of the cross-sectional structure of muscle (from McComas 1996, with permission).

2. It transmits force and movement from the muscle fibres to the tendinous attachments.

3. It resists passive stretching of a muscle.

4. It enhances muscle strength by controlling muscle pressure and muscle volume. Cutting the epimysium of a dog hind limb results in a 15% reduction in muscle force and a 50% reduction in intracompartmental pressure (Garfin et al 1981). In the lumbar spine, the thoracolumbar fascia has been estimated to enhance the strength of the back muscles by 30% (Hukins et al 1990).

5. It provides a channel for blood vessels and nerves.

Connective tissue is also the major constituent of fascia, which is divided into superficial and deep. Superficial fascia lies just below the skin and allows skin movement; it is thick on the plantar aspect of the hands and thin on the dorsum of the hands and feet. Deep fascia acts as retinacula, intermuscular septa, intermuscular aponeurosis and attachment for muscle. In the thoracic and abdominal cavities deep fascia covers and supports the viscera, for example, the pleura, pericardium and peritoneum. The flexor and extensor retinacula of the wrist and foot are deep fascia arranged as a transverse thickening to retain tendons deep to it. The intermuscular septa pass between groups of muscles and attach to bone. Muscles can take attachment from the intermuscular septa, which may then be better named intermuscular aponeurosis, for example the rectal sheath. The deep fascia can be a point of attachment for muscle to bone and from muscle to muscle. For example, the tensor fascia lata and gluteus maximus attach to the iliotibial tract (fascia), which then passes down the leg and attaches to the tibia. Deep fascia in the lower leg connects the peroneus longus to the biceps femoris, and in the upper arm, pectoralis minor to the short head of biceps. Fascial connections around the pelvis have been recognized as important by Vleeming et al (1997) and have been explored by Myers (2001) who has coined the phrase 'myofascial meridians'.

Musculotendinous (or myotendinous) junction

This is the junction between the muscle and the tendon. The contact area is characterized by the muscle cells forming finger-like projections in which the collagen fibres of the tendon insert (Fig. 5.5). This arrangement increases the surface area of the contact region and so reduces the tensile force applied to the tissue (Eisenberg & Milton 1984, Kvist et al 1991). Interestingly, this is reflected in difference in surface area between type I and type II muscle fibres. The area is greater for type II fibres, which are involved in powerful voluntary movements, than for type I fibres, which generate lower forces and are involved largely in postural control (Kvist et al 1991). There is a high density of glycosaminoglycans, which are thought to increase the adhesive forces between the two regions and thus help to strengthen the region (Jozsa et al 1992). Despite this arrangement, the region is the weakest part of the tendon–muscle unit and is susceptible to strain injuries (Garrett 1990, Garrett et al 1989, Nikolaou et al 1987, Tidball 1991).

Osteotendinous junctions

This is where tendon attaches to bone. Tendons usually attach directly to bone, that is, there is an abrupt well-defined area of attachment with a clear demarcation of tendon and bone; examples include supraspinatus, where it attaches to the superior facet on the greater tuberosity of the humerus, and the medial collateral ligament to the medial condyle of the femur (Woo et al 1988). Tendons with direct attachments have a superficial layer which blends with periosteum, and a larger deep layer which inserts directly into bone via a thin layer of fibrocartilage (Cooper & Misol 1970, Woo et al 1988). Sometimes tendons attach rather more indirectly, such that there is a more gradual and less distinct area of attachment (Woo et al 1988). The superficial layer in this case provides the predominant attachment, blending with the periosteum and bone via Sharpey's fibres (Woo et al 1988), while the deep layer attaches directly to the bone.

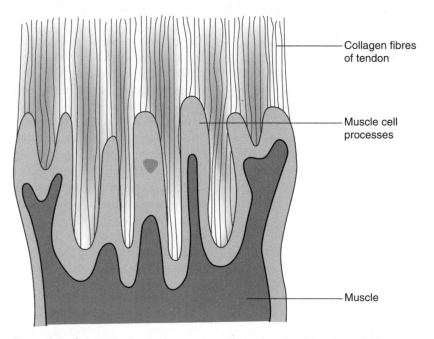

Figure 5.5 Schematic figure of musculotendinous junction (after Jozsa & Kannus 1997, with permission).

Collagen fibres of tendon

Muscle cell processes

Muscle

Tendons

Tendons are designed to transmit high tensile force from muscle to bone, and they allow muscles to lengthen and bend around bone. They are therefore flexible, relatively inextensible and able to withstand large tensile forces (Elliott 1965, Jozsa & Kannus 1997). Tendons are made up of approximately 70% of longitudinally arranged collagen tissue, with some elastin tissue, embedded in a proteoglycan–water matrix (Hess et al 1989). They have a sparse blood supply and so are white in appearance. Between the collagen fibres (the basic unit of tendon) there is loose connective tissue; this provides a channel for vessels and nerve.

Tendons sometimes contain a sesamoid bone (named because of the resemblance to sesame seed) which the ancient Hebrews believed was the resting place of the soul (McBryde & Anderson 1988). Their function is rather more mundane: they increase the mechanical advantage of the muscle and decrease friction between adjacent tissues. They are covered with hyaline cartilage. Examples include the pisiform bone within flexor carpi ulnaris tendon, the patella within the quadriceps tendon and the sesamoid bone within the flexor hallucis brevis tendon. The existence and shape of sesamoid bones varies between individuals (McBryde & Anderson 1988).

During a muscle contraction, tendon moves on adjacent tissue, the frictional resistance to this movement is minimized by bursae and sheaths which can be classified as fibrous, synovial and paratenon sheaths.

1. A bursa may lie adjacent to tendon to aid gliding movement of the tendon on adjacent tissue; for example, the infrapatellar bursae facilitates gliding movements of the patella.

2. A fibrous sheath may surround a tendon, as in the tendons around the ankle. Bony grooves and notches contain a layer of fibrocartilage, and superficially the tendon is held in place by retinaculum.

3. A synovial sheath may surround a tendon where ease of movement with adjacent tissue is of paramount importance, as in the tendons of the hand and feet. Synovial sheaths are composed of an outer fibrotic sheath and an inner synovial sheath. A thin film of synovial fluid, rich in hyaluronic acid, fills the space between the sheaths and acts as a lubricant reducing frictional resistance (Jozsa & Kannus 1997) and enhancing tendon nutrition (Lundborg 1976, Matthews 1976).

4. A paratenon sheath (or peritendinous sheet) may surround a tendon – for example, the tendocalcaneus tendon. The paratenon is made up of collagen fibres, elastic fibrils and synovial cells, and acts as an elastic sleeve, facilitating movement between the tendon and its surrounding tissues (Hess et al 1989, Jozsa & Kannus 1997). The paratenon and epitenon are sometimes referred to as the peritendon.

The tendon itself is covered in a fine connective tissue sheath called the epitenon (Fig. 5.6) which lies underneath the synovial or paratenon. Most of the fibres that make up the epitenon are arranged at about 60 degrees to the direction of the tendon fibres, but when the tendon is lengthened this angle reduces to about 30 degrees, so that the fibres lie more in line with the direction of stress; this is thought to help protect against overstrain (Jozsa & Kannus 1997).

Underneath the epitenon is the endotenon, which covers tertiary, secondary and primary bundles of collagen fibres together (Elliott 1965, Jozsa & Kannus 1997). These layers of connective tissue enable the fibres to glide on each other, and provide a channel for blood vessels, lymphatics and nerves into the deep portions of the tendon (Elliott 1965, Hess et al 1989). Collagen fibres are made up of collagen fibrils which are orientated longitudinally, transversely and horizontally to withstand forces from a variety of directions during movement (Jozsa & Kannus 1997). The longitudinal collagen fibrils have a wavy or crimped appearance (Jozsa & Kannus 1997) and cross each other to form spirals and plaits (Fig. 5.7) (Elliott 1965, Jozsa et al 1991); this is thought to increase the tensile strength of tendon (Jozsa & Kannus 1997). The crimped appearance of the collagen fibril varies within and between collagen fibres (Nicholls et al 1983, Rowe 1985).

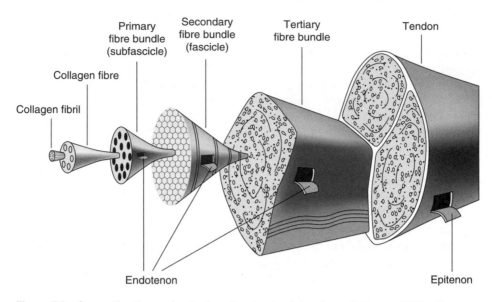

Figure 5.6 Connective tissue sheaths investing tendon (after Jozsa & Kannus 1997, with permission).

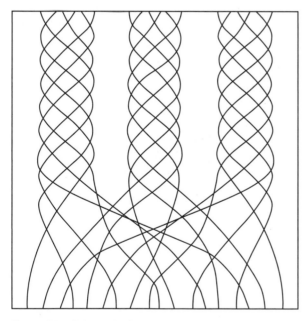

Figure 5.7 Schematic drawing of the interweaving of tendon bundles near its insertion (from Elliott 1965, with permission).

Like other tissues in the body, form and function go hand in hand. Tendon tissue is plastic (Brown & Hardman 1987) and so will alter its composition and construction according to the physical demands placed upon it (Elliott 1965). For example, with exercise, there is an increase in tendon thickness (Inglemark 1948); when a muscle is immobilized in a lengthened position there is an increase in tendon thickness (Elliott 1965), and exercise causes an increase in strength of the tendon at its insertion site (Woo et al 1988). The stimulus for tendon growth is the tension that is applied and does not appear to be related to the size or strength of the muscle (Elliott 1965).

Tendons have viscoelastic properties; the load–displacement curve for a tendon is shown in Figure 5.8. The toe region is concave and is considered to reflect the straightening of the wavy collagen fibres shown in Figure 5.9 (Hirsch 1974, Rigby et al 1959). Little force is required to lengthen the tendon in this region. This region is considered to be responsible for the ability of tendon to absorb shock (Wood TO et al 1988). With continued lengthening, the wave pattern straightens and the tendon behaves like a stiff spring; this occurs with about 3% elongation (Herzog & Gal 1999). As the force increases, there is an increase in the stiffness of the tendon, producing the linear part of the curve; this occurs at about 4% elongation (Wainwright et al 1982). Both toe and linear regions are temporary and,

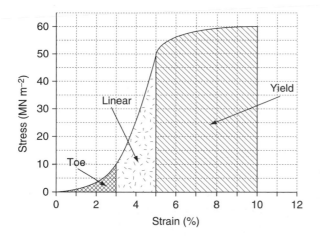

Figure 5.8 Load–displacement (stress–strain) curve for tendon (from Herzog & Gal 1999, with permission).

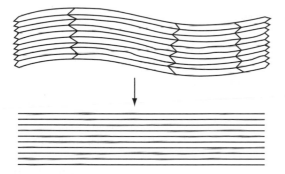

Figure 5.9 The wavy pattern of a tendon in a relaxed state straightens out when it is stretched (from Jozsa & Kannus 1997, with permission).

on removal of the force, the tendon will return to its resting length. During normal everyday activities, tensile forces on tendon are thought to lie within the toe and linear region and are thought to be less than 4% strain (Fung 1993). If the force continues to elongate beyond this there is a permanent deformation in the yield region of the curve, up to a maximum of approximately 8–15% elongation, where failure occurs (Fung 1993, Rigby et al 1959). During the yield region, a relatively small increase in force will produce a relatively large increase in displacement. Temperatures of up to 37° C make no difference to the force–displacement curve of tendon; however, by 40° C (104–105° F) displacement of 3–4% will result in breakage of the tendon (Rigby et al 1959).

The stiffness of tendon is not the same throughout its length. Tendon is stiffest in the middle of its length and least stiff at its insertion. So when a tendon is lengthened there is greatest displacement at the insertion region (Woo et al 1988).

Blood supply of tendon. Tendons receive their blood supply at the osteotendinous junction, from vessels within bone and periosteum. At the musculotendinous junction it receives blood from vessels within muscle and from the surrounding vessels within the paratenon, mesotenon and synovial sheath (Jozsa & Kannus 1997). The blood supply at the osteotendinous junction is fairly sparse and is limited to where the tendon attaches to bone. Blood vessels are present only in the distal third of the tendon (Jozsa & Kannus 1997). At the musculotendinous junction the blood vessels from within the muscle pass into, and supply, the proximal third of the tendon (Peacock 1959). There is therefore a fairly marked transition between the highly vascular muscle tissue and the relatively poor vascular supply of tendon. The blood vessels around the outer covering of tendons perforate both the epitenon and endotenon, and so supply the superficial and deep portions of the tendon.

Some tendons have an area of poor vascularity; for example, the tendocalcaneus tendon has an avascular area 2–6 cm proximal to its distal attachment (Carr & Norris 1989), the extensor pollicis longus tendon has an area of poor vascularity where it lies underneath the dorsal carpal ligament of the wrist (Jozsa & Kannus 1997), the posterior tibial tendon has an area of poor vascularity posterior and distal to the medial malleolus (Frey et al 1990), and the supraspinatus tendon has poor vascularity where it inserts onto the humerus (Chansky & Iannotti 1991, Lohr & Uhthoff 1990). Interestingly, the area of poor vascularity in supraspinatus tendon does not increase with age (Lohr & Uhthoff 1990).

Biomechanics of the muscle–tendon unit

It is useful to consider the biomechanical behaviour of the muscle–tendon unit as a single unit. The strength of the muscle–tendon unit with respect to tensile loading can be depicted on a force–displacement curve as shown in Figure 5.10; this curve was obtained from the whole tibialis anterior muscle–tendon unit of a rabbit (Taylor et al 1990). The load or force is plotted against the stretch or deformation. The slope of the curve is the modulus of elasticity, measured in Pa or N/m^2, and is a measure of the 'stiffness' of the muscle–tendon unit (Panjabi & White 2001). It can be seen in Fig. 5.10 that only a little force is initially required to deform the muscle–tendon unit, a region referred to as the 'toe' region (Threlkeld 1992) or 'neutral zone' (Panjabi & White 2001). Stiffness then increases, so that greater force is required to deform the muscle–tendon unit; this region is referred to as the elastic zone (Panjabi & White 2001). Forces within the elastic zone will result in no permanent change in length; as soon as the force is released the muscle–tendon unit will return to its pre-load shape and size (Panjabi & White 2001). The neutral zone and elastic zone fall within normal physiological range of forces and deformation on the muscle–tendon unit during everyday activities (Nordin & Frankel 1989). Heating muscle beyond 43° C causes a 170% increase, and cooling muscle to +10° C causes a 30% decrease in its viscoelastic properties (Talishev & Fedina 1976). Thus, heating muscle will cause it to be less stiff and cooling muscle will cause it to be more stiff.

The strength of a muscle or tendon is measured by stress (force per unit area, measured in Pa or N/m^2), and strain (percentage change in length, from the resting length). The stress–strain properties of muscle and tendon are compared to bone, cartilage, ligament and nerve in Table 5.1. The ability of muscle to resist lengthening reduces with age (Panjabi & White 2001). Failure occurs at 58% elongation in the 7th decade compared to 65% elongation in a teenager (Panjabi & White 2001).

A muscle–tendon unit is viscoelastic, that is, it has time-dependent mechanical properties. These properties affect the behaviour of the muscle–tendon unit to movement and forces and are therefore important principles for clinicians. They can be summarized as:

- elastic nature
- viscous nature
- creep phenomena
- stress relaxation
- loading rate
- hysteresis.

The muscle–tendon unit has elastic properties; it will stretch and return to its original shape like an elastic band.

The muscle–tendon unit has viscous properties; that is, it will gradually elongate over a period of time when a constant force is applied – a phenomenon known as creep.

The muscle–tendon unit undergoes load (or stress) relaxation. In Figure 5.11, the muscle–tendon unit of extensor digitorum longus was lengthened repeatedly 10 times to 78 N. The

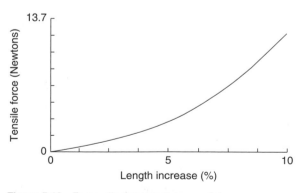

Figure 5.10 Force–displacement curve of the muscle–tendon unit (after Taylor et al 1990, with permission).

Table 5.1 Tensile properties of muscle and tendon compared to bone, cartilage, ligament and nerve (Panjabi & White 2001)

Tissue	Stress at failure (MPa)	Strain at failure (%)
Muscle (passive)	0.17	60
Tendon	55	9–10
Cortical bone	100–200	1–3
Cancellous bone	10	5–7
Cartilage	10–15	80–120
Ligament	10–40	30–45
Nerve roots	15	19

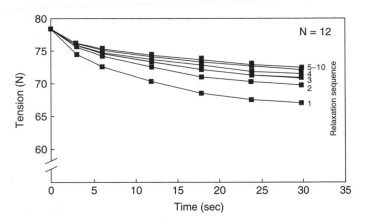

Figure 5.11   Load relaxation of extensor digitorum longus muscle–tendon unit of the New Zealand white rabbit (from Taylor et al 1990, with permission). A gradual decrease in tension occurs with the first two repetitions with a force of 78 N.

reduction in tension is indicated by the gradient of the curve. There is a significant ($P < 0.05$) reduction in tension between the first two stretches (Taylor et al 1990).

The muscle–tendon unit will elongate on loading and is dependent on the rate of loading. When the muscle–tendon unit of tibialis anterior is loaded quickly it will be stiffer and deform less than when it is loaded more slowly (Fig. 5.12). This is relevant when applying therapeutic force,

as a slower rate will result in less resistance and more movement. An additional effect is that the failure point of the muscle–tendon unit will be higher with a higher loading rate; in other words, it will be stronger and less likely to rupture when the force is applied at a faster rate.

The muscle–tendon unit demonstrates the phenomenon of hysteresis, which is the energy loss during loading and unloading (Fig. 5.13). These data are taken from the tibialis anterior

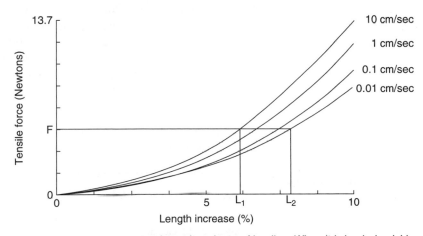

Figure 5.12   The muscle–tendon unit and rate of loading. When it is loaded quickly it will be stiffer and will sustain a higher force before breaking than when it is loaded more slowly. For example, a given force, if applied at 10 cm/sec, will cause a displacement L_1, but if applied more slowly, at 0.01 cm/sec, will cause a greater displacement to L_2. These data are from the tibialis anterior muscle–tendon unit from New Zealand white rabbits. (After Taylor et al 1990, with permission.)

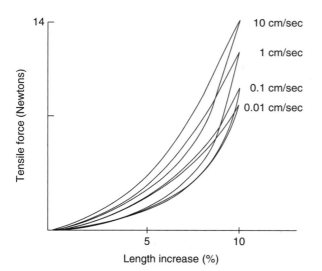

Figure 5.13 The muscle–tendon unit demonstrates the phenomenon of hysteresis (from Taylor et al 1990, with permission). The graph was produced from the tibialis anterior muscle–tendon unit of New Zealand white rabbits. The loading rate used was 0.01, 0.1, 1 and 10 cm/sec.

muscle–tendon unit of rabbits (Taylor et al 1990). The unloading curve lies below the loading curve and reflects a greater energy expenditure on loading compared with the energy regained during unloading. This results in a loss of energy known as hysteresis loss (Panjabi & White 2001). It can also be seen that hysteresis produces an elongation of the muscle–tendon unit.

The muscle belly is less stiff than the tendon, so when a muscle is passively lengthened most of the length change occurs in the muscle belly and the tendon is minimally affected (Jami 1992). Muscle length refers to the length of the muscle

through the available range of joint movement. During normal daily activities muscle lengthens and shortens to allow movement. Muscle length reduces with age (Gajdosik et al 1996).

Types of muscle fibre

Muscle fibres can be classified in various ways (Table 5.2). Initially, muscle fibres were described according to the speed of shortening and were identified by staining for myoglobin concentration (myoglobin binds oxygen). Muscles were divided into (i) slow muscles (type I), which stained red owing to a high concentration of myoglobin enabling aerobic energy metabolism, and (ii) fast muscles (type II), which stained white owing to a low concentration of myoglobin enabling anaerobic energy metabolism (Pette & Staron 1990). Fast-twitch fibres (type II) contract more quickly, generate higher forces but fatigue more quickly than slow-twitch (type II) fibres (Table 5.3).

An alternative classification system identified type I and type II myofibrillar actomyosin adenosine triphosphate (mATP) which related to different contractile properties (Pette & Staron 1990). When this classification was combined with the myoglobin classification a metabolic enzyme-based classification was developed (Table 5.2). This classification describes three types of muscle fibre: slow-twitch oxidative (SO), fast-twitch oxidative (FOG) and fast-twitch glycolytic (FG) (McComas 1996, Pette & Staron 1990). Fibres that fall between slow-twitch (type I) and fast-twitch (type IIb) are termed interme-

Table 5.2 Classification of muscle fibre types (Scott et al 2001, Staron 1997). The question mark beside FOG and FG indicates that muscle fibre types IIA and IIB do not always rely on aerobic/oxidative and anaerobic/glycolytic metabolism (McComas 1996)

Myosin ATPase	Myosin ATPase hydrolysis rate	Myosin heavy chain (MHC)	Biochemical identification of metabolic enzymes
I	I	MHC1	Slow-twitch oxidative (SO)
	IC	MHC1 and MHCIIa	
	IIC	MHC1 and MHCIIa	
	IIAC	MHC1 and MHCIIa	
IIA	IIA	MHCIIa	? Fast-twitch oxidative (FOG)
	IIAB	MHCIIa and MHCIIb	
IIB	IIB	MHCIIb	? Fast-twitch glycolytic (FG)

diate (type IIa) (Pette et al 1999). The characteristics of these types of muscle fibre are summarized in Table 5.3.

While it is convenient to classify muscle fibres into three types, the reality is more of a continuum between fast-twitch and slow-twitch muscles (Pette et al 1999, Pette & Staron 1990). A third type of fast fibre has since been identified and is known as IID or IIX (Pette et al 1999).

More recent advances in staining techniques have led to the identification of seven types of muscle fibre: I, IC, IIC, IIAC, IIA, IIAB and IIB. The types of muscle fibre can also be classified according to the protein composition of myosin (Staron 1997). Myosin consists of two myosin heavy chains and four myosin light chains (Pette & Staron 1990).

It is worth remembering that these classification systems relate to individual muscle fibres and not to whole muscle. While a few muscles do have a high percentage of type I fibres (80% in adductor pollicis, 86–89% in soleus, 73% in tibialis anterior) or type II fibres (85% in orbicularis oculi, 71% lateral head of rectus femoris), the vast majority of whole muscle contains a range of types of muscle fibre with a large variation between individuals (Johnson et al 1973). For this reason the classification of individual muscle fibres cannot be applied to whole muscle; that is, generally speaking, whole muscles cannot be classified as fast twitch or slow twitch.

For any one motor unit, the characteristic of the muscle fibre type is mirrored by the motor nerve supply (Box 5.1). All muscle fibres that are innervated by the same motor neurone are of the same type; that is, the conduction rate of a motor neurone innervating fast-twitch fibres is faster than that for slow-twitch fibres (Buller et al 1960). The motor neurone determines the characteristic of a muscle fibre and is described as a phasic or tonic motor neurone. In animals, large, phasic high-threshold motor neurones discharge at the high frequency of 30–60/sec compared to small, tonic low-threshold motor neurones with a lower frequency of 10–20/sec (Granit et al 1957). The nerve is so influential on muscle fibre type that if the motor neurones to fast- and slow-twitch fibres are experimentally switched, the muscle fibre types will also switch characteristics (Buller et al 1960, Lomo et al 1980).

The size of the motor unit varies between muscles and within a muscle. There is a tendency for smaller motor units to be composed of slow-twitch fibres and larger motor units to be composed of fast-twitch fibres (Wuerker et al 1965). The motor neurone of a slow-twitch motor unit

---

Box 5.1 Characteristics of motor neurone and muscle fibre type (Newham & Ainscough-Potts 2001)

Nerve:	*Nerve:*
Large motor neurone	Small motor neurone
Phasic	Tonic
High threshold	Low threshold
High frequency	Low frequency
Muscle fibres:	*Muscle fibres:*
Fast twitch	Slow twitch
Type IIa – FOG	Type I – SO
Type IIb – FG	
Large motor unit supplies 300–800 muscle fibres	Small motor unit supplies 12–180 muscle fibres

---

Table 5.3 Characteristics of skeletal muscle and motor neurones (Newham & Ainscough-Potts 2001)

Characteristic	Type I	Type IIa	Type IIb
Muscle fibre type	Slow oxidative (SO)	Fast oxidative glycolytic (FOG)	Fast glycolytic (FG)
Motor unit type	Slow	Fast fatigue resistant	Fast fatigable
Motor unit size	Small	Medium	Large
Conduction rate of motor neurone	Slow	Fast	Fast
Twitch tension	Low	Moderate	High
Speed of contraction	Slow	Fast	Fast
Resistance to fatigue	High	High	Low
Mitochondrial enzyme activity	High	Medium	Low
Myoglobin content	High	Medium	Low
Capillary density	High	Medium	Low

innervates 12–180 muscle fibres compared to 300–800 muscle fibres of a fast twitch motor unit. The fewer number of slow-twitch muscle fibres supplied by a motor neurone enables greater control of muscular contraction. For example, the motor neurone supplies only approximately 12 muscle fibres in the eye (Bors 1926), allowing for the fine control needed. The greater number of fast-twitch muscle fibres supplied by a motor neurone will cause a greater speed and force of contraction of fast-twitch motor units.

The fact that any one muscle contains both small and large motor units providing fine control of muscle contraction, as well as great speed and force of contraction, attests to the multiplicity of muscle functions.

Nerve supply of muscles

Sensory nerve endings in the muscle–tendon units include muscle spindles, golgi tendon organs and free nerve endings. Large-diameter myelinated group Ia and II fibres supply the muscle spindles, slightly smaller myelinated IIb fibres supply golgi tendon organs, and fine myelinated A delta (or group III fibres) and unmyelinated C (or group IV) fibres supply the free nerve endings.

Muscle spindles

Muscle spindles are proprioceptors acting as stretch receptors controlling the length (or tension) and rate of change in length of muscle. They are sensitive to static and dynamic length changes and are affected by the velocity, acceleration or deceleration of the length change.

Muscle spindles lie within the muscle belly, parallel to extrafusal fibres, and near the musculotendinous junction (Boyd 1976). The muscle spindle consists of intrafusal fibres to distinguish it from the rest of muscle which, in turn, consists of a non-contractile central portion within a capsule with contractile ends. The muscle spindle typically consists of one nuclear bag 1 and one nuclear bag 2 (Fig. 5.14), distinguished by differences in ATP concentration, and about four or more nuclear chain fibres (Hunt 1990). The nuclear bag fibres extend beyond the fibrous capsule of the muscle spindle while the nuclear

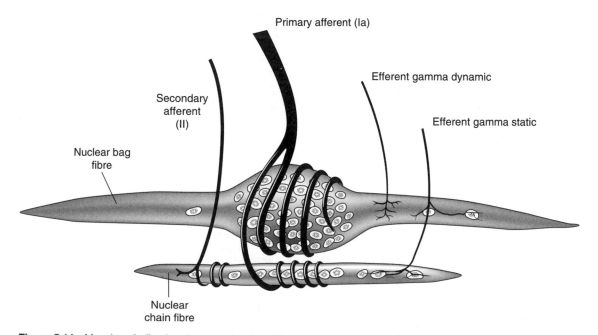

Figure 5.14 Muscle spindle showing a nuclear bag fibre and a nuclear chain fibre. Group 1a and II afferent fibres supply the muscle spindle. (After Shumway-Cook & Woollacott 1995, with permission.)

chain fibres are contained within the capsule. The nuclear bag fibres are more elastic and less stiff than the nuclear chain fibres.

The group Ia primary afferents terminate in annulospiral endings on all of the intrafusal fibres (nuclear bag and nuclear chain) in the spindle (Hunt 1990). The group Ia afferents have a low threshold to stretch, and they respond to both static and dynamic stretches (Shumway-Cook & Woollacott 1995). Even a small change in length will trigger a steep rise in the discharge rate (Hasan & Houk 1975). The group II secondary afferents terminate in 'flower spray' endings on both the nuclear chain fibre and nuclear bag 2 fibres (Hunt 1990). Group II fibres have a higher threshold, responding only to changes in muscle length, and they therefore act as position detectors with little to no dynamic response (Hunt 1990, Shumway-Cook & Woollacott 1995).

The behaviour of muscle spindle to stretch is often identified by stretching a muscle at a constant velocity, then holding it at a new increased length and then releasing the muscle, a procedure known as the ramp-and-hold stretch. When a muscle is stretched at a constant velocity, the primary endings initially have a burst of activity (Hunt 1990). The rate of activity depends on the velocity of the stretch; increased velocity results in an increased rate of activity (Hunt 1990). If the lengthened muscle is then maintained at its new length, there is a reduction in the rate of discharge. The sensitivity of static length is related to muscle length; there is greater sensitivity at greater lengths, although the discharge rate is still relatively small. While the lengthened muscle is maintained at its new length the nuclear bag fibres within the muscle spindle exhibit creep, that is, they lengthen (Boyd 1976). The discharge rate from the secondary group II fibres increases with a maintained position, and so appear to act as position detectors (Hunt 1990). On release from a lengthened position, the discharge rate from the primary endings reduces, and may stop, and then resume at the rate associated with the new length. Because the intrafusal fibres lie parallel to the extrafusal fibres, the discharge from the sensory fibres in the muscle spindle diminishes or ceases when the muscle contracts and increases when the muscle is lengthened (Hunt 1990). In addition to group Ia and II afferent nerve supply, muscle spindles in the cat have been found to receive a sympathetic innervation (Barker & Saito 1981); however, the effect of this is unclear (Hunt 1990).

The nuclear bag and nuclear chain fibres have a motor nerve supply via the gamma motor neurone (or fusimotor) fibres. Nuclear bag 1, sensitive to dynamic lengthening, is supplied by dynamic-gamma fibres, whereas nuclear bag 2 and nuclear chain fibres, sensitive to static length, are supplied by static-gamma fibres (Hunt 1990, Shumway-Cook & Woollacott 1995). Whenever the alpha motor neurone causes contraction of the extrafusal fibres there is, at the same time, gamma motor neurone activity (static- and dynamic-gamma activity) causing contraction of the intrafusal fibres. The contraction of the intrafusal fibres causes increased tension of the nuclear bag and nuclear chain fibres and thus maintains the sensitivity of the muscle spindle. If the gamma motor neurone activity did not occur then muscle contraction would shorten the intrafusal fibres and switch off sensory information from the muscle spindle. This enables continuous information of the length of muscle to be relayed to the sensory cortex of the brain. The gamma efferent system is under central nervous system control by the cerebellum, basal ganglia and cerebral cortex.

Stretch of the muscle spindle causes excitation of the alpha motor neurones leading to contraction of the extrafusal muscle fibres in which the spindle is situated, and inhibition of the antagonistic muscles. This phenomenon is known as the spindle stretch reflex (Fig. 5.15). This phenomenon is used clinically with the reflex hammer to apply a brisk tap to a tendon to produce a reflex contraction of the muscle; for example, a tap to the quadriceps tendon causes a contraction of the quadriceps muscle. Muscle spindles protect and limit the muscle from excessive lengthening by an external force. Clearly, this is a useful protective mechanism to regulate movement and maintain posture (Hunt 1990). Where a muscle becomes shortened, treatment may be directed to lengthen it; slow movements to lengthen a muscle would

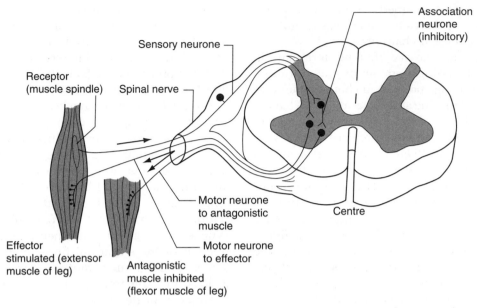

Figure 5.15 Spindle stretch reflex. Excitation of the muscle spindle causes a reflex contraction of the muscle in which the spindle lies and inhibition of the antagonistic muscle (from Crow & Haas 2001, with permission).

seem more effective to minimize this protective response.

The density of muscle spindles varies between different muscles. The suboccipital muscles and the muscles of the hand contain a rich density of muscle spindles whereas the large muscles of the arm and leg contain much fewer. The suboccipital muscles, such as the superior oblique and rectus capitus posterior major, have 43 and 30 spindles per gram respectively, the small muscles of the hand such as the lumbricals and opponens pollicis have 16 and 17 spindles per gram respectively, whereas pectoralis major, triceps brachii and latissimus dorsi have only about 1.4 spindles per gram (McComas 1996). The difference in density is probably related to the need for rapid and accurate movements (McComas 1996).

Summary of the muscle spindle

Each muscle spindle lying within a muscle belly and the musculotendinous junction is a stretch receptor. A statically maintained muscle length will cause stimulation of group 1a and particularly group II afferents. An increase in muscle length will cause stimulation of group Ia afferents with a reflex contraction of the extrafusal fibres of that muscle and inhibition of the antagonist muscle.

Golgi tendon organs

Golgi tendon organs lie in the musculotendinous or musculo-aponeurotic junction (Barker 1974); they are not found, as their name implies, in the tendon (Jami 1992). They are encapsulated corpuscles containing collagen fibres, lying in series with 15 to 20 muscle fibres (Houk & Henneman 1967, Shumway-Cook & Woollacott 1995) (Fig. 5.16). Golgi tendon organs are stimulated only by the tension in these muscle fibres in series (Houk & Henneman 1967).

Golgi tendon organs are proprioceptors, particularly sensitive to changes in muscle tension and to the rate of change of this tension produced by active muscle contraction (Houk & Henneman 1967). Golgi tendon organs can be stimulated by passive lengthening of the muscle–tendon unit; however, the threshold for discharge is very high and rarely persists with a maintained muscle

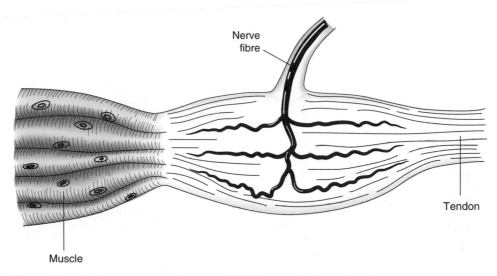

Figure 5.16 Golgi tendon organ in series with 15–20 muscle fibres (from Shumway-Cook & Woollacott 1995, with permission).

stretch (Houk et al 1971, Jami 1992). Each tendon organ is innervated by a large fast-conducting Ib afferent fibre. The continuous steady state of firing from the golgi tendon organ is proportional to the muscle tension (Crow & Haas 2001). When the muscle fibres contract there is a lengthening of the musculotendinous junction with approximation of the collagen fibres within the golgi tendon organ; this compresses the nerve terminals and causes firing of the Ib afferent fibre.

Stimulation of golgi tendon organs leads to inhibition of the muscle in which it is situated (inhibition of both alpha and gamma motor neurones), a mechanism known as autogenic inhibition, and excitation of the antagonist muscles (Fig. 5.17). So, for example, when lifting a weight, such that the muscle contraction and the weight cause excessive force that may damage musculotendinous junction, the golgi tendon organs will be stimulated, producing inhibition of the agonist muscles and stimulation of the antagonist. This is a protective mechanism to avoid injury to the musculotendinous junction. However, this mechanism is not seen during competitive sport – for example, wrist wrestling can result in ruptured muscles and tendons. In this case the highly motivated athlete disinhibits the process (Brooks & Fahey 1987).

Summary of the golgi tendon organ

Golgi tendon organs lie in the musculotendinous junction and help to protect this region from excessive tension brought about by muscle contraction.

Free nerve endings

Free nerve endings have been investigated in the gastrocnemius and soleus muscle of the cat and rat, and it is thought that similar findings are to be found in humans (Reinert & Mense 1992, Stacey 1969). Free nerve endings lie throughout the muscle, in the connective tissue, between intrafusal and extrafusal fibres, in arterioles and venules, in the capsule of muscle spindles and tendon organs, in tendon tissue at the musculotendinous junction and in fat cells (Reinert & Mense 1992, Stacey 1969). This is summarized in Box 5.2. Free nerve endings are supplied by myelinated A delta (group III) and unmyelinated C (group IV) fibres.

Type III afferents act as low-threshold mechanical pressure receptors, contraction-sensitive receptors and nociceptors (Mense & Meyer 1985). Most type IV afferents are mainly nociceptors (to both noxious mechanical and chemical stimulation), with a smaller proportion being low-threshold

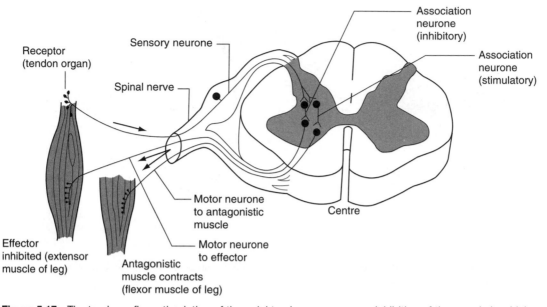

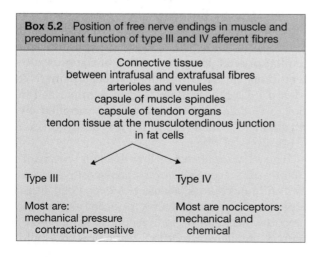

Figure 5.17 The tendon reflex: stimulation of the golgi tendon organ causes inhibition of the muscle in which it lies and excitation of the antagonistic muscle (from Crow & Haas 2001, with permission).

mechanical pressure receptors, contraction-sensitive receptors and thermo-receptors (Kniffki 1978, Mense & Meyer 1985).

Mechanoreceptors. Mechanoreceptors respond to pressure, active muscle contraction and muscle lengthening. The majority of group III fibres respond to local pressure stimulation (Iggo 1961, Kaufman et al 1984a, Paintal 1960), while very few of the group IV fibres respond to low-threshold innocuous pressure (Franz & Mense 1975).

Group III and IV fibres are activated in a linear fashion to the force of a muscle contraction or the force of a stretch on a muscle (Kaufman et al 1983, Mense & Meyer 1985, Mense & Stahnke 1983), the greater the force the greater the response. Approximately half of the afferents respond to both contraction and lengthening, and half are specific to one or other stimulus (Mense & Meyer 1985).

Afferents responsive to active contraction are often also chemical receptors responsive to bradykinin (Mense & Meyer 1985), a chemical released with inflammation. Group III afferents appear to be stimulated by the mechanical effects of the contraction, whereas group IV receptors seem to be stimulated by the metabolic products produced by the muscle contraction (Kaufman et al 1982, 1983, Kniffki et al 1978). Receptors that respond to the metabolic products have been named ergoreceptors (erg is a unit of work or energy) as they are thought to be involved in alterations to the cardiorespiratory system during physical activity (Kao 1963).

Box 5.2 Position of free nerve endings in muscle and predominant function of type III and IV afferent fibres

Connective tissue
between intrafusal and extrafusal fibres
arterioles and venules
capsule of muscle spindles
capsule of tendon organs
tendon tissue at the musculotendinous junction
in fat cells

Type III

Type IV

Most are:
mechanical pressure
  contraction-sensitive

Most are nociceptors:
mechanical and
  chemical

Chemical receptors. Some free nerve endings are sensitive to muscle pH, concentrations of extracellular potassium and sodium chloride, and changes in oxygen and carbon dioxide. They help to regulate the cardiopulmonary system during exercise or activity (Laughlin & Korthuis 1987, McCloskey & Mitchell 1972). Group IV afferents in muscle are thought to be primarily responsible for producing the reflex changes in cardiorespiratory function with exercise (Kaufman et al 1982, 1983, Kniffki et al 1978). Other group IV afferents are activated in the presence of chemicals released with inflammation, such as bradykinin, 5-hydroxytryptamine and potassium ions (Franz & Mense 1975, Kaufman et al 1982, Kumazawa & Mizumura 1977, Mense 1981). Chemically induced muscle pain in humans is thought to be due to activation of these free nerve endings (Mense 1996).

Thermal receptors. Some group IV receptors respond to small changes of temperature in muscle (Iggo 1961, Kumazawa & Mizumura 1977, Mense 1996). Others have been identified to have a high threshold for thermal stimulation and are thus thermal nociceptors (Iggo 1961, Mense & Meyer 1985). A high proportion of thermoreceptors has also been found to be sensitive to noxious mechanical pressure (Mense & Meyer 1985).

Nociceptors. Muscle nociceptors have a high mechanical threshold and some also have a high thermal threshold. The vast majority of group IV afferents in the cat have been found to be high-threshold mechanoreceptors and thus thought to be nociceptors (Franz & Mense 1975). It is also thought that group III muscle afferents may also be capable of acting as nociceptors and thus mediating pain (Paintal 1960). Bradykinin, a chemical released with inflammation, has been found to sensitize muscle and tendon nociceptors (Mense & Meyer 1985). This sensitization lowers the firing threshold such that an innocuous mechanical stimulus, for example movement or a light touch, causes excitation, a phenomenon known as allodynia (Raja et al 1999).

Summary of free nerve endings in muscle

The presence of nociceptors indicates that muscle has the potential to be a primary source of symptoms, and this could be brought about by noxious mechanical, chemical or thermal stimulation.

Efferent nerve fibres

Generally, the efferent fibres to muscle consist of the large myelinated alpha motor neurones that supply the extrafusal fibres, and the small myelinated gamma (or fusimotor) fibres that supply the intrafusal fibres within the muscle spindle. Type 1 muscle fibres are innervated by small, low-threshold, slowly conducting motor nerves while type 2b fibres are innervated by large higher-threshold, fast-conducting motor nerves.

The efferent fibres enter the muscle around the centre of the muscle belly, a region known as the motor point. Motor nerves divide into small branches to supply each muscle fibre; the presynaptic terminal synapses at the neuromuscular junction, with the motor end plate (Fig. 5.18). When an action potential arrives at the presynaptic terminal, a chain of chemical reactions is initiated which causes diffusion of acetylcholine across the synaptic cleft to the postsynaptic membrane. This chemical causes an increase in the permeability of sodium ions which, if sufficient, will initiate an action potential along the muscle fibre.

Each muscle fibre is supplied by a motor neurone. The motor neurone, and the muscle fibres it innervates, is termed a motor unit and is the functional unit of a muscle. Stimulation of the motor neurone initiates and maintains a series of complex events leading to either shortening (concentric contraction) or active lengthening (eccentric contraction) of muscle, and the development of muscle tension. Muscle contraction ceases when the stimulation of the motor nerve stops.

Muscle contraction is thought to be produced by the sliding of myosin and actin filaments so that the length of the sarcomere is shortened; this is termed the sliding filament theory (Fig. 5.19). The length of actin and myosin filaments does not change appreciably when a muscle contracts. Myosin contains proteins that extend towards the actin filaments, in the form of a tail and a head. The head contains a binding site for actin

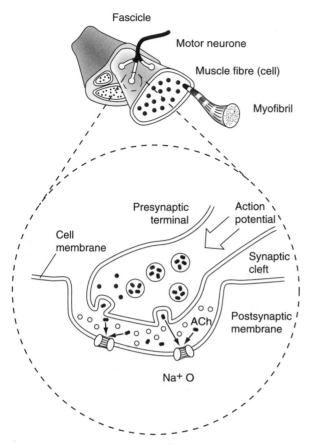

Figure 5.18 Neuromuscular junction formed by the motor nerve and the motor end plate (after Herzog 1999, with permission).

(Fig. 5.20) and forms the cross-bridge between myosin and actin. The reader is directed to a physiology textbook for a more detailed description of the sliding filament theory.

Muscle and proprioception

Several lines of research support the view that muscle has an important proprioceptive function (Grigg 1994). Isolated movement of a tendon, so as to stretch its muscle, gives a sensation of joint movement (Matthews & Simmonds 1974). In the hand of man, it has been found that isolated stimulation of individual spindle afferents is insufficient to cause a perception of joint movement. However, the spatial summation of a number of muscle spindles provides sufficient information for proprioception (Macefield et al 1990).

In addition, vibration of muscle produces a sensation of joint movement and a sense of joint position (Goodwin et al 1972). The movement is in the direction that would stretch the muscle being vibrated, so it is the muscle being stretched that provides a sense of joint movement. For example, on elbow extension the elbow flexor muscles will be stretched and give a sense of the extension movement. Because muscle spindles are more sensitive to vibration than golgi tendon organs it is thought that the illusion of movement is produced by stimulation of the muscle spin-

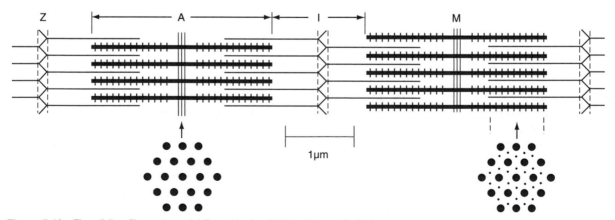

Figure 5.19 The sliding filament model (from Huxley 2000, with permission).

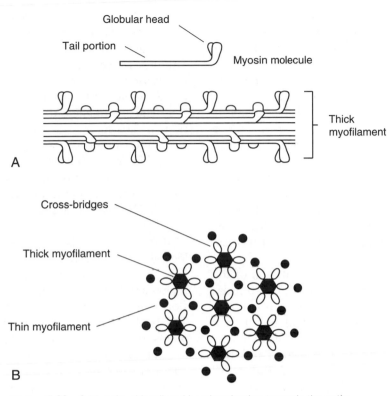

Figure 5.20 **A** Myosin with tail and head projecting towards the actin filaments (from Herzog 1999, with permission). **B** Cross-sectional arrangement of actin and myosin (after Herzog 1999, with permission).

dles (Goodwin et al 1972). Further evidence comes from the fact that, if muscle afferent activity is abolished during joint movement, proprioception is less accurate (Gandevia et al 1983, Gandevia & McClosky 1976) and, conversely, when skin and joint receptor activity is abolished the sense of proprioception remains (Clark et al 1979, Gandevia & McClosky 1976, Goodwin et al 1972), albeit poor (Clark et al 1979, Moberg 1983). Additionally, increased tension in a muscle increases the sensitivity of muscle spindles, and increased muscle tension has been found to enhance proprioception (Gandevia & McClosky 1976, Goodwin et al 1972, Macefield et al 1990).

The nerve supply to the skin is also relevant as this will be involved in any movement caused by muscle contraction; details of skin sensation can be found under nerve function in Chapter 8.

Muscle contraction

The strength of a muscle contraction depends on the following factors.

1. The type and number of motor units recruited. The recruitment of muscle fibres is directly related to the size of the motor neurone (Milner-Brown et al 1973). There is an initial recruitment of small motor neurones and then recruitment of large motor neurones as more force is required (Henneman & Olson 1965, Henneman et al 1965). Thus, small motor units are recruited first and then large motor units. The greater the stimulus the greater the number of muscle fibres stimulated and the greater the strength of contraction. The fact that all muscles contain both type I and II muscle fibres enables graded levels of muscle contraction to occur.

2. The initial length of the muscle. The resting length of a muscle fibre affects its strength of contraction. The optimal length is where there is maximum overlap between actin and myosin. Where a muscle fibre is less or more than the optimal length, fewer cross-bridges between actin and myosin are formed and the tension is lessened. This phenomenon produces a length–tension relationship in muscle which can be depicted on a graph (Fig. 5.21). When a single muscle fibre is lengthened there is an uneven lengthening such that the central portion of the muscle fibre lengthens more than the ends of the muscle; so while there is a reduction in the cross-bridges in the central portion there are still cross-bridges at the ends (Huxley 2000).

3. The nature of the neural stimulation of the motor unit. The frequency of the neural stimulation affects the strength of the muscular contraction. A single neural stimulus will result in a muscle twitch. A muscle twitch consists of a brief latent period, then a muscle contraction and then a relaxation period. The total time this takes varies between 10 and 100 ms (Ghez 1991). The strength of the contraction and the total time will depend on the type of muscle fibre, with fast-twitch fibres contracting more quickly, and with more force, than slow-twitch fibres. If a series of neural stimuli are used, (1–3 ms apart) (Ghez 1991), the muscle has not had time to relax and so an increase in muscle tension is produced due to the summation of each twitch. If the frequency of the neural stimuli is increased still further individual contractions are blended together in a sin-gle sustained contraction known as fused tetanus (Ghez 1991). This contraction will continue until the neural stimuli is stopped or the muscle fatigues. Muscular contractions that occur during normal body movements are the result of these tetanic contractions.

4. The age of the patient. Age causes a reduction in isokinetic calf strength (Gajdosik et al 1996) and isometric quadriceps strength (Grimby 1995, Heyley et al 1998, Young et al 1982a). Between the 4th and 7th decade there is a 14% reduction in isokinetic quadriceps strength per decade (Hughes et al 2001).

Muscle strength is proportional to the physiological cross-sectional area of the muscle, reflecting the number of sarcomeres in parallel (Newham 2001). As a muscle contracts, the tension at adjacent sarcomeres is equal and opposite and is therefore not transmitted to the attachments at the end of the muscle. The attachments to bone or fascia are subject to tension from the adjacent sarcomere only. For this reason force is independent of fibre length (Newham 2001). The cross-sectional area of muscle has been found to reduce with age. The quadriceps femoris cross-sectional area for 20-year-olds compared to 70-year-olds has been found to reduce by 27% in both men and women (Trappe et al 2001) and 35% in women (Young et al 1982a). This decrease in cross-sectional area is thought to be mainly responsible for the decrease in muscle strength with age (Akima et al 2001).

Muscle power

Muscle power is calculated from the force of contraction and the speed of contraction (force multiplied by velocity). Muscle power is determined by the number of sarcomeres in series (muscle length), the angle of pennation of the muscle fibres (the more parallel to the direction of force the greater the speed of contraction) as well as the biochemical properties of the muscle (Sacks & Roy 1982). For a given muscular force, the speed of movement is greater in muscles that contain a higher percentage of fast-twitch fibres (Fig. 5.22). For both fast- and slow-twitch muscle

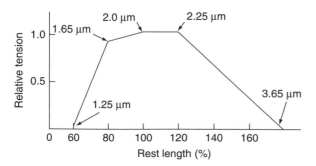

Figure 5.21 Length–tension relationship in skeletal muscle (from Powers & Howley 1997, with permission).

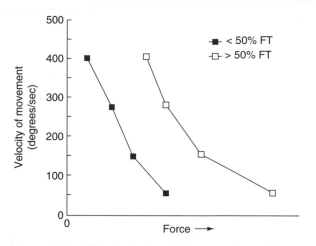

Figure 5.22 Difference in muscular force and speed of movement between muscles predominantly with fast-twitch and with slow-twitch muscle fibres (from Powers & Howley 1997, with permission).

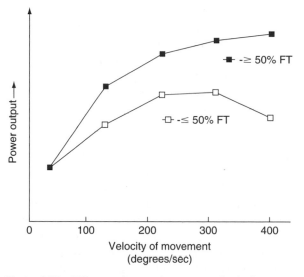

Figure 5.23 Difference in muscle power and velocity between muscles with predominantly fast-twitch (FT) and slow-twitch muscle fibres (from Powers & Howley 1997, with permission).

fibres, the maximum speed of active contraction occurs with the lowest force (Kojima 1991). Fast-twitch fibres are capable of producing greater force at a faster speed than slow-twitch fibres, hence muscles with predominantly fast-twitch fibres have greater power than muscles with predominantly slow-twitch fibres. Speed of contraction is also related to neuromuscular coordination (Kerr 1998). Muscle power reduces with age (Gajdosik et al 1996).

The relationship of muscle power and velocity is depicted in Figure 5.23. For a given velocity the peak power generated is greater in muscle that contains a high percentage of fast-twitch fibres than in muscle that contains a high percentage of slow-twitch fibres (Powers & Howley 1997). The peak power generated by any muscle increases with increasing speed of movement, up to a movement speed of 200–400 degrees/second.

In vitro muscle studies have demonstrated that the type of muscle contraction affects the force generated by a muscle. The greatest force is produced by an eccentric contraction (Katz 1939), the least force by a concentric contraction; an isometric contraction lies somewhere between the two (Hill 1938, Wilkie 1950). Increased speed of eccentric contraction further increases the force generated (Katz 1939), whereas increased speed

of concentric contraction reduces the force generated (Hill 1938). This relationship is depicted in Figure 5.24. In vivo muscle function behaves in a similar, but not identical, fashion (Newham 1993).

Muscle endurance

Muscle endurance is the ability of a muscle to continue an activity over time. It includes all types of muscle contraction and so may include

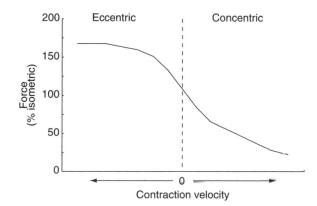

Figure 5.24 Force–velocity relationship for skeletal muscle (from Newham 1993, with permission).

repetitive movement, for example walking, or it may involve holding an isometric contraction over a period of time, for example using the rings in gymnastics. Muscle strength affects the endurance of a muscle. A muscle that is relatively weak, when required to contract during a functional activity, will do so at a proportionally greater level of maximum contraction than a muscle that is relatively strong. Other factors affecting muscle endurance include the energy store and circulation within the muscle (De Vries & Housh 1994).

There is a variety of ways to measure muscle endurance, and they depend on what specific type of muscle contraction is being tested. Measuring muscle endurance involves measuring the resultant muscle fatigue. Holding an isometric contraction at 60% maximum voluntary contraction (MVC) will increase the pressure within the muscle such that there will be no blood flowing into the muscle (Royce 1958). The ability then to continue holding the contraction will depend on the energy store within the muscle. A contraction at less than 60% MVC will enable the contraction to be held for longer, and a contraction at more than 60% MVC will result in the contraction being held for less time. An alternative method for measuring isometric endurance is to measure the increase in EMG activity that accompanies muscle fatigue (De Vries & Housh 1994).

Measurement of a muscle to repeated isotonic contractions can be obtained by using an ergograph, whereby a constant force is provided through a range of movement and the decrease in endurance is reflected in a reduction in range (De Vries & Housh 1994). Measurement of isokinetic endurance can be measured by the strength decrement index, which measures the decline in peak torque during repeated maximal isokinetic contractions. In the clinical situation, muscle endurance may be measured by identifying the length of time a patient can continue to perform a specific activity.

Measurement of more general cardiovascular endurance activity, such as distance running, swimming or cycling, involves measurements of heart rate, volume and composition of expired air to reflect oxygen uptake. An improvement in endurance is reflected, for the same relative amount of work:

- in reduced oxygen uptake and reduced heart rate
- in a reduced sense of effort (Borg 1982)
- in an ability to continue for longer
- in an ability to increase the number of repetitions in the same time period (Newham 2001).

Normal motor control

Normal control of movement occurs as a result of incoming sensory information of position and movement and is integrated at all levels of the nervous system. Automatic and simple reflex movements occur in the spinal cord. Postural and balance reactions occur at the level of the brain stem and basal ganglia. More complicated movements are initiated and controlled at the motor/sensory cortices, and the cerebellum controls and coordinates movement (Crow & Haas 2001). A schematic diagram of these levels of control of voluntary movement is shown in Figure 5.25. Motor control depends 'on the spatial and temporal integration of vestibular, visual, and somatosensory information about the motion of the head and body, and the generation of appropriate responses to that motion' (Speers et al 2002).

Posture and gait are organized at two levels (Allum et al 1998). The first level provides direction-specific patterns of movement determining activation, timing and sequencing of muscle. It is formed from hip and trunk proprioceptive input and vestibular input. The second level allows for particular adaptation for specific tasks, on the basis of the total afferent input from the body. For example, standing and moving one arm forward quickly to 90 degrees flexion causes activation of ipsilateral hamstrings and gluteus maximus. Contralaterally, an increase in activation of tensor fascia lata and gluteus maximus prior to activation of the shoulder flexors is seen. No such anticipatory activation occurs if the arm movement is

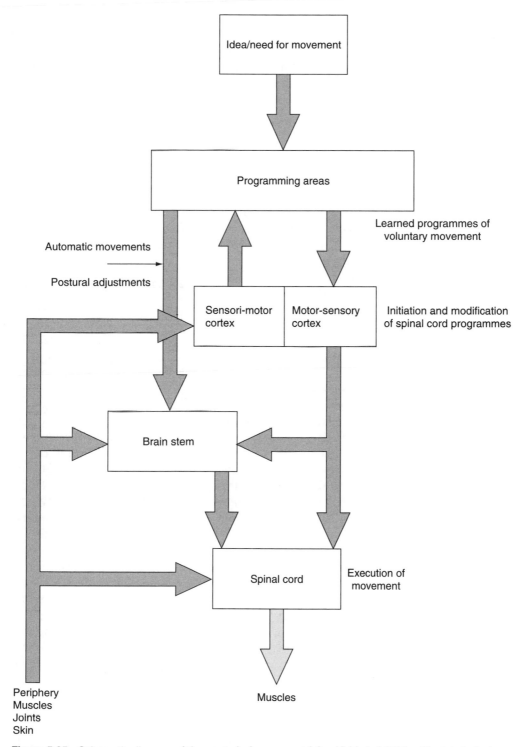

Figure 5.25 Schematic diagram of the control of movement (after Kidd et al 1992, with permission).

produced passively (Bouisset & Zattara 1981, Zattara & Bouisset 1988).

Similar anticipatory muscle activity (Hortobagyi & DeVita 2000) has been found during unsupported rapid elbow flexion where increased activation of gastrocnemius (Cordo & Nashner 1982) and biceps femoris and erector spinae (Friedli et al 1984) preceded biceps brachii activity. The activation of biceps femoris and erector spinae was reduced if the body was supported (strapped against a wall), reducing the threat to equilibrium (Friedli et al 1984). Rapid elbow extension causes activation of rectus abdominis, prior to activation of triceps brachii (Friedli et al 1984). Activation of the rotator cuff muscles and biceps brachii has been found to occur prior to both concentric and eccentric internal and external rotation of the glenohumeral joint (David et al 2000). Similarly, activation of the deep abdominal muscles and multifidus has been found to occur prior to rapid leg and arm movements in standing (Hodges & Richardson 1997a, b, c).

Automatic postural adjustments are constantly being made with functional activities. When a subject stands unsupported, with arms at the side, on a surface that suddenly translates forward, there is increased activity of tibialis anterior to counteract the backward sway, and so maintain equilibrium. If this is repeated with arm support there is very little activity in tibialis anterior but a large increase in activity of biceps brachii (Cordo & Nashner 1982). From this observation, it appears that any muscle may be automatically activated to maintain equilibrium (Cordo & Nashner 1982).

This anticipatory muscle activity is thought to enhance balance and reduce postural disturbance (Bouisset & Zattara 1981, Cordo & Nashner 1982, Friedli et al 1984, Horak et al 1984, Zattara & Bouisset 1988).

Muscle length

Muscle length can be measured by lengthening muscle fully through joint movement and measuring the final joint angle, using a goniometer or by visual estimation. The passive resistance of a muscle to lengthening is more difficult to measure. The clinician can passively lengthen the muscle and estimate the 'feel' of the resistance to movement, or length can be more objectively measured using isokinetic equipment.

Both the non-contractile and contractile components of muscle will each contribute to the resistance felt when passively lengthening a muscle. The muscle–tendon unit is viscoelastic, as discussed earlier. Initial lengthening will be achieved with a relatively small force, but as the muscle is stretched out this resistance will increase. The rate at which a muscle is lengthened will affect the resistance felt: increasing the speed will increase the resistance.

Classification of muscle function

There are a number of classification systems of muscle function. Each is useful in understanding muscle, but they each have limitations. Classification systems separate out and make distinct that which is often inseparable and indistinct. Enhanced knowledge often tends to produce a blurring of the categories, and a multidimensional continuum is often a more accurate representation. An obvious example is the change in the understanding of pain, which Descartes described as a signal of tissue damage (Descartes 1985), and has been developed as having physiological, sensory, affective, cognitive, behavioural, socio-cultural and ethno-cultural dimensions (Ahles & Martin 1992, McGuire 1995). Each of the systems below is not complete in itself but, taken as a whole, these systems provide insight into muscle function. An overview of the current classification systems is given in Figure 5.26.

The architecture of a muscle, the monoarticular/polyarticular and the spurt, shunt and spiral classification systems together cover anatomical and biomechanical aspects of muscle function. The phasic and tonic classification describes an aspect of muscle physiology. The use of agonist, antagonist, fixator and synergist describes the function of a muscle contraction in relation to a specific movement. The final two classification systems of local and global, and local stabilizers,

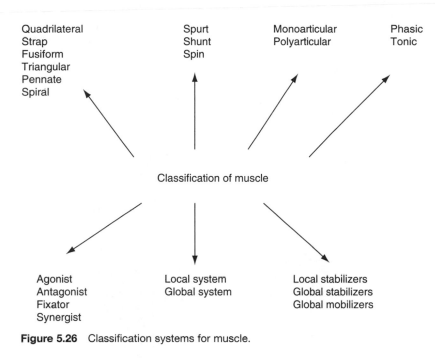

Figure 5.26 Classification systems for muscle.

global stabilizer and global mobilizer go one step further and attempt to identify the overall predominant function of a muscle. Each of these classification systems is discussed below.

Muscle architecture

Aspects of architecture include the fibre length, muscle length and pennation angle; each of these aspects will influence the function of the muscle. Each muscle fibre is capable of shortening to approximately half its total length (Norkin & Levangie 1992). Thus, a long muscle is able to shorten over a greater distance than a short muscle, so in terms of joint movement a long muscle will produce more movement of the bone than a short muscle. Long muscles usually lie more superficially than shorter muscles, giving them a greater leverage with which to move bone. Shorter muscles generally lie more deeply and often function to stabilize the joint. The shapes of muscles have been categorized as quadrilateral, strap, fusiform, triangular, pennate and spiral (Fig. 5.27).

The direction of the muscle fibres differs with each shape and so affects the direction of force during muscle contraction. A quadrilateral muscle, as the name suggests, is flat and square. The muscle fibres run parallel and extend the length of the muscle. Muscles of this shape, such as pronator quadratus and quadratus lumborum, are well designed to support and stabilize underlying bones and joints.

Strap muscles are long and rectangular in shape, with fibres running the full length of the muscle. They are able to produce movement through a large range, for example, sartorius. Rectus abdominis is a strap muscle, but is unusual in that it has three fibrous bands running across it.

Fusiform muscles are in the shape of a spindle with fibres running almost parallel to the line of pull. The two ends of the muscle converge onto a tendon. Biceps brachii consists of two fusiform-shaped muscles, while triceps brachii has three fusiform-shaped muscles.

Triangular muscles have a tendon at one end, and at the other end the muscle attaches to bone

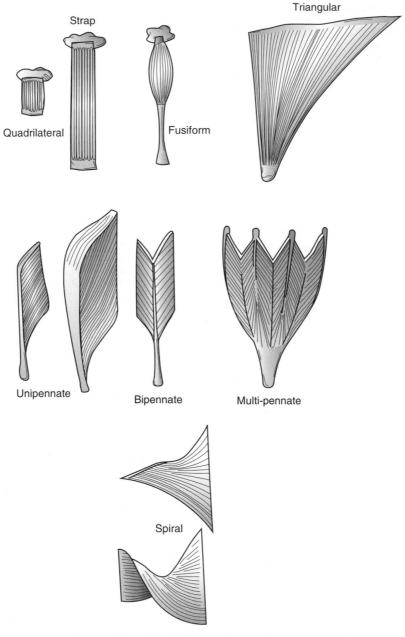

Figure 5.27 Shapes of muscles: quadrilateral, strap, fusiform, triangular, pennate, and spiral (from Williams et al 1995).

via either a flat tendon or an aponeurosis. The shape of the muscle means that some muscle fibres run at quite an oblique angle to the line of pull of the tendon, thus reducing its potential force of contraction. At its flat attachment though, the force of pull is across a broad area. Lower trapezius is an example of a triangular muscle.

Pennate muscles appear like a feather and may be unipennate (fibres attach to only one side of the tendon), bipennate (to both sides of the tendon) or multipennate (a number of bipennate arranged fibres). Examples include flexor pollicis longus (unipennate), rectus femoris (bipennate) and deltoid (multipennate). The oblique direction of the muscle fibres to the line of pull means that the force will be relatively less than if they were parallel; only a component of the force (the cosine of the angle) is available to move the bone. Pennate muscles have shorter and more numerous muscle fibres than do fusiform muscles. The greater number of muscle fibres give pennate muscles, such as deltoid and gluteus maximus, a greater strength compared with fusiform muscles.

Spiral muscles twist on themselves, and often de-twist on muscle contraction, thus producing a rotation force. Examples include latissimus dorsi twisting 180 degrees through its length to rotate the humerus medially (Lockwood 1998).

These architectural arrangements provide valuable insight into the function of a muscle and have been shown to have more effect on the force-generating capability of a muscle than its fibre type composition (Bodine et al 1982, Burkholder et al 1994, Sacks & Roy 1982).

Monoarticular and polyarticular

Monoarticular muscles cross only one joint while polyarticular muscles cross more than one joint. This classification system describes the relationship of muscle to joint, and so provides insight into the movement that will be produced by the muscle. For example, the rectus femoris is a polyarticular muscle crossing the anterior aspect of the hip and knee and therefore causing hip flexion and knee extension on concentric contraction. Muscles crossing more than one joint will be longer, and will produce more movement, than a muscle crossing just one joint. This classification system closely relates to the architecture of muscle and, together, they describe anatomical aspects of muscle.

Spurt, shunt and spin

This system describes the biomechanical aspect of muscle function, highlighting the leverage of muscle force on bone. In a spurt muscle the proximal attachment of the muscle lies at a distance from the joint axis, and the distal attachment lies close to the joint axis – for example, the biceps brachii (Fig. 5.28). With this arrangement the predominant effect of muscle contraction will be

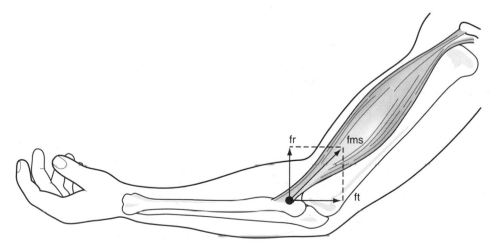

Figure 5.28 Biceps brachii is acting as a spurt muscle on flexion of the elbow where the force of contraction is fms; one component of this force (fr) causes a large flexion force, and the other, smaller component (ft), causes joint compression (from Norkin & Levangie 1992, with permission).

rotation of the bone, i.e. flexion of the elbow, rather than translation of the radius on the humerus.

The direction of the force, however, changes as the bone rotates (Fig. 5.29). When the biceps brachii contracts with the elbow at 35 degrees flexion there will be a relatively stronger compression force. At 70 degrees there will be a greater rotational force. At 90 degrees flexion there will be maximum rotational force with no translatory force. Finally, at 145 degrees flexion there will be a relatively greater amount of translatory force that will cause distraction of the joint surfaces. From elbow extension to flexion, then, biceps brachii acts as a shunt (35 degrees), spurt (70 and 90 degrees) and a shunt (145 degrees).

An additional consideration is that, as a muscle contracts, there is a change in the muscle architecture, that is, the muscle fibres change direction relative to the angle of pull (Fukunaga et al 1997, Kawakami et al 1998, Maganaris et al 1998), so this also will alter the angle of pull on the bone.

A shunt muscle is the reverse of this; the proximal attachment is close to the joint axis and the distal attachment lies at a distance from the joint axis – the popliteus at the knee or brachioradialis at the elbow are examples of this arrangement (Fig. 5.30). These muscles are positioned in such a way as to apply a predominantly compression force through the joint rather than a rotational force on the bone.

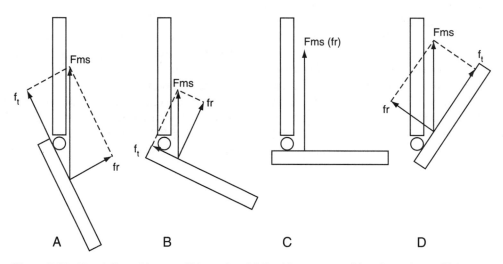

Figure 5.29 Resolution of forces of biceps brachii (fms) into rotatory (fr) and translatory (f_t) forces at elbow flexion angles of **A** 35 degrees, **B** 70 degrees, **C** 90 degrees and **D** 145 degrees (from Norkin & Levangie 1992, with permission).

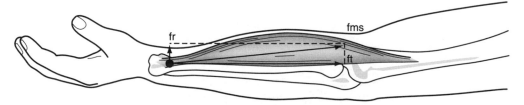

Figure 5.30 Brachioradialis is acting as a shunt muscle; where the force of contraction is fms, one component of this force (fr) causes a very small flexion force, and the other larger component (ft) causes joint compression (from Norkin & Levangie 1992, with permission).

Brachioradialis can be analysed in the same way (Fig. 5.31). At all angles, it can be seen that the translatory force is always greater than the rotational force so that the muscle predominantly acts as a shunt muscle (Norkin & Levangie 1992). Maximum rotation force occurs at 90 degrees flexion.

The line of force of a spin muscle is on the tangent of the long axis of the moving bone, so that contraction causes a rotation about its axis. For example, pronator quadratus is positioned to rotate the radius on its longitudinal axis (Fig. 5.32).

The classification of a muscle as a spurt, shunt or spin is rather simplistic. The force of a muscle contraction on bone follows simple mechanics and can be resolved into two planes: along the long axis of the bone (Fcos theta) and at right angles to the long axis (Fsin theta), where theta is the angle between the muscle force and each plane (Fig. 5.33). The component of the force along the axis will produce a compression force at the joint; the component of the force at right angles to the long axis will produce rotation of the bone. Hence, for any muscle contraction, there will be both a rotational and compression force applied. The rotational force will produce the spurt function and the compression force will produce the shunt function. Furthermore, if the muscle attaches to one side of the long axis of movement it will produce spin, such as pronator teres. Some muscles may be described as predominantly spurt or shunt, but with the emphasis on predominant – as most muscles will act as both spurt and shunt. For example, pronator teres combines all three types of muscle action: spurt, shunt and spin. It is positioned such that it weakly flexes the elbow, applies a compression force of the radius on the humerus, and pronates the forearm.

This simplistic classification is further highlighted on analysing a muscle when it reverses its action, that is, when it acts from the distal attachment. In this situation, a muscle that acted as a spurt muscle now acts as a shunt muscle, and vice versa (Norkin & Levangie 1992). For example, when the foot is taken off the ground the hamstring muscle group acts as a spurt muscle to the knee joint and as a shunt extensor muscle to the hip. On returning the foot to the ground, hamstring acts as a shunt flexor muscle to the knee and as a spurt extensor muscle to the hip (Kidd et al 1992).

The forces applied by the majority of muscles in the body have a greater translatory force (causing joint compression) than a rotational

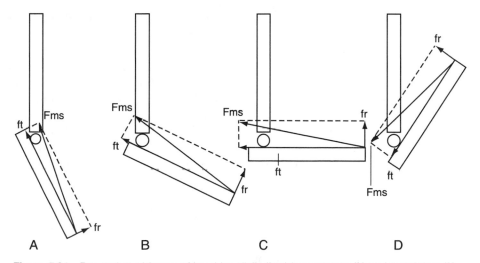

Figure 5.31 Resolution of forces of brachioradialis (fms) into rotatory (fr) and translatory (ft) forces at elbow flexion angles of **A** 35 degrees, **B** 70 degrees, **C** 90 degrees, and **D** 145 degrees (from Norkin & Levangie 1992, with permission).

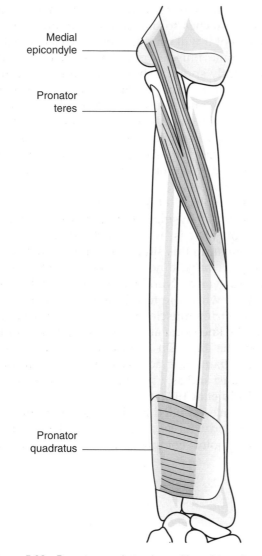

Figure 5.32 Pronator quadratus is positioned to act predominantly as a spin muscle, while pronator teres combines spurt, shunt and spin functions (from Palastanga 2002, with permission).

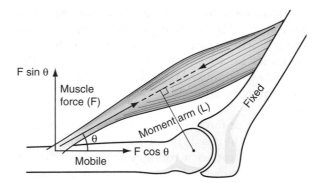

Figure 5.33 Resolution of force of contraction into a vertical force (Fsin θ) and a horizontal force (Fcos θ) (after Williams 1995, with permission).

force, which aids joint stability (Norkin & Levangie 1992).

Phasic and tonic

This classification system attempts to distinguish muscles according to their predominant type of fibre (Norkin & Levangie 1992) or their predominant function (Janda 1985). If a muscle contains a high proportion of type II muscle fibres it is a phasic muscle, and if it contains a high proportion of type I muscle fibres it is a tonic muscle. This system therefore makes the logical assumption that the characteristics of a muscle will reflect the predominant characteristic of its muscle fibre.

There is some overlap between this classification system and that of the spurt, shunt and spin classification system (Norkin & Levangie 1992). Broadly, muscles that are classified as phasic would also be classified as spurt muscles, and muscles that are tonic would also be shunt muscles (Table 5.4).

There are a number of difficulties in attempting to distinguish muscles according to their predominant type of fibre. Orbicularis oculi, sternocleidomastoid and the lateral head of rectus femoris may be considered phasic muscles under this classification system as they each contain a high proportion of type II fibres, and this has been found consistently between individuals (Johnson et al 1973). Similarly, soleus and tibialis anterior have been found consistently to contain a high proportion of type I fibres (87% and 73% respectively) and can therefore be categorized as having a tonic or postural function. Apart from these few exceptional muscles, the vast majority of muscles contain more or less equal proportions of type I and type II fibres (Johnson et al 1973).

The proportion of type I and II fibres is surprising in some muscles. The erector spinae mus-

Table 5.4 Characteristics of phasic (spurt) and tonic (shunt) muscles (Janda 1985, Norkin & Levangie 1992)

	Phasic/spurt	Tonic/shunt
Fibre type	High proportion of type II	High proportion of type I
Fibre arrangement	Strap, fusiform	Pennate
location	Superficial	Deep
	Cross more than one joint	Cross one joint
Function	Mobility	Stability
Action	Flexion	Extension
	Adduction	Abduction
	Medial rotation	Lateral rotation
	Tibialis anterior the vasti glutei rectus abdominis lower stabilizers of the scapula deep neck flexors extensors of the upper extremity	Tibialis posterior Rectus femoris Iliopsoas Tensor fascia lata Hamstrings Short hip adductors Quadratus lumborum Piriformis Part of Paravertebral back Muscles Pectoralis major Sternocleidomastoid Upper trapezius Levator scapula

cles might be expected to have a predominantly postural role and thus have a higher proportion of type 1 fibres; however, this has not been found consistently. The percentage of type I fibres in erector spinae between individuals ranges from 27 to 100% (Johnson et al 1973) with regional differences such that, in the thoracic spine, there is about 74% type I fibres compared to the lumbar spine, which has about 57% (Sirca & Kostevc 1985). Lumbar multifidus may also be expected to have a postural role and contain a large proportion of type I fibres; however, at L3 they have been found to contain about 63% of type I fibres (Sirca & Kostevc 1985).

Another limitation is that the proportion of types of muscle fibre in any one muscle varies widely between individuals (Johnson et al 1973) and is considered to be genetically determined (Simoneau et al 1986), related to gender (Brooke & Engel 1969), and may be related to age and occupation (Johnson et al 1973). For example, the superficial erector spinae contained 100% type 1 fibres in one individual but 27% in another individual (Johnson et al 1973).

The situation is further complicated by the fact that, in some individuals, there is a wide variation in the proportion of fibre types within any one muscle; for example, there are more type II fibres in the superficial layer than in the deep layer of deltoid, biceps brachii, adductor magnus, vastus medialis and vastus lateralis, rectus femoris muscles and lateral head of gastrocnemius (Johnson et al 1973). Additionally, the superficial and deep portions of multifidus have been found to contain 4% and 62.6% respectively of type I fibres at the L4/5 level (Rantanen et al 1994).

The vast majority of muscles contain more or less equal proportions of type I and type II fibres (Johnson et al 1973); this is thought to be due to the required variation in muscle activity during functional activities (Saltin et al 1977, Scott et al 2001).

There are difficulties in determining the predominant function of a muscle. Muscles can function in a variety of ways. For example, the hamstring group consists of two joint muscles acting over the hip and knee, and will be active during walking or running. In these activities the endurance of the hamstring muscle group is being challenged. However, during the high jump and triple jump it will be strength and power that is required. In gymnastics, on the beam, or in ballet, the hamstring muscle group is required to act with strength, power, control and precision. In the same way, a monoarticular muscle, such as brachialis muscle, is considered to act as a stabilizer. Any suggestion that this muscle functions only to stabilize and fine-tune movement seems rather limited, especially when one considers fast ballistic movements of the upper limb when boxing and weight lifting.

All muscles contribute to joint stability, including the large polyarticular muscles (Norkin & Levangie 1992). During gait, for example, the hamstring muscle group acts as a shunt extensor muscle to the hip when the foot is taken off the ground, and on returning the foot to the ground the hamstrings act as shunt flexor muscle to the knee (Kidd et al 1992). The cross-sectional area of the hamstring muscles is much greater than the small muscles around the hip and knee and therefore the strength of hamstrings is greater. The component of the contraction force of hamstrings compressing the hip and knee joints will therefore be greater than that of the local muscles and may have a significant impact on joint stability.

There are exceptions to this classification system. The internal oblique muscle is considered a global stabilizer, yet it is also thought to act as a local stabilizer (Hodges & Richardson 1997a). Serratus anterior is active during forceful shoulder girdle protraction against resistance, in reaching and pushing (Williams et al 1995), requiring concentric muscle activity. It also contracts isometrically to stabilize the scapula during the early phase of glenohumeral joint abduction. Therefore the suggestion that serratus anterior is a global stabilizer seems too limited.

The scalenii muscles are categorized as global mobilizers yet the position and direction of the muscle fibres would suggest that they will also provide a compression force to the cervical spine and therefore could act as stabilizers. Interestingly, Leonardo da Vinci first suggested this stability function of the cervical spine as early as the 16th century (Gombrich et al 1989), comparing them to the mast of a ship: 'such a convergence of the muscles of the spine holds it erect as the ropes of a ship supports its mast, and the same ropes, tied to the mast, also support in part the framework of the ships to which they are attached'. He also argued that the muscles will be most effective when they are attached to the ribs further from the axis of the spine, which is, of course, where all the scalene muscle attach. This suggestion – that the neck muscles stabilize the spine in much the same way as ropes attached to a mast of a ship – was also used in a rather more modern review of spinal muscles (Newman 1968).

In conclusion, this classification system seems to be inaccurate and therefore unhelpful in describing the function of muscle.

Prime mover, antagonist, fixator and synergist

This classification system describes the way in which a muscle functions in relation to a specific movement. Any one muscle may act as a prime mover (or agonist), antagonist, fixator or synergist (Williams et al 1995). The way in which a muscle acts depends on a number of factors which include the start position, the direction and speed of the movement, the phase of the movement and the resistance to movement.

Prime mover and antagonist. When a muscle is active in initiating and maintaining a movement it is acting as a prime mover. A muscle that opposes the prime mover is considered to be the antagonist.

Co-contraction of agonist and antagonist. It might be assumed that when the prime mover is contracting the antagonist is silent. However, there are numerous examples of co-contraction of agonist and antagonist. During maximal voluntary knee extension, the flexors of the knee are also contracting, albeit to a lesser degree (Baratta et al 1988). When extending the trunk during a lifting task, there is co-contraction of the trunk flexors and extensors (Granata & Marras 1995). When biceps brachii contracts eccentrically, to control extension of the elbow, there is activation of the triceps muscle (Norman & Komi 1979). The antagonistic contraction measured by EMG activity may not be indicative of an opposing torque, as there is a time delay between EMG activity and torque production (Corser 1974, Norman & Komi 1979). With a rapid voluntary movement there is a triphasic pattern of muscle activity, with bursts of activity initially in the agonist, then the antagonist, and then the agonist (Friedli et al 1984). In snow skiing, the hip, knee and ankle medial and lateral rotators have been found to co-contract and this is thought to provide postural control during this highly skilled movement (Louie et al 1984). The effect of co-contraction is to increase stiffness and thus stability of a joint, which is likely to be needed in stressful and complex movements (Fig. 5.34). There is therefore activity of the agonist and antagonist muscles during active movements.

Interestingly, the amount of co-contraction can be altered by activity. Athletes who strongly exercised the quadriceps and not the hamstrings had reduced co-contraction of the hamstrings on active knee extension compared to those who exercised both groups of muscles (Baratta et al 1988). The amount of co-contraction is related to motor control; co-contraction is greater when motor skill is poor and reduces when motor skill is improved (Osu et al 2002).

The amount of co-contraction increases with age: elderly women compared to young women were found to have over 100% greater activity of hamstring muscles just before and during a step-down movement (Hortobagyi & Devita 2000) and both men and women were found to have greater co-contraction of biceps femoris during a maximum isometric contraction and one-repetition maximum of quadriceps femoris muscle (Tracy & Enoka 2002).

This increased co-contraction functions to increase joint stiffness and is thought to compensate for the neuromotor impairments associated with the elderly (Hortobagyi & Devita 2000). The neuromotor impairments include: reduced muscle strength (Hortobagyi et al 1995), increased time to develop muscle torque (Thelen et al 1996), reduced proportion and cross-sectional area of type II muscle fibres (Larsson et al 1979), and poorer proprioception (Heyley et al 1998, Skinner et al 1984). It has been found that quadriceps isometric and concentric muscle strength reduces with age much faster than eccentric muscle strength (Hortobagyi et al 1995).

Fixators. As the name applies, this is when muscles contract to fix a bone. Muscles on either side of a joint sometimes contract together to create a fixed base on which another muscle can contract. For example, the muscles acting around the wrist contract together to fix the wrist when a strong fist is made. The particular wrist muscles in this case are acting as fixators.

Synergists. When a muscle acts over two or more joints, but the required movement is only over one joint, other muscles contract to eliminate the movement. When a muscle acts in this way it is said to act as a synergist (derived from syn, together, and ergon, work). Contraction of the finger flexors would produce flexion at both the wrist and fingers. The wrist extensors contract to eliminate the wrist flexion during a power grip and thus act as a synergist. Similarly, during elbow flexion with a pronated forearm,

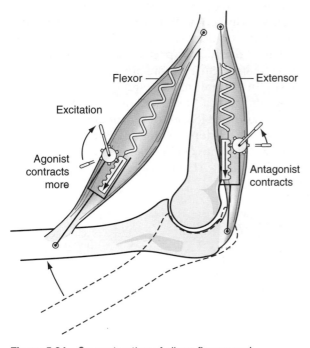

Figure 5.34 Co-contraction of elbow flexors and extensors to increase joint stiffness and stability (from Ghez 1991, with permission).

the contraction of biceps brachii will produce both elbow flexion and supination. To maintain the pronated forearm, the pronator quadratus and pronator teres contract and thus act as synergists. In the same way, when muscles around the shoulder contract to produce movement at the glenohumeral joint, muscles around the cervical spine, thoracic spine and scapula must contract to prevent unwanted movement and are therefore acting as synergists.

Any clinician attempting to analyse muscle activity during movement will immediately appreciate the difficulty in doing this. Visual and palpatory cues are simply inadequate to sense whether a particular muscle is active and in what way it is active. The classification system of prime mover, antagonist, fixator or synergist can be used to give a crude and probably inaccurate analysis of muscle activity. A Pressure Biofeedback Unit (PBU, Chatanooga, Australia), ultrasound imaging (Hides et al 1995) and EMG biofeedback (Richardson et al 1999) provide information on muscle activity, albeit limited.

Global and local systems

This classification system is very similar to the monoarticular and polyarticular classification systems. It has been used to create a mechanical model of the lumbar spine in order to identify the function of muscle in spinal stability (Bergmark 1989). Muscles were identified as a local system of muscles attaching directly onto the lumbar vertebra and a global system that consists of muscles that attach to the thoracic cage and pelvis (Box 5.3). The global system functions to transfer load between the thoracic cage and the thorax and to move one on another. The local system controls the curvature of the lumbar spine and provides sagittal and lateral stiffness to intervertebral segments of the lumbar spine.

The system evaluates muscle specifically in terms of the effect of a muscle on lumbar spine stability and is not attempting to provide a comprehensive description of the function of each of these muscles. For this reason, caution needs to be taken in generalizing not only the function of these muscles into global and local systems but in widening this to all muscles in the body. For example, the latissimus dorsi muscle is classified as a global muscle (Bergmark 1989) – and this is supported by the movement it produces at the glenohumeral joint; yet it can also act as a stabilizer of the scapula (Williams et al 1995). Psoas major is categorized as a global muscle, as it actively flexes the hip, yet it also provides a compression stabilizing force to the lumbar spine (Adams et al 2002). Finally, the internal oblique muscle is considered to be a global muscle, yet it is closely linked anatomically with transversus abdominis, which is considered part of the local system; it might be expected that where there is a close anatomical relationship there would be a close functional relationship. Some evidence supports a local function of internal oblique, which has been found to be activated along with transversus abdominis in a feedforward manner prior to hip movements, suggesting a possible stabilizing role (Hodges & Richardson 1997a).

Box 5.3 Classification of muscles into local and global muscle systems (Bergmark 1989)	

Global system
Global erector spinae:
longissimus thoracis pars thoracis iliocostalis lumborum
    pars thoracis
	Local system
	Local erector spinae:
	longissimus thoracis pars lumborum iliocostalis lumborum
	    pars lumborum
	Multifidus
	Interspinales
	Intertransversarii

Quadratus lumborum (lateral fibres) Abdominal muscles: rectus abdominus internal and external obliques	Quadratus lumborum (medial fibres) Abdominal muscles: internal oblique (via thoracolumbar fascia) transversus abdominis

These examples further highlight the difficulty in categorizing muscle according to function.

Local stabilizers, global stabilizers and global mobilizers

The two classification systems, the monoarticular system and polyarticular system, and the local and global system, have been combined by Comerford and Mottram (2001a, 2001b). Muscle function, in this system, is divided into local stabilizers, global stabilizers and global mobilizers.

Local stabilizers. Local stabilizers function to control the underlying joint movement. These muscles are sometimes referred to as postural or tonic muscles. Transversus abdominis has been described as a local stabilizer, and this has been supported by a number of research studies. Transversus abdominis has been found, using needle EMG, to contract a few milliseconds prior to rectus femoris, tensor fascia lata, and gluteus maximus during rapid hip flexion, abduction and extension respectively (Hodges & Richardson 1997a). This pre-emptive contraction has been demonstrated prior to deltoid muscle activity during rapid arm flexion, extension and abduction (Hodges & Richardson 1997b, 1997c). Transversus abdominis has also been found to be the major abdominal muscle responsible for increasing intra-abdominal pressure (Cresswell 1993, Cresswell et al 1992, Cresswell & Thorstensson 1994). The anticipatory activity of transversus abdominis, and its ability to raise intra-abdominal pressure, provides evidence to suggest that it functions as a local stabilizing muscle for the trunk (Cresswell 1993, Cresswell et al 1992, Cresswell & Thorstensson 1994, Hodges & Richardson 1997a, 1997b, 1997c). This is supported by the observation that low back pain patients have been found to have a delayed activation of transversus abdominis (Hodges & Richardson 1996).

In the lower limbs vastus medialis oblique and vastus lateralis may also act to stabilize the knee. In prone lying the EMG activity of vastus medialis oblique and vastus lateralis did not alter with active knee flexion and extension movements, nor with increasing speeds of movement – unlike rectus femoris and hamstring muscle groups which were activated according to the cycle of the movement and with increase in activity with increasing speed (Richardson & Bullock 1986). Vastus medialis oblique and vastus lateralis appeared therefore to be continually contracting and not in relation to the knee movement, suggesting a possible stabilizing function.

Throughout the body, small muscles often contract alongside much larger muscles to fine-tune the gross movement produced by the larger muscles (Peck et al 1984). Examples include supination produced by the larger biceps brachii and the smaller supinator; extension of the spinal column with the larger erector spinae and multifidus and the smaller occipital muscles, interspinales and intertransversarii. In all cases, the smaller muscles contain appreciably more muscle spindles than longer muscles (Abrahams 1977, 1981, Cooper & Daniel 1963, Peck et al 1984) and are thus thought to provide proprioceptive input (Adams et al 2002, Bastide et al 1989, Peck et al 1984).

Global stabilizers. The global stabilizers are considered to generate force to control movement through eccentric control, particularly of the inner and outer range of joint movement (Comerford & Mottram 2001a, 2001b). They are thought to provide rotational control during functional movements. Stabilizer muscles have been referred to as monoarticular muscles (Comerford & Mottram 2001b). Eccentric muscle contraction is considered to provide shock absorption by decelerating the body during activities such as walking and running (Stauber 1989). Examples of muscles in this category are the internal and external oblique muscles, spinalis, gluteus medius, serratus anterior and longus colli (M Comerford personal communication, 2000).

Global mobilizers. The global mobilizers are considered to generate force to produce movement through concentric contraction, particularly in the sagittal plane (Comerford & Mottram 2001a, 2001b). These muscles are often long superficial muscles, strap or fusiform in shape, and could be also categorized as spurt, phasic or polyarticular muscles designed for power and speed (Mitchell 1993). Examples could include rectus abdominis, iliocostalis, hamstrings, latissimus dorsi, levator scapula, and the scalenii.

This classification system attempts to identify the overall predominant function of a muscle, with the suggestion that global (polyarticular) muscles control movement and alignment while local (monoarticular) muscles provide stability (Comerford & Mottram 2001b). The limitations of this system are similar to that of the phasic and tonic classification: there are major difficulties in suggesting that a muscle has a predominant function.

Summary of classification of muscle function

Each of the classification systems provides insight into muscle function. The theory of motor control provides a valuable context in which to consider these functions. Muscle contraction is not an isolated event in the body, it is controlled by various levels of the central nervous system (CNS). The motor cortex that initiates muscle contraction does not function in relation to individual muscles; rather, it controls the coordinated contraction of a large number of muscles to control movement. The CNS is thus concerned with movement, and it can be argued that analysis should focus more on gross movement than on individual muscle activity. This is reinforced by the fact that muscle is in a constant state of change; muscle activity per se is highly unstable and is being constantly altered by the CNS to maintain balance and coordinate movements.

Because almost all muscles contain similar proportions of type I and type II muscle fibres, it can be presumed that the characteristics of whole muscles reflect both characteristics. That is, all muscles can contract slowly and gently for a long period of time, exhibiting endurance. All muscles can contract quickly and strongly, exhibiting strength and power; the actual amount will depend on factors such as the cross-sectional area of the muscle, leverage and architecture. It seems reasonable to suggest that all muscles will have a role in posture and balance, and all muscles will have a role in movement. The CNS will activate type I fibres in all types of muscle in order to pro-

vide the necessary posture and balance and will activate the type II fibres in all types of muscle in order to provide strength and power. The relative amounts of activation, and in which muscles, will depend on the specific position and movement that is being carried out.

MUSCLE DYSFUNCTION

Just as the function of muscles depends on the function of joints and nerves, so dysfunction of muscles can lead to dysfunction of joints and nerves. They are dependent on each other in both normal and abnormal conditions; this is depicted in Figure 5.35. The following examples may help

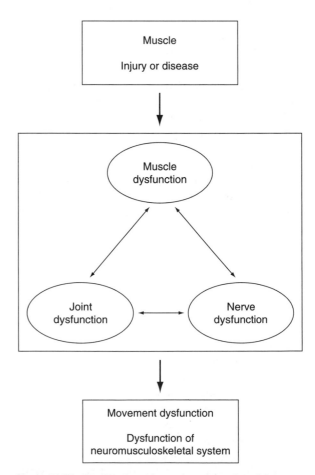

Figure 5.35 Dysfunction of muscle can produce joint and/or nerve dysfunction, and can lead to movement dysfunction.

to highlight how muscle dysfunction will often be accompanied by joint and/or nerve dysfunction.

Dysfunction in muscle and joint often occur together. For example, abnormality of the eccentric muscle force of the quadriceps muscle may be a contributing factor in anterior knee pain (Bennett & Stauber 1986, Hughston et al 1984), and lateral epicondylitis is associated with tears of the lateral collateral ligament of the elbow (Bredella et al 1999). This evidence highlights the close relationship of muscle and joint dysfunction.

There is overwhelming evidence that weakness of a muscle occurs with joint pathology and dysfunction. This has been demonstrated in the knee in the presence of a variety of pathologies: rheumatoid arthritis (deAndrade et al 1965), osteoarthritis (deAndrade et al 1965, Hurley & Newham 1993), ligamentous knee injuries (DeVita et al 1997, Hurley et al 1992, 1994, Kennedy et al 1982, Newham et al 1989, Snyder-Mackler et al 1994, Urbach & Awiszus 2002) and following meniscectomy (Hurley et al 1994, Shakespeare et al 1985, Stokes & Young 1984, Suter et al 1998a); in the elbow in the presence of rheumatoid arthritis (Hurley et al 1991); and in the glenohumeral joint in the presence of anterior dislocation (Keating & Crossan 1992). The inhibition of muscle is thought to be due to inhibitory input (Iles et al 1990, Suter & Herzog 2000, Torry et al 2000) or abnormal input (Hurley & Newham 1993, Hurley et al 1991) from joint afferents. Thus, joint pathology leads to altered neural activity, which alters muscle activity. A muscle that is inhibited will, over time, weaken and this may make the joint vulnerable to further injury (Stokes & Young 1984, Young et al 1982b). For example, it is thought that weakness of the posterior rotator cuff muscles may make the glenohumeral joint vulnerable to recurrent anterior dislocation (Keating & Crossan 1992). This sequence of events is outlined in Figure 5.36.

Another example of the close relationship between joint, nerve and muscle is the effect of joint immobilization. Following 3 weeks of finger and thumb immobilization there is reduced maximal voluntary contraction of the muscles around the joint and a decrease in the maximal

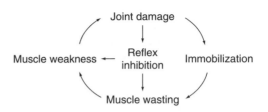

Figure 5.36 Effect of joint damage and/or immobilization on muscle and nerve tissues. (Reproduced, with permission, from Stokes M, Young A 1984 Clinical Science 67:7–14. © The Biochemical Society and the Medical Research Society.) (After Stokes & Young 1984, with permission).

firing rate of motor neurones supplying the muscles (Seki et al 2001).

Muscle activity around a joint is altered in the presence of ligament insufficiency and joint instability. During throwing, EMG activity of the elbow muscles is altered with ligament insufficiency of the elbow (Glousman et al 1992). Similarly, during throwing, the EMG activity around the shoulder region is altered with shoulder instability (Glousman et al 1988). In the lower limb, the EMG activity of quadriceps and hamstring muscle groups is altered with anterior cruciate ligament deficiency during knee movement (Solomonow et al 1987) and during gait and functional activities (Berchuk et al 1990, Ciccotti et al 1994). Figure 5.37 identifies a proposed cycle of events of progressive knee instability following an initial ligament injury (Kennedy et al 1982).

Muscle activity is directly affected by joint nociceptor activity. Pain around the knee causes a nociceptive flexor withdrawal response: hip and knee flexion and ankle dorsiflexion. There is increased alpha motor neurone excitability of the muscles to produce this movement (Stener & Peterson 1963) and reciprocal inhibition of the knee extensors (Stener 1969, Stener & Peterson 1963, Young et al 1987). For example, pressure or tension on a partially ruptured medial collateral ligament results in an increased activity of sartorius and semimembranosus (knee flexors) with inhibition of the vastus medialis (extensor) (Stener and Peterson 1963). Pain over the lateral

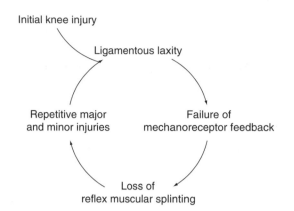

Figure 5.37 A proposed cycle of progressive knee instability following an initial ligament injury (from Kennedy et al 1982, with permission).

femoral epicondyle leads to inhibition of the vastus medialis and lateralis, both knee extensors (Stener 1969). In the lumbar spine, pain from the zygapophyseal joint causes increased activity of the hamstring muscle group (Mooney & Robertson 1976).

Interestingly, activation of type I, II and IV receptors in the zygapophyseal joints of the cervical spine have more widespread effects than just on the muscles around the neck: they also influence the muscles around the eye and mandible (Wyke & Polacek 1975). This research clearly indicates that nociceptor activity increases the activation of some muscles and decreases the activation of others.

Nociceptor activity is thought to influence muscle activity via the alpha motor neurone (Wyke & Polacek 1975). Nociceptor activity is thought to have a greater inhibitory effect upon the low-threshold motor units supplying type 1 muscle fibres than on the high-threshold motor units supplying type II fibres (Gydikov 1976). If this is true, it might be speculated that a muscle containing a relatively higher proportion of type I fibres, such as soleus and tibialis anterior, may be more affected by nociceptor activity than a muscle that has a more equal proportion of type I and II fibres.

The functions of a muscle are essentially to produce and allow movement to occur. That is, it will contract with strength, power and endurance, it will lengthen and shorten with movement and, under the control of the central nervous system (motor control), it will produce coordinated movement. The signs and symptoms of muscle dysfunction are related to these functions, that is, there may be one or more of the following: reduced muscle strength, reduced muscle power, reduced muscle endurance, altered motor control, reduced muscle length, or production of symptoms. Box 5.4 highlights these characteristics of muscle function and dysfunction. A particular mix of these signs and symptoms occurs with a muscle or tendon injury, and these are discussed at the end of the chapter.

Reduced muscle strength

Reduced muscle strength can occur as a result of disuse such as immobility (Berg et al 1997), immobilization (Labarque et al 2002, Sargeant et al 1977, Vaughan 1989), trauma (DeVita et al 1997, Hurley et al 1992, Newham et al 1989, Snyder-Mackler et al 1994, Urbach & Awiszus 2002), weightlessness (Edgerton et al 1995, Fitts et al 2000, 2001), and pathology (Sirca & Kostevc 1985, Yoshihara et al 2001, Zhao et al 2000). As will be seen later, a reduction in muscle strength will produce a reduction in muscle power and a reduction in endurance.

A body of knowledge is emerging on the effects of space flight on the musculoskeletal system in anticipation of a manned mission to Mars (Fitts et al 2000, 2001). While the reader is unlikely to be managing patients recovering from the effects of space flight(!), the effects on

Box 5.4 Signs and symptoms of muscle dysfunction
Reduced muscle strength
Reduced muscle power
Reduced muscle endurance
Altered motor control
Reduced muscle length
Production of symptoms

muscle are of interest in furthering our understanding of the plastic nature of the muscle. Space flight causes a reduction in muscle strength and power (Edgerton et al 1995, Fitts et al 2000, 2001). Initially, space flight causes greater atrophy and weakness of the leg extensors, but after 110 days there is a similar 30% loss in dorsiflexion and plantarflexion strength (Greenleaf et al 1989). It is thought that the rate of muscle atrophy plateaus such that little further atrophy will occur beyond this period of time (Antonutto et al 1999, Fitts et al 2000).

With microgravity, atrophy of human soleus muscle is greater than the atrophy of gastrocnemius (Fitts et al 2001, Widrick et al 2001). This might be expected as microgravity will affect type I fibres more than type II fibres; moreover, as soleus has such a high proportion of type I fibres, this muscle may be affected more than gastrocnemius with a lower percentage of type I fibres (H Fiddler, personal communication, 2004). Within the human soleus muscle, two studies (Edgerton et al 1995, Widrick et al 2001) have found greater atrophy of type II than type 1 fibres, while one study found similar degrees of atrophy for both types of fibre (Fitts et al 2001). The results of these studies are not conclusive as the number of subjects was small and there was a large variation between individuals. Microgravity has also been found to cause a 50% reduction in muscle power (Antonutto et al 1999), which is thought to be caused by an alteration in the recruitment of motor units (Antonutto et al 1999, Fitts et al 2000).

Muscle atrophy has been found to occur with pathology. For example, in patients who underwent surgery for a chronic lumbar disc herniation there was atrophy of the multifidus and longissimus muscles (Sirca & Kostevc 1985). In another similar study a biopsy of multifidus at L4/5 and L5/S1 levels also revealed muscle atrophy on the side of herniation, with smaller type I and type II fibres (Zhao et al 2000). Patients with a L4/5 disc herniation and L5 nerve root compression (identified at surgery) were found to have atrophy of multifidus with a 6.4% reduction in cross-section area of type I fibres and a 9.8% reduction in type II fibres at the level of the

herniation; interestingly, no atrophy was found at the L4 level (Yoshihara et al 2001).

It should be remembered that there are normal age-related changes in muscle strength. For instance, there is a reduction in isokinetic calf strength (Gajdosik et al 1996) and isometric quadriceps strength (Grimby 1995, Heyley et al 1998, Young et al 1982a). Between the 4th and 7th decade there is a 14% reduction in isokinetic quadriceps strength per decade (Hughes et al 2001).

Muscle strength is profoundly affected by immobilization. Immobilization also affects the non-contractile portion of muscle, the musculotendinous junction and the tendon and these are discussed below.

Immobilization

Immobilization affects the contractile portion of muscle, the non-contractile portion of muscle, the musculotendinous junction and the tendon. The reduced strength resulting from immobilization is thought to be due to muscle atrophy, that is, reduced fibre area and diameter (Berg et al 1997, Sargeant et al 1977, Young et al 1982b) and reduced neural input to the muscle (Berg et al 1997). The effects of immobilization on muscle depend on the length of time, the position of the muscle when immobilized, and the predominant muscle fibre type within the muscle.

Time of immobilization. If a muscle does not contract at all muscle strength will decrease by approximately 5% a day, but one contraction at half maximum contraction (0.5 repetition maximum (RM)) is considered sufficient to prevent this reduction (Muller 1970). Normally, some degree of muscle contraction may occur while a muscle is immobilized, giving a more realistic estimate of 2–3% reduction in muscle strength per day (Appell 1990, Muller 1970); bed rest is estimated to cause a 1–1.5% reduction per day (Muller 1970).

Following 2 weeks of elbow immobilization, subjects developed a significant decrease ($P < 0.01$) in elbow flexion strength; interestingly, there was no significant decrease in extensor strength (Vaughan 1989). It appears that if the elbow is immobilized for a longer period of time, 5–6 weeks, reduction of extensor strength occurs and decreases by 41% (MacDougall et al 1980). With knee immobilization there is uniform atrophy of all the heads of quadriceps (Lieb & Perry 1968). It is sometimes suggested that there is selective wasting of muscle groups; however, there is no research evidence to support this.

Position of the muscle. The effects of immobilization on muscle depend on the position in which the muscle is held, whether it is in a shortened or lengthened position.

The effects of immobilization in a shortened position are summarized in Box 5.5. The changes in muscle demonstrate the plastic nature of muscle, which changes its structure as a consequence of a change in function. The decrease in the number of sarcomeres and increase in length of each sarcomere ensure that the muscle is able to contract maximally in the shortened immobilized position. The connective tissue loss, due to immobilization, occurs at a lower rate than the loss of contractile tissue, resulting in a relative increase in connective tissue (Goldspink & Williams 1979); this can occur as early as 2 days after immobilization (Williams & Goldspink 1984). In addition, the connective tissue remodels during immobilization to produce a thicker perimysium and endomysium (Goldspink &

Williams 1979). These changes produce an increased stiffness to passive lengthening, which is thought to occur to prevent the muscle from being overstretched (Goldspink & Williams 1979, Tabary et al 1972).

The increase in connective tissue associated with immobilization in a shortened position can be prevented by 15 minutes of passive stretch on alternative days (Williams 1988). This intermittent stretching regime, however, does not influence the reduction in muscle fibre length and subsequent reduction in range of movement (Williams 1988).

The muscle spindle is also affected by immobilization. Three weeks of immobilization of rat calf muscle caused a 40% reduction in the cross-sectional area of the intrafusal fibres of the muscle spindle, and a marked increase in the thickness of the capsule surrounding the muscle spindle (Jozsa et al 1988). The effect of these changes on muscle function is unclear.

When the immobilization ceases the muscle will be weak, shortened and will have an increased resistance to passive lengthening. The plastic nature of muscle is further demonstrated by the fact that the changes to immobilized muscle (in cat and mouse), revert to normal with removal of the immobilization (Tabary et al 1972, Williams & Goldspink 1973). It has been demon-

---

Box 5.5 Effects of immobilization on muscle in a shortened position

Decrease in muscle weight and fibre size	Williams & Goldspink 1978
	Witzmann 1988
Decrease in the number of sarcomeres	Goldspink et al 1974
	Goldspink 1976
	Tabary et al 1972
	Tabary et al 1987
	Williams & Goldspink 1973
	Williams & Goldspink 1978
Increase in the sarcomere length	Tabary et al 1987
	Williams & Goldspink 1978, 1984
Increase in amount of perimysium	Williams & Goldspink 1984
Increase in ratio of collagen concentration	Goldspink & Williams 1979
	Williams & Goldspink 1984
Increase in ratio of connective tissue to muscle fibre tissue	Goldspink & Williams 1979
	Williams & Goldspink 1984
Reduction in the cross-sectional area of the intrafusal fibres of the muscle spindle	Jozsa et al 1988
Increase in the thickness of the capsule surrounding the muscle spindle	Jozsa et al 1988

strated that the new sarcomeres on remobilization are added at the ends of the muscle fibres (Williams & Goldspink 1973).

Two weeks' immobilization of the human knee held in almost full extension (shortened position for knee extensors and relative lengthened position for knee flexors) resulted in a 27% reduction in knee extensor torque and an 11% reduction in knee flexor torque (Labarque et al 2002). The reduction in knee extensor torque agrees with the estimate of 2–3% reduction per day in muscle strength (Appell 1990, Muller 1970).

The effects of immobilization of muscle in a lengthened position are summarized in Box 5.6. There is an increase in the number of sarcomeres that lie in series, thus lengthening the muscle (Goldspink 1976, Tabary et al 1972, 1987, Williams & Goldspink 1973, 1976, 1978). The length of the sarcomeres is reduced (Tabary et al 1972, 1987, Williams & Goldspink 1978, 1984). There is hypertrophy, which may then be followed by atrophy (Tabary et al 1987, Williams & Goldspink 1984). Functionally the muscle has a greater capacity to generate tension. There is no change in the muscle stiffness to passive lengthening (Tabary et al 1972, Williams & Goldspink 1978).

Predominant type of muscle fibre within the muscle. There is some suggestion that the effect of immobilization on a muscle is affected by its proportion of type I and type II muscle fibres. The effect of immobilization in near-resting length of a guinea-pig soleus (predominantly type 1 muscle fibres) has been compared to immobilization of gastrocnemius (predominantly type II muscle fibres) (Maier et al 1976). In both muscles type 1 fibre atrophied to a greater extent than type II fibres, and interestingly this was greater in soleus than in gastrocnemius (Maier et al 1976). The capacity of gastrocnemius to create tension was significantly (P <0.05) reduced, whereas in soleus there was no significant reduction (Maier et al 1976). In contrast, another study found that type II fibres atrophied more than type I fibres (MacDougall et al 1980). Following 5–6 weeks of elbow immobilization there was a 30% reduction in cross-sectional area of type II fibres and a 25% reduction in type I fibres (MacDougall et al 1980).

Effect of immobilization on the musculotendinous junction and the tendon

Immobilization has widespread effects on the musculotendinous junction and the tendon (Box 5.7). At the musculotendinous junction, 3 weeks of immobilization of the rat gastrocnemius–soleus–tendon unit in a shortened position resulted in over 40% reduction in the contact area between the muscle and the tendon (Kannus et al 1992). Other changes included an increase in scar tissue in the area, reduced glycosaminoglycans, and an increase in weaker type III collagen fibres (Kannus et al 1992).

Collectively, these changes will reduce the tensile strength of the musculotendinous junction. An experimental muscle strain and 2 days of immobilization resulted in a significant (P < 0.001) reduction in tensile strength and stiffness at the musculotendinous junction (Almekinders & Gilbert 1986). In addition, a 30% reduction in blood vessels in the musculotendinous junction has also been observed following immobilization (Kvist et al 1995). Three weeks of immobilization of rat calf muscle caused a marked increase in the thickness of the capsule surrounding the golgi tendon organ (Jozsa et al 1988); the effect of this on muscle function is unclear.

In tendons it has been found that 5 weeks of disuse of rat achilles tendon resulted in a reduc-

Box 5.6 Effects of immobilization on muscle in a lengthened position	
Increase in the number of sarcomeres in series	Goldspink 1976 Tabary et al 1972 Tabary et al 1987 Williams & Goldspink 1973, 1976, 1978
Decrease in the length of sarcomeres	Tabary et al 1972 Tabary et al 1987 Williams & Goldspink 1978, 1984
Muscle hypertrophy that may be followed by atrophy	Tabary et al 1987 Williams & Goldspink 1984

Box 5.7 Effects of immobilization on the musculotendinous junction and tendon	
Musculotendinous junction	
Reduction in the contact area between muscle and tendon	Kannus et al 1992
Increase in scar tissue	Kannus et al 1992
Reduced glycosaminoglycans	Kannus et al 1992
Increase in the weaker type III collagen fibres	Kannus et al 1992
Reduced tensile strength	Almekinders & Gilbert 1986
	Kannus et al 1992
Reduced stiffness	Almekinders & Gilbert 1986
Reduction in blood vessels	Kvist et al 1995
Increase in the thickness of the capsule of the golgi tendon organ	Jozsa et al 1988
Tendon	
Reduced collagen fibres	Nakagawa et al 1989
Reduced energy supply, oxygen consumption and enzyme activity	Jozsa & Kannus 1997

tion in the number of collagen fibres, causing a reduction in tensile strength (Nakagawa et al 1989). There is also reduced energy supply, oxygen consumption and enzyme activity within the tendon following a period of immobilization (Jozsa & Kannus 1997).

The effect of remobilization of tendon following a period of immobilization is still largely unclear. The 30% loss of vascularity at the musculotendinous junction can be restored following remobilization (Kvist et al 1995). There is acceleration of collagen synthesis and enzyme activity (Karpakka et al 1990). However, the collagen content and orientation of remobilized tendon may continue to be inferior despite remobilization (Jozsa & Kannus 1997).

Measurement of muscle strength

Muscle strength is often clinically assessed using manual muscle testing with a scale from 0 (no contraction) to 5 (normal strength). The value of this is severely limited as the accuracy and sensitivity are very poor (Newham 2001). In one study a muscle which was only 8% of normal strength was rated as grade 4, clearly underestimating true muscle strength (Agre & Rodriquez 1989).

Quadriceps muscle wasting has been measured clinically by using a tape measure around the circumference of the thigh. There are difficulties with this measure as it includes the subcutaneous fat and hamstring muscle group, which can conceal the quadriceps muscle wasting (Young et al 1982b). The measurement has been found to underestimate the extent of the quadriceps muscle atrophy (Arangio et al 1997, Sargeant et al 1977, Young et al 1980, 1982b, 1983) and is of questionable value in the clinical environment (Arangio et al 1997).

Muscle strength can be more objectively tested by measuring muscle cross-sectional area, or by measuring muscle force or pressure during active contraction. Physiological cross-sectional area (PCSA) can be measured by ultrasound, computerized axial tomography (CAT) and magnetic resonance imaging (MRI). The physiological cross-sectional area, however, underestimates muscle strength; Young et al (1983) found a 15% increase in isometric strength of the quadriceps following a training period, but only a 6% increase in PSCA. Force or pressure can be measured using devices such as the hand-held dynamometer for grip strength and the large isotonic or isokinetic dynamometers for larger muscle groups (Watkins et al 1984). Where strength is measured by an active contraction, muscle length and the motivation and effort by an individual will affect the force measurement. Muscle strength testing is further complicated by the fact that asymptomatic subjects have been found to vary the maximal voluntary contraction over different days of testing (Allen et al 1995, Suter & Herzog 1997).

Reduced muscle power

Muscle power is a function of force and velocity and if either is reduced there will be a subsequent reduction in power. Where there is a reduction in muscle strength, there will be, by definition, a reduction in muscle power. Velocity is a function of force and distance and therefore any reduction in muscle length or any reduction in the speed of contraction will result in a reduction in muscle power. It has already been identified that immobilization in a shortened position causes a reduction in strength and a reduction in length; both of these changes will cause a reduction in muscle power.

The velocity of a contraction is determined, in part, by the proportion of fibre types within the muscle – the greater the proportion of type II fibres the greater the power (Newham 2001). Any reduction in type II fibres within a muscle would potentially reduce its power.

No difference in atrophy of type I and type II fibres in vastus lateralis was found in healthy volunteers confined to 6 weeks' bed rest (Berg et al 1997). Any reduction in muscle power would not be as a result of a reduction in type II fibres; however, all subjects had an 18% reduction in cross-sectional area of the muscle and this would reduce muscle strength, and hence power.

A number of studies have investigated the effect of knee immobilization on the proportion of type I and type II fibres in vastus lateralis (Haggmark et al 1981, Hortobagyi et al 2000, MacDougall 1986, MacDougall et al 1980, Sargeant et al 1977). Three weeks of knee immobilization resulted in a 13% reduction in type I fibres and a 10% reduction in type II fibres (Hortobagyi et al 2000). Following a lower limb fracture and knee immobilization for up to 7 weeks there was a 46% reduction in type I fibres and a 37% reduction in type II fibres (Sargeant et al 1977). Following knee surgery and 5 weeks of knee immobilization there was a reduction only in the cross-sectional area of type I fibres with no alteration in type II fibres (Haggmark et al 1981). The studies suggest that knee immobilization causes a greater atrophy of type I fibres than of type II fibres in vastus lateralis.

The effect of immobilization on the atrophy of type I and type II fibres has also been investigated in triceps muscle (MacDougall 1986, MacDougall et al 1980). Two studies have investigated type I and II atrophy following elbow immobilization and found greater reduction in type II fibres (MacDougall 1986, MacDougall et al 1980). Following 6 weeks of elbow immobilization there was a 38% reduction in cross-sectional area of type II fibres and a 31% reduction in type I fibres (MacDougall 1986). In a similar study, 5–6 weeks of elbow immobilization resulted in a 33% reduction in type II fibres and a 25% reduction in type I fibres (MacDougall et al 1980). In the triceps muscles it appears that immobilization causes greater atrophy in type II fibres than in type I fibres.

From the above studies on vastus lateralis and triceps muscles it appears that muscle fibre types in different muscles respond slightly differently to immobilization. While the proportional atrophy of type I fibres and II fibres differs in vastus lateralis and triceps, the magnitude of the difference is, in all cases, less than 9%, which seems quite a small difference.

Reduced muscle endurance

Reduced muscle endurance may be manifested by a reduced ability to repeat a contraction, or a reduced ability to hold an isometric contraction over a period of time (McArdle et al 2000). In order to avoid testing muscle strength it is suggested that the resistance is sufficiently low to allow 15–20 repetitions.

More general cardiovascular endurance training such as distance running, swimming or cycling, involves measurements of volume and composition of expired air to reflect oxygen uptake and heart rate. An improvement in endurance is reflected, for the same relative amount of work:

- in reduced oxygen uptake and reduced heart rate

- a reduced sense of effort (Borg 1982)
- an ability to continue for longer
- an ability to increase the number of repetitions in the same time period (Newham 2001).

Altered motor control

Aspects of altered motor control include:

- muscle inhibition
- timing of onset
- increased muscle activation
- altered activation of agonist and antagonist.

Muscle inhibition

Muscle inhibition may be identified by the clinician by visual and/or palpatory cues. While these methods are clearly practical in the clinical setting and require no special equipment, they may have questionable reliability. Some muscles are superficial and may be relatively easy to identify – for example sternocleidomastoid; the vast majority of muscles overlap with other muscles or lie deep underneath a whole muscle, so that identification of these muscles is extremely difficult, if not impossible. This has led to the development of instrumentation to help the clinician identify muscle inhibition; it includes ultrasound imaging (Hides et al 1995) and EMG biofeedback (Richardson et al 1999). In research, voluntary muscle activity can be measured using the interpolated twitch technique (ITT) and involuntary muscle activity by a reduction in the Hoffman (H)-reflex.

The ITT involves applying a single electrical twitch to a nerve during a maximal isometric contraction and indicates the motor unit activity (Gandevia et al 1998, Hales & Gandevia 1988, Rutherford et al 1986), although a high-frequency train of stimuli is considered to be a more sensitive measure than the single twitch (Kent-Braun & Le Blanc 1996). A dynamometer measures muscle torque during the active contraction, and if there is full motor unit activity then the addition of nerve stimulation will not produce any increase in torque. Any increase in torque (referred to as 'interpolated twitch torque' (Suter & Herzog 2000)) indicates muscle inhibition due to incomplete activation.

In asymptomatic subjects, the ITT will produce, on average, a 4% increase in isometric quadriceps muscle torque at 90 degrees flexion (Suter et al 1996). It should be noted that the extent of muscle inhibition measured by the ITT is dependent on the joint angle; at 60 degrees, knee flexion muscle inhibition is three times greater than with the knee in extension (Suter & Herzog 1997).

Involuntary muscle activity is measured by a reduction in the Hoffman (H)-reflex, indicating an inhibition of the alpha motor neurone pool (Iles et al 1990, Spencer et al 1984). The H-reflex is a small muscle contraction (via alpha motor neurones) in response to low-intensity stimulation of a mixed nerve (via stimulation of group 1a fibres from muscle spindles). This reflex inhibition continues to be present during active contraction of the muscle (Iles et al 1990).

Both acute and chronic joint pathology, effusion, pain and immobilization have been found to lead to inhibition of the overlying muscle, a response sometimes referred to as arthrogenous muscle inhibition (Stokes & Young 1984). All of the research studies identified in Box 5.8 have been carried out on the knee, apart from those on rheumatoid arthritis of the elbow joint. The muscle inhibition of an active voluntary contraction seems to be related to the extent of the joint damage: the greater the injury the greater the inhibition of muscle (Newham et al 1989, Urbach & Awiszus 2002).

The presence of pain can cause muscle inhibition (Arvidsson et al 1986, Rutherford et al 1986), although the mechanism is not fully understood. It has been suggested that muscle inhibition can be due to inhibitory input (Iles et al 1990, Shakespeare et al 1985, Snyder-Mackler et al 1994, Suter & Herzog 2000, Torry et al 2000) or abnormal input (Hurley & Newham 1993) from joint afferents, which reduces the motor drive to muscles acting over the joint.

The presence of effusion can cause muscle inhibition. This inhibition has been found by measuring a voluntary active contraction (deAndrade et al 1965, Wood L et al 1988), using

Box 5.8	Possible causes of arthrogenic muscle inhibition

Causes	Reference
Rheumatoid arthritis of knee	deAndrade et al 1965
Rheumatoid arthritis of the elbow	Hurley et al 1991
Osteoarthritis (knee joint) with no pain or effusion	deAndrade et al 1965, Hurley & Newham 1993
Articular cartilage	Suter et al 1998a
Degeneration of the patellar or tibial plateau	
Sub-periosteal tumour of the femur	Stener 1969
Anterior knee pain	Suter et al 1998b
	Suter et al 1998a
Muscle pain	Rutherford et al 1986
Ligamentous knee injuries without pain or effusion	DeVita et al 1997
	Hurley et al 1992
	Hurley et al 1994 Newham et al 1989 Snyder-Mackler et al 1994 Urbach & Awiszus 2002
Post-meniscectomy (knee joint)	Hurley et al 1994
	Shakespeare et al 1985
	Stokes & Young 1984
	Suter et al 1998a
Presence of pain	Arvidsson et al 1986
	Rutherford et al 1986
Effusion of the knee joint	deAndrade et al 1965 Fahrer et al 1988
	Iles et al 1990 Jones et al 1987 Kennedy et al 1982
	Spencer et al 1984
	Stratford 1981
	Wood L et al 1988
Anterior cruciate ligament	Hurley et al 1994 Newham, Hurley & Jones 1989
Deficiency of the knee joint	Snyder-Mackler et al 1994
	Suter et al 1998a
	Suter et al 1998b
Immobilization	Vaughan 1989

the H-reflex (Iles et al 1990, Spencer et al 1984), measuring EMG activity (Torry et al 2000), and by using the interpolated twitch technique (Fahrer et al 1988). One study found that a knee effusion had no effect on quadriceps strength or power (McNair et al 1994).

The effect of knee joint effusion and muscle inhibition has a marked effect on gait (Berchuck et al 1990, Torry et al 2000). This inhibition is thought to be due to increased intra-articular pressure causing an increase in tension in the joint capsule that stimulates mechanoreceptors in the intra-capsular receptors and causes a reflex inhibition of the alpha motor neurone pool (Iles et al 1990, Spencer et al 1984, Torry et al 2000). The inhibition is thought to affect both the voluntary and involuntary muscle activity.

In experimentally produced effusion there is a linear relationship between the volume of the effusion and the reduction in the H-reflex amplitude, that is, the greater the effusion the greater the muscle inhibition (Iles et al 1990, Spencer et al 1984). In chronic effusions, associated with arthritis, the degree of effusion is not related to the amount of inhibition (Jones et al 1987). In one study an effusion immediately caused inhibition of rectus femoris (Iles et al 1990), while 50–60 ml was needed in another study to inhibit rectus femoris and vastus lateralis and between 20 and 30 ml to inhibit vastus medialis (Spencer et al 1984).

With experimentally induced knee joint effusion, aspiration reduces the muscle inhibition (Spencer et al 1984), whereas in chronic or recurrent knee joint effusions muscle inhibition remains the same post-aspiration (Jones et al 1987). The amount of inhibition of the muscle is related to the angle of the joint, with greater inhibition occurring with the knee in extension than in flexion (Jones et al 1987, Krebs et al 1983, Shakespeare et al 1983, Stokes & Young 1984). This is thought to be due to the difference in intra-articular pressure, which is greater in full extension than in a few degrees of flexion (Levick 1983).

There has been some suggestion that the heads of a muscle are inhibited separately, that is, there is selective inhibition. One study found greater inhibition of vastus medialis than vastus lateralis or rectus femoris following effusion of the knee joint, although only 10 subjects were investigated (Kennedy et al 1982). Another study found all heads of the quadriceps inhibited following knee joint effusion (Spencer et al 1984).

Interestingly, a number of studies have found that muscle inhibition is not just restricted to the local muscles but also occurs in the contralateral limb (Hurley & Newham 1993, Hurley et al 1994, Newham et al 1989, Suter et al 1998a, 1998b, Urbach & Awiszus 2002). The clinician needs to be aware of this when comparing muscle function on the side of injury with the unaffected side as the degree of inhibition may be underestimated. The reason for the change on the unaffected side is unclear, it has been suggested to be due to altered movement patterns (Berchuck et al 1990, Frank et al 1994). Another explanation may be the connection of nerve pathways in the spinal cord.

In rats, experimental injury to one paw produces hyperalgesia and swelling on the opposite side (Levine et al 1985a), a response known as reflex neurogenic inflammation (Levine et al 1985b). It should be noted that research in this area has been restricted to rats, and the effects have not yet been demonstrated in humans.

Timing of onset

The timing of onset of muscles activation during movement and functional activities has been identified in patients. Patients with chronic low back pain have exhibited delayed activation of transversus abdominis muscle when asked to perform rapid arm movements (Hodges & Richardson 1996). There was also a significant ($P <0.05$) delayed activation found in the internal oblique, external oblique and rectus abdominis muscles during rapid shoulder flexion (Hodges & Richardson 1996).

Altered timing of the vastus medialis oblique relative to the vastus lateralis has been identified in patients with anterior knee pain (Cowan et al 2002, Voight & Wieder 1991). It was found that, in normal subjects, the reflex response of vastus medialis preceded the vastus lateralis but in the patient group this was reversed: vastus lateralis was activated before vastus medialis oblique (Voight & Wieder 1991, Witvrouw et al 1996).

It should be noted that there are normal age-related changes in the activation of muscles. For example, with age there is increased coactivation of quadriceps and hamstring muscle groups during a step-down movement (Hortobagyi & DeVita 2000). In addition, older subjects have been found to have a delay in muscle activation in the lower limb when stepping to regain balance during a fall (Thelen et al 2000).

Increased muscle activation

Increased muscle activation is brought about by an increase in the activation of the alpha motor neurone pool supplying the muscle. The alpha motor neurone pool can be activated by the central nervous system, as part of motor control, or by peripheral input from muscle spindles, skin, joint, nerve and muscle afferents, including nociceptors. The underlying causes are therefore wide-ranging, and could include the perception of pain, as well as joint, nerve or muscle dysfunction.

Baseball players with known elbow medial collateral ligament insufficiency have been found to have increased EMG activity of extensor carpi radialis longus and brevis and reduced EMG activity of triceps, flexor carpi radialis (FCR) and pronator teres compared to a control group (Glousman et al 1992). Flexor carpi radialis and pronator teres might have been expected to demonstrate increased activity to compensate for the ligamentous insufficiency but this was not the case.

Baseball players with known anterior shoulder instability have been found to have reduced EMG activity of pectoralis major, subscapularis, latissimus dorsi and serratus anterior and increased activity of biceps and supraspinatus compared to a control group (Glousman et al 1988). The authors postulate that the reduced muscle activity exacerbates the anterior shoulder instability while the increased activity of biceps and supraspinatus compensates for the anterior instability.

This compensation or protective mechanism has also been suggested in another study that found increased EMG activity of biceps femoris, vastus lateralis and tibialis anterior in patients with an ACL-deficient knee (Cicotti et al 1994).

Experiments on the rabbit, cat and rat have identified that sympathetic efferent activity causes an increase in muscle tone (Passatore et al 1985). There was an increase in activity, and decrease in position sensitivity, of the muscle spindle. This suggests that the increase in muscle tone was due to contraction of the intrafusal fibres of the muscle spindle and some extrafusal fibres.

Altered activation of agonist and antagonist

This alteration in the relative activation of agonist and antagonist can result from the above consequences of increased or decreased muscle activation. In addition to these dysfunctions, there is also evidence of a specific alteration in the agonist and antagonist activation patterns.

Pain around the knee causes a nociceptive flexor withdrawal response: hip and knee flexion and ankle dorsiflexion. To produce this movement there is increased alpha motor neurone excitability of the hip and knee flexors and ankle dorsiflexors (Stener & Peterson 1963) and reciprocal inhibition of the knee extensors (Stener 1969, Stener & Peterson 1963, Young et al 1987). Stener and Peterson (1963) observed that pressure or tension on a partially ruptured medial collateral ligament resulted in increased muscle activity of sartorius and semimembranosus (knee flexors) with inhibition of vastus medialis (knee extensor). Stener (1969) found that pain over the lateral femoral epicondyle caused inhibition of the vastus medialis and lateralis.

Patients with more chronic ACL deficiency (16 months–21 years) have been found to have less quadriceps and gastrocnemius activity and greater hamstring activity during the stance

phase, and increased hamstring activity during the swing phase of gait (Branch et al 1989). In another study of patients with chronic ACL deficiency (2–3 years), horizontal walking failed to show any difference in EMG activity of quadriceps and hamstrings but on walking uphill the hamstring muscle was activated much earlier compared to control subjects (Kalund et al 1990). Patients with a ACL-deficient knee following 6 months' rehabilitation continued to have increased EMG activity of vastus lateralis, biceps femoris and tibialis anterior muscles during functional movements, compared to a control group (Ciccotti et al 1994).

A number of studies have demonstrated that chronic anterior cruciate ligament (ACL) deficiency and post-ACL reconstruction causes an alteration of the motor control around the knee (Beard et al 1996, Berchuck et al 1990, Branch et al 1989, Ciccotti et al 1994, DeVita et al 1997, Kalund et al 1990). Patients who have had an ACL reconstruction were found to have an altered gait pattern such that, compared to control subjects, the knee was in more flexion at heel contact and mid stance, and a greater range of extensor torque was present during the stance phase (DeVita et al 1997). Patients with chronic ACL deficiency, longer than 6 months without repair, were found to walk with the knee in more flexion at heel contact and mid-stance and this correlated with an increased duration of hamstring activity (Beard et al 1996).

A clinical observation of the reaction of muscle to pain has been described (Janda 1985). It has been suggested that postural (or tonic) muscles become hypertonic and short, while phasic muscles are thought to become hypotonic and weak. Muscle shortness describes a muscle which, when inactive, has a length less than normal and limits the full range of joint movement (Schmid & Spring 1985). Janda (1985), however, uses the classification system that a muscle is either postural or phasic (Box 5.9), which is difficult because it is a rather flawed classification system. The vast majority of muscles contain equal proportions of type I and type II muscle fibres and therefore cannot easily be divided into these two categories.

Box 5.9 The reaction of postural and phasic muscles to pain (Janda 1985)

Postural muscles which become tight, short or hypertonic	Phasic muscles which become inhibited, weak and hypotonic
Soleus	
Gastrocnemius	Tibialis anterior
Tibialis posterior	The vasti
Rectus femoris	Glutei
Iliopsoas	Rectus abdominis
Tensor fascia lata	Lower stabilizers of the scapula
Hamstrings	Deep neck flexors
Short hip adductors	Extensors of the upper extremity
Quadratus lumborum	
Piriformis	
Part of paravertebral back muscles	
Pectoralis major	
Sternocleidomastoid	
Upper trapezius	
Levator scapula	

There is, nevertheless, some evidence to support the muscle reaction proposed by Janda (1985). For example, pain around the knee has been found to cause increased activation of the hip flexors, which might be assumed to include rectus femoris and iliopsoas (Stener & Peterson 1963), and increased activation of the knee flexors (Stener & Peterson 1963), which would mean the hamstring group, and inhibition of the knee extensors (Stener 1969, Stener & Peterson 1963, Young et al 1987), which can be assumed to include the vasti. This research therefore supports the contention that rectus femoris, iliopsoas and hamstrings tend to react to pain by becoming hypertonic and the vasti react by being hypotonic.

Research supports the observation that the deep neck flexor muscles become hypotonic and weak (Janda 1985). Patients with recurrent headaches were found to have reduced isometric strength and endurance of the deep neck flexors, compared to a control group (Watson 1994).

Finally, arm pain produced by an upper limb tension test (ULTT2a, Butler 2000) in asymptomatic subjects was found to be associated with an increase in EMG activity of the upper fibres of trapezius (van der Heide, Allison & Zusman 2001). This provides further support to the observation of Janda (1985) that the upper trapezius muscle reacts to pain by becoming hypertonic.

Altered muscle length

The most obvious reduction in muscle length is seen following immobilization of a joint, with the muscle held in a shortened position. In this situation the muscle will be shortened and will have an increased resistance to passive lengthening (Goldspink 1976, Goldspink & Williams 1979, Tabary et al 1972). Upon removal of the immobilization, in the cat soleus muscle, the muscle returns to its original length within 4 weeks (Goldspink 1976, Tabary et al 1972).

When muscle is immobilized in a lengthened position it increases the number of sarcomeres and thus becomes longer; there is no change in resistance to passive lengthening. Again, on removal of the immobilization, in the cat and mouse, the muscle quickly returns to its original length (Tabary et al 1972, Williams & Goldspink 1976).

Muscle length can be measured by lengthening muscle fully and measuring the final joint angle using a goniometer, or by visual estimation. The passive resistance of muscle to lengthening is more difficult to measure. The clinician can passively lengthen the muscle and estimate the 'feel' of the resistance to movement or the muscle can be more objectively measured using isokinetic equipment.

Production of symptoms

Symptoms from muscle dysfunction are commonly a pain or an ache. Symptoms may be felt when the muscle is at rest, when it is lengthened or when it contracts. The clinician attempts to obtain an accurate assessment of the behaviour of symptoms with each of these tests (palpation, length and contraction) so that they can be used as a sensitive measure on reassessment of the patient. If symptoms are produced when a muscle is lengthened, the detailed behaviour of when the symptom is first produced during the movement P_1, and what happens to its intensity with any continued movement P_2 or P', can be depicted on a movement diagram (Petty & Moore 2001). The symptom may be sufficiently intense to be the cause of the limitation in range, depicted as P_2 on a movement diagram (Fig. 5.38A), or may reach a particular intensity at the limit of range P', spoken as 'p prime' (Fig. 5.38B). Symptoms may be produced in muscle with 'normal' or hypomobile range of movement, with or without altered quality of movement.

Before discussing muscle pain a distinction needs to be made between nociception and pain. Nociception is the transmission of impulses from nociceptors that occurs with tissue damage. This activation, however, does not necessarily lead to pain being felt. The perception of pain occurs within the central nervous system (Grieve 1994) and is more than simply the sensation and physiological effects of tissue damage (Fig. 5.39); it also includes affective factors such as mood and emotion, cognitive factors such as beliefs and knowledge, behavioural factors such as posture and analgesic intake, and socio-cultural factors such as age, gender and ethnicity (Ahles & Martin 1992, McGuire 1985).

Pain has therefore been defined as 'an unpleasant sensory and emotional experience associated with actual or potential tissue damage, or described in terms of such damage' (Merskey et al 1979). This is not an entirely new idea: Descartes (1985) in the 17th century recognized that pain was accompanied by sadness. He wrote that the body is 'ill-disposed when I feel pain', while unclear of the relationship between 'the thing which causes pain and the sense of sadness to which this feeling gives rise'. In 1940 the classical Christian scholar C.S Lewis attempted to unravel the meaning of pain (Lewis 1998), describing it as 'any experience, whether physical or mental, that the patient dislikes and is

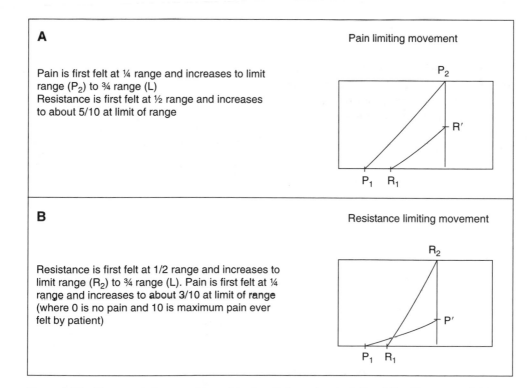

Figure 5.38 Movement diagram of hamstring length in supine depicting **A** P_2 with some resistance and normal range, and **B** P' and resistance limiting movement.

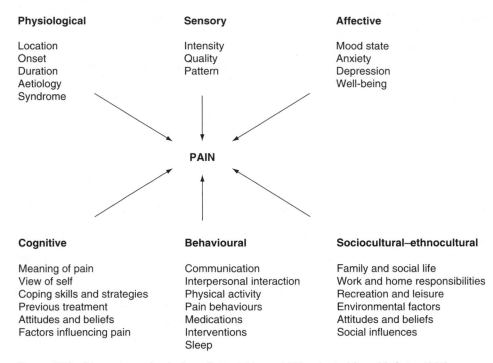

Figure 5.39 Dimensions of pain (from Petty & Moore 2001, adapted from McGuire 1995).

synonymous with suffering, anguish, tribulation, adversity and trouble'; he clearly associated pain with effects on emotion and thought. Indeed, what person has ever felt indifferent when experiencing pain? Most, if not all, of us will be able to testify to the sense of suffering and to an emotional response that goes hand in hand with the experience of pain. Pain is an extensive subject and cannot be covered comprehensively in this text. The reader is referred to a number of excellent books on pain, most notably a text by Wall and Melzack (1999). What follows here is an overview of how tissue damage in a joint can cause nociception and potentially cause a person to perceive pain.

The perception of pain affects the sympathetic nervous system, which has widespread effects on the respiratory, cardiovascular, gastrointestinal and genitourinary systems, and endocrine and metabolic function (Cousins & Power 2002); these effects are summarized in Box 5.10.

Box 5.10 The effect of acute pain on respiratory, cardiovascular, gastrointestinal and genitourinary systems, and endocrine and metabolic function (Cousins & Power 1999)	
Respiratory	Splinting of abdominal and thoracic muscles
	Grunting on expiration
	Small tidal volume
	Rapid respiratory rate
Cardiovascular	Increased heart rate
	Increased blood pressure
	Increased cardiac output
	Decreased blood flow in the limbs
Gastrointestinal and genitourinary	Increased intestinal secretions
	Increased smooth muscle tone
	Reduced intestinal motility
	Urinary retention
Endocrine and metabolic function	Nausea, vomiting
	Altered metabolic rate

Free nerve endings supplied by group III and IV afferents can be found throughout muscle. They lie in the connective tissue, in between the intrafusal and extrafusal fibres, in arterioles and venules, in the capsule of muscle spindles and tendon organs, in tendon tissue at the musculo-tendinous junction and in fat cells (Reinert & Mense 1992, Stacey 1969). Muscle can therefore be a primary source of pain. Both A delta and C fibres can be activated by noxious thermal, mechanical and chemical stimuli (Kaufman et al 1982, Kumazawa & Mizumura 1977, Mense 1996). The latter two, noxious mechanical and chemical forms of irritation, are the probable causes in patients with muscle pain seen in the musculoskeletal field. The pain from muscle can therefore be classified as mechanical or chemical nociceptive pain (Gifford 1998).

Mechanical pain occurs where certain movements stress injured tissue, increasing the mechanical deformation and activation of nociceptors; other movements may reduce the stress on injured tissue, reducing the mechanical deformation and activation of nociceptors (Box 5.11). Thus, with mechanical pain, there are particular movements which aggravate and ease the pain, sometimes referred to as 'on/off' pain. The magnitude of the mechanical deformation may be directly related to the magnitude of nociceptor activity; this has been found in the skin of the cat where greater forces cause greater nociceptor activity (Garell et al 1996).

Chemical nociceptive pain can be produced by the chemicals released as a result of inflamma-tion, ischaemia or sympathetic nervous system activity (Gifford 1998).

Experimentally induced inflammation of muscle in the cat and rat has been shown to cause an increased irregular resting discharge in both group III and IV afferents in muscle (Berberich et al 1988, Diehl et al 1988). This increased resting discharge or sensitization produces primary hyperalgesia (Raja et al 1999). In addition, inflammation was found to lower the mechanical threshold of group IV afferents and is the probable cause of muscle tenderness on palpation (Berberich et al 1988, Diehl et al 1988), a response known as allodynia (Raja et al 1999). An increase in the levels of substance P from muscle afferent fibres has been found to initiate background activity of muscle nociceptors (Reinert et al 1992); thus, with muscle injury, substance P may, in part, be responsible for muscle pain (Mense 1996, Reinert et al 1992).

Clinical features of inflammatory pain are: redness, oedema and heat, acute pain and tissue damage, a close relationship of stimulus response and pain, a diurnal pattern with pain and stiffness worst at night and in the morning, signs of neurogenic inflammation (redness, swelling or symptoms in the neural zone) and a beneficial effect of anti-inflammatory medication (Butler 2000).

Ischaemic nociceptive pain in muscle is not yet fully understood (Mense 1996). It may be related to chemical irritation (Moore et al 1934), build-up of potassium ions (Harpuder & Stein 1943), lack

---

Box 5.11 Clinical features of mechanical, inflammatory and ischaemic nociceptive pain (Butler 2000)

Mechanical pain	Particular movements that aggravate and ease the pain, sometimes referred to as 'on/off pain'
Inflammatory pain	Redness, oedema and heat
	Acute pain and tissue damage
	Close relationship of stimulus response and pain
	Diurnal pattern with pain and stiffness worst at night and in the morning
	Signs of neurogenic inflammation (redness, swelling or symptoms in neural zone)
	Beneficial effect of anti-inflammatory medication
Ischaemic pain	Symptoms produced after prolonged or unusual activities
	Rapid ease of symptoms after a change in posture
	Symptoms towards the end of the day or after the accumulation of activity
	Poor response to anti-inflammatory medication
	Absence of trauma

of oxidation of metabolic products (Pickering & Wayne 1933–1934) or the presence of bradykinin (Nakahara 1971). Experimentally induced ischaemia of muscle activated only 10% of muscle nociceptors. However, when a muscle contracts under ischaemic conditions there is much stronger activation of group IV nociceptors (Kaufman et al 1984b, Mense & Stahnke 1983). With muscle hypoxia there is an increase in group III and IV mechanoreceptor and nociceptor afferent activity (Kieschke et al 1988). The underlying mechanism of ischaemic contraction causing nociceptor activity appears to be related to chemical sensitization of muscle nociceptors (Mense 1996).

Clinical features of ischaemic pain are thought to be: symptoms produced after prolonged or unusual activities, rapid ease of symptoms after a change in posture, symptoms towards the end of the day or after the accumulation of activity, a poor response to anti-inflammatory medication and sometimes absence of trauma (Butler 2000).

The sympathetic nervous system can cause pain. Increased concentrations of adrenaline (epinephrine) in muscle causes an increased discharge frequency of muscle nociceptors, and this response is enhanced with the addition of noxious mechanical stimulation (Kieschke et al 1988). In the presence of tissue injury or inflammation, sympathetic nervous system activity can maintain the perception of pain or enhance nociception in inflamed tissue (Raja et al 1999). Sympathetically maintained pain can occur with complex regional pain syndromes and may play a part in chronic arthritis and soft-tissue trauma (Raja et al 1999). Thus, it appears that the sympathetic nervous system can cause muscle pain.

The effect of nociceptor activity by a mechanical or chemical stimulus alters the physiology of the nociceptor itself; in this way the nociceptor is plastic: it alters according to its environment. Nociceptor activity causes an increased sensitivity of the nociceptors so there is a lower threshold for response, an increased response to a supra-threshold stimuli, and spontaneous activity (Raja et al 1999). For example, 5-hydroxytryptamine and prostaglandin E_2 cause sensitization of group IV afferents that are sensitive to these substances (Mense 1981). This increased sensitivity of nociceptors leads to a decreased pain threshold, an increased pain to supra-threshold stimuli, and spontaneous pain – changes collectively referred to as primary hyperalgesia. If a stimulus is applied which would normally not provoke pain, such as movement or a light touch, and pain is provoked, then this is termed allodynia (Raja et al 1999). In addition, mechanoreceptors in adjacent uninjured tissue develop the ability to evoke pain, a phenomenon known as secondary hyperalgesia (Raja et al 1999). It is thought to be due to an increase in the responsiveness of second-order nociceptor neurones in the spinal cord that become activated by mechanoreceptor activity, a response known as central sensitization (Raja et al 1999).

Constant experimentally induced muscle pain in humans has been found to cause an increase in the stretch reflex of the relaxed muscle, suggesting that muscle pain increases the sensitivity of the muscle spindle to stretch (Matre et al 1998). In the same study, muscle pain did not alter the H-reflex, suggesting that muscle pain does not directly alter the sensitivity of alpha motor neurone activity, although it may have an indirect effect by causing a reduction in descending inhibition on the alpha motor neurone activity and thus cause an increase in the stretch reflex (Matre et al 1999). Inducing muscle pain also increases the stretch reflex of the antagonist muscle group; pain in tibialis anterior increases the stretch reflex of soleus (Matre et al 1998). The increased stretch reflex induced by muscle pain is present only when the muscle is relaxed – there is no change in stretch reflex during an isometric muscle contraction or during walking (Matre et al 1999).

Muscle pain is thought to have a greater inhibitory effect upon low-threshold motor units supplying type I fibres than high-threshold motor units supplying type II muscle fibres (Gydikov 1976). If this is correct then it can be speculated that pain over the soleus muscle, for example, which has a high proportion of type I fibres, would have a greater effect than pain in a muscle that has a more even distribution of fibre types.

It should be noted that the information given here has focused on pain from muscle tissue only. Clearly, pain may be felt from a number of tissues, including the skin, joint and nerve overlying the joint. Joint pain is discussed in the chapter on function and dysfunction of joints, and pain from skin and nerve is discussed in the chapter on function and dysfunction of nerves.

Referral of pain from muscle

In the upper and lower limbs, muscle pain is often felt over the joint that the muscle moves, provided that the joint has the same segmental innervation as the muscle (Kellgren 1939). Some generalizations can be made about the pattern of pain referral from muscle. The segmental distribution of muscle is given in Figure 5.40.

An early investigation of referred pain from muscle was made by Kellgren in 1938. Observations of pain referral were made following noxious injection of saline into muscle in three asymptomatic co-workers. The chart of pain referral for various muscles is shown in Figure 5.41. The study investigated differences in the quality of pain from muscle, from tendon and from fascia. Fascia and tendon tended to produce sharp localized pain, while muscle tended to produce some localized pain and a diffuse referred pain with tenderness of structures deep to the skin.

The limb muscles are generally innervated by more than one spinal segment; for example, infraspinatus is supplied by C5 and C6 and this produces more widespread area of referral than the dermatome areas for skin (Kellgren 1938). Pain from muscle appears to be referred to regions corresponding to the spinal segments from which it obtains its motor supply; this is clearer in the upper limb than in the lower limb (Kellgren 1938).

Pain from muscle may be poorly localized to muscle; for example, pain from flexor digitorum profundus may refer to the metacarpophalangeal joint, and when this joint is injected the pain is considered to be very similar to that from the muscle (Kellgren 1938). In the same way, pain from the lumbar erector spine muscle produces pain similar to that caused by injection of the gluteal fascia. Some muscles, such as rectus abdominis and muscles in the hand, are much more sensitive and produce more severe pain than biceps brachii and glutei muscles. Metabolic muscle disease, in contrast, typically causes pain that the patient is able to locate as 'in the muscle'; it is not vague and does not refer (Petty 2003).

Referred pain from muscle has also been investigated by another group of researchers (Feinstein et al 1954). Injection of saline (6%) into the paravertebral muscles (immediately on either side of the mid-line) at each segmental level of the spine resulted in referral maps obtained from five subjects (Fig. 5.42). The pain was described as a deep ache that was 'boring', 'heavy', 'crampy' or 'lumpy'. The intensity of pain was related to the amount of saline that was injected – greater amounts caused more pain. Injection of the thoracic paravertebral muscles was also accompanied by autonomic symptoms of pallor and sweating, and sometimes bradycardia, reduced blood pressure, faintness and nausea.

Injection of saline (6%) into peripheral muscles was also carried out on three to four subjects (Fig. 5.43). The muscles injected were serratus anterior, infraspinatus, pectoralis major, brachialis, flexor carpi ulnaris and extensor digitorum. The area of pain spread variable distances from the injection site. In most cases of spinal and peripheral injection the pain was accompanied by deep tenderness and skin hypoalgesia (diminished pin prick sensation) and in some cases by muscle spasm.

Referred pain from muscle has been more recently investigated by stimulating the median nerve fascicles innervating muscles in the forearm and hand (Torebjork et al 1984). Intraneural stimulation of the median nerve at the elbow gave rise to an aching cramp-like pain deep in the forearm and thumb, and in 50% of cases (13 of 26) superficial pain over the hand. In some subjects there was also referred pain, that is, pain felt outside the innervation area of the median nerve, with deep cramp-like pain felt in the upper arm, axilla or mammillary region (Torebjork et al 1984). The results of this study support the existence of

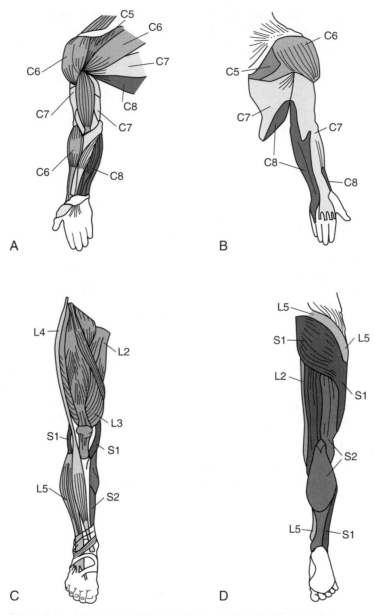

Figure 5.40 Myotomes of **A** upper limb, anterior view, **B** upper limb, posterior view, **C** lower limb, anterior view, and **D** lower limb, posterior view (after Inman & Saunders 1944, Referred pain from skeletal structures. Journal of Nervous and Mental Disease 99:660–667, with permission).

myotomes (Inman & Saunders 1944). This study also provided the interesting observation that dysfunction of the median nerve at the elbow may refer pain proximally to the upper arm, axilla and mammillary region.

In a similar study, stimulation of muscle nociceptors of the common peroneal nerve also produced a deep cramp-like pain (Simone et al 1994). Stimulation of tendon nociceptors produced a sharp and localized pain (Simone et al 1994).

Text continues on page 208

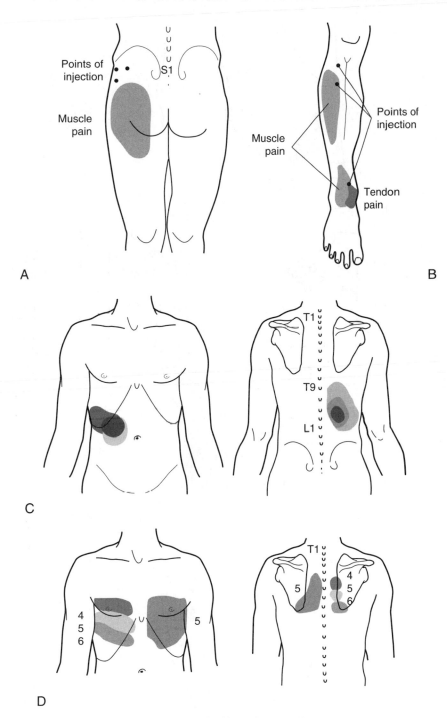

Figure 5.41   Referred pain from muscle. (Reproduced, with permission, from Kellgren J H 1938 Clinical Science 3:175–190 © The Biochemical Society and the Medical Research Society.) **A** Gluteus medius. **B** Tiblalis anterior; stippling is tendon pain. **C** Horizontal hatching from multifidus, vertical hatching from intercostals & stippling from rectus abdominis. **D** From 4th, 5th and 6th intercostal muscles.

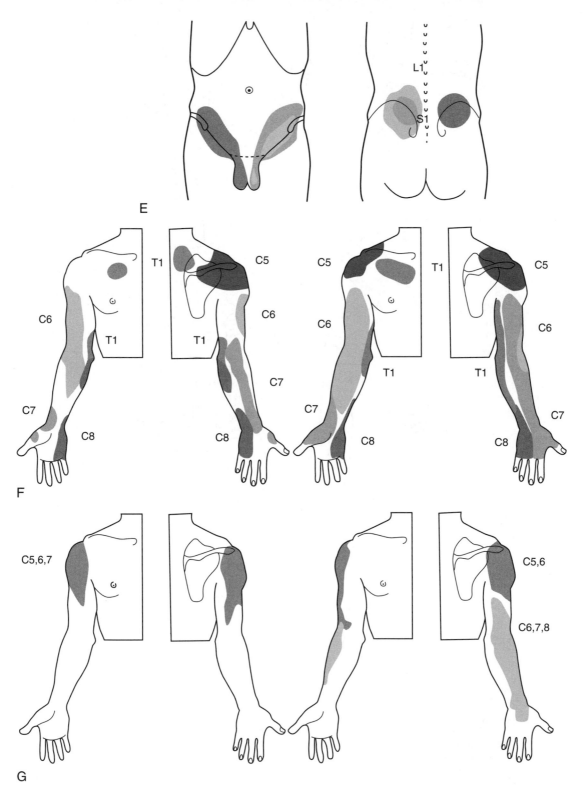

Figure 5.41 *(Cont'd)*

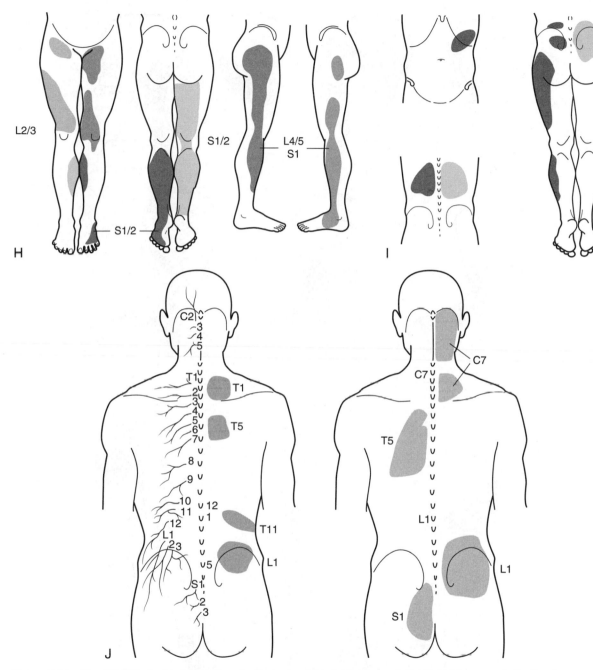

Figure 5.41 *(Cont'd)* **E** Vertical hatching from testis, horizontal hatching from abdominal obliques and stippling from multifidus. **F** Crosses from rhomboids, oblique hatching from flexor carpi radialis, stippling from abductor pollicis longus, vertical hatching from third dorsal interosseous, horizontal hatching from first intercostals space. **G** Vertical hatching from serratus anterior, oblique hatching from infraspinatus & stippling from latissimus dorsi. **H** Left leg with oblique hatching from adductor longus from, right leg with oblique hatching from sartorius, vertical hatching from gastrocnemius, horizontal hatching from first interosseous, crosses from tensor fascia lata and stippling from peroneus longus. **I** Vertical hatching from erector spinae & horizontal hatching from multifidus stimulated opposite T9 and L5. **J** Left figure represents anterior aspect of erector spinae and right figure posterior aspect of erector spinae at the spinal level indicated.

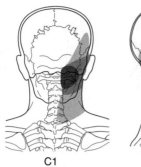
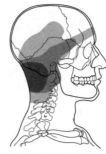
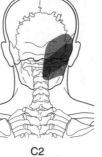
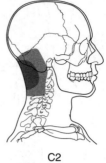

C1   C1   C2   C2

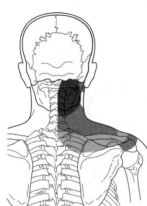
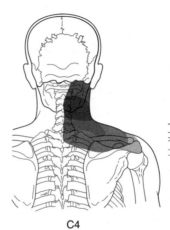

C3   C4   C5

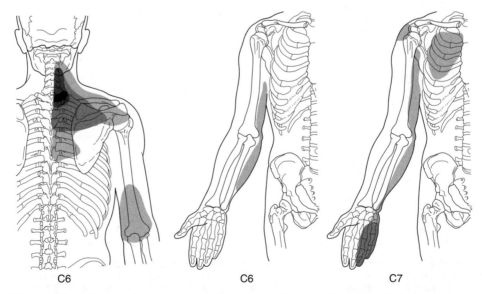

C6   C6   C7

Figure 5.42 Referred pain from paravertebral muscle. The area of pain from five subjects is superimposed. (From Feinstein et al 1954, Experiments on pain referred from deep somatic tissues. Journal of Bone and Joint Surgery 36(A)5:981–997, with permission, © The Journal of Bone and Joint Surgery, Inc.)

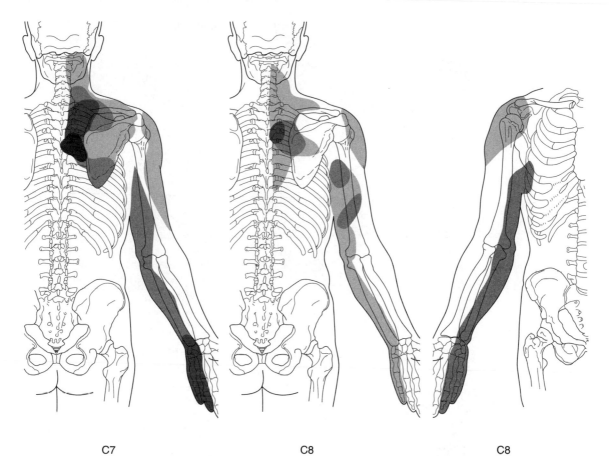

C7   C8   C8

Figure 5.42   (*Cont'd*)

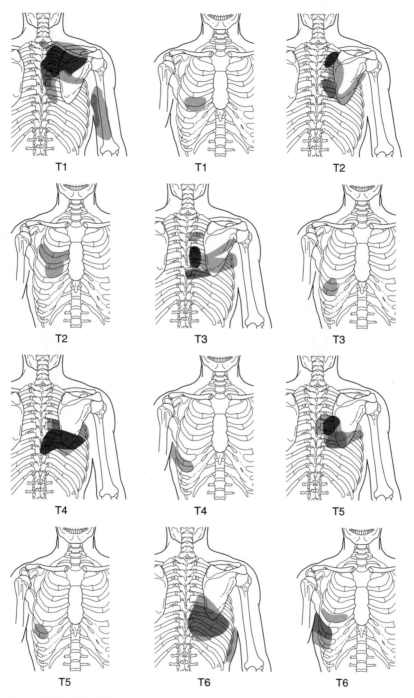

T1 T1 T2

T2 T3 T3

T4 T4 T5

T5 T6 T6

Figure 5.42 (Cont'd)

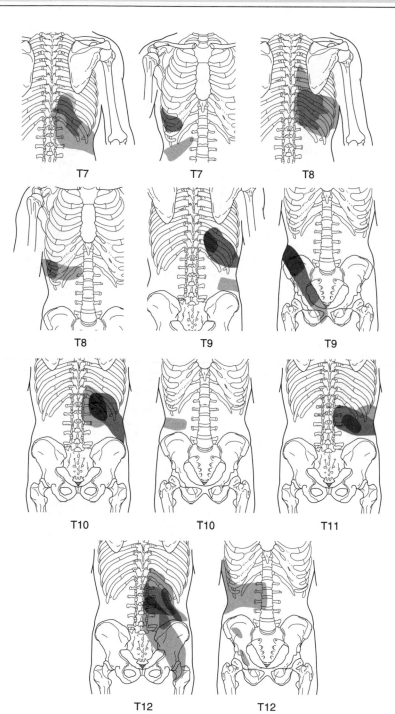

Figure 5.42 *(Cont'd)*

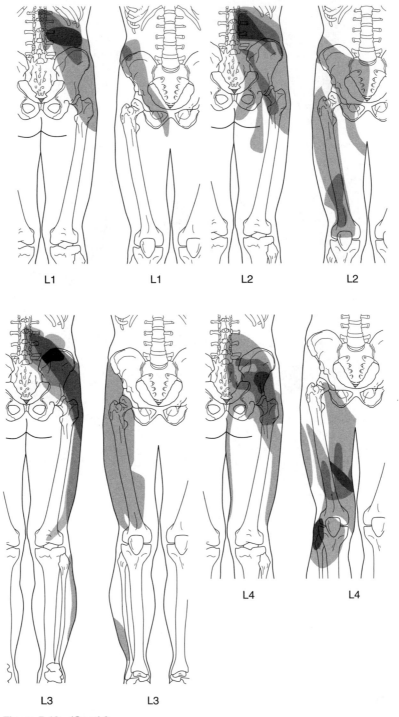

L1   L1   L2   L2

L3   L3   L4   L4

Figure 5.42 (Cont'd)

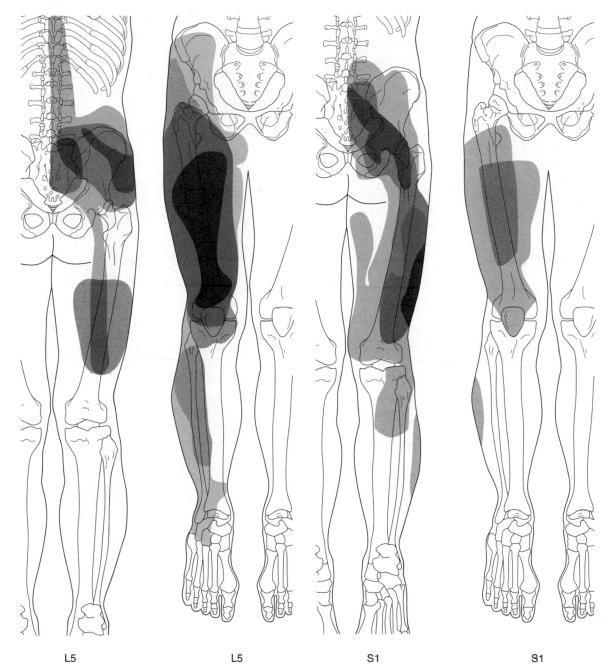

L5   L5   S1   S1

Figure 5.42   (*Cont'd*)

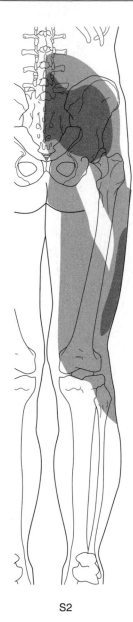
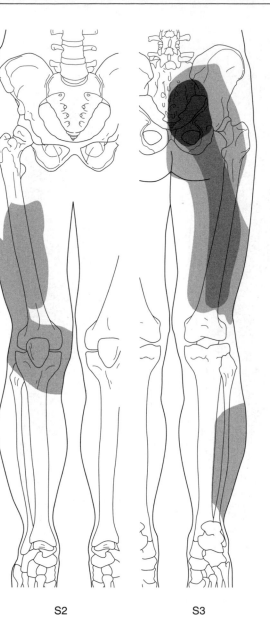
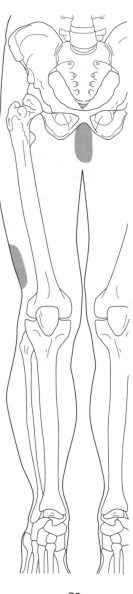

S2   S2   S3   S3

Figure 5.42   (Cont'd)

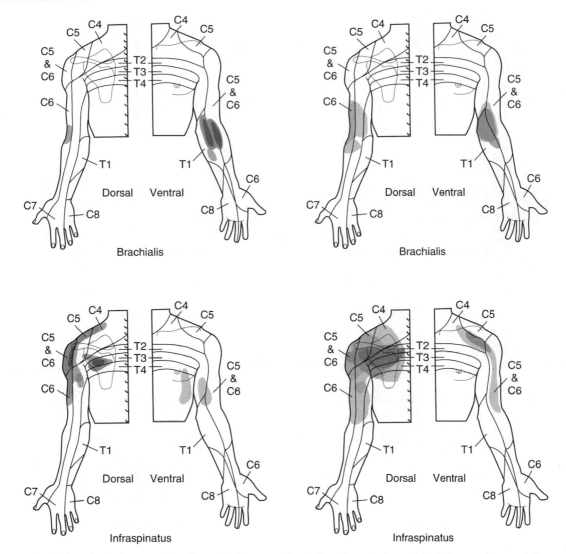

Figure 5.43 Referred pain from peripheral muscle. The area of pain from three to four subjects is superimposed. Cross hatch represents deep pain, and vertical hatching cutaneous hypoalgesia. (From Feinstein et al 1954, Experiments on pain referred from deep somatic tissues. Journal of Bone and Joint Surgery 36(A)5:981–997, with permission, © The Journal of Bone and Joint Surgery, Inc.)

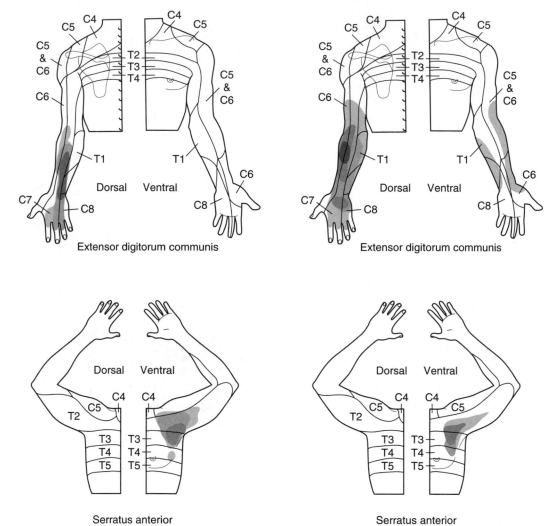

Extensor digitorum communis

Extensor digitorum communis

Serratus anterior

Serratus anterior

Figure 5.43 *(Cont'd)*

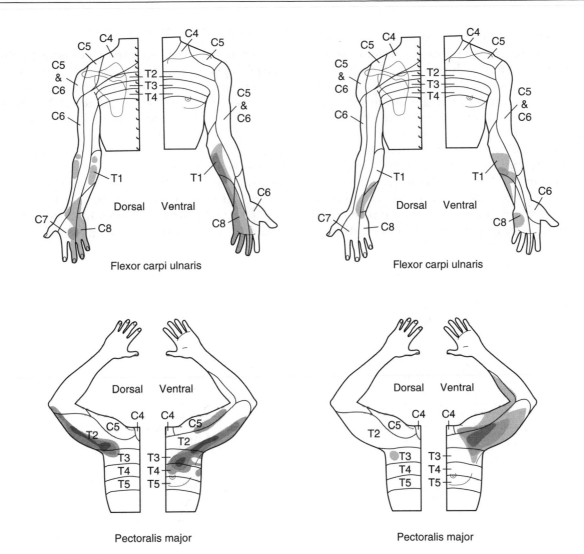

Flexor carpi ulnaris

Flexor carpi ulnaris

Pectoralis major

Pectoralis major

Figure 5.43 (Cont'd)

The mechanism of referred pain is thought to be due to the convergence of afferents in the periphery and in the dorsal horn (Torebjork et al 1984). This is depicted in Figure 5.44. In the periphery, proximal to the spinal cord, sensory neurones from skin and muscle converge (Wells et al 1994). In the dorsal horn, there is convergence of skin afferents and group III and IV muscle afferents onto wide dynamic range cells (Foreman et al 1979). In both cases, activation of nociceptors from the muscle, for example, is perceived by the brain to come from the skin; the brain thus misinterprets the information.

Summary of symptom production

The commonest symptom from a muscle is pain. The perception of pain occurs in the central nervous system and is multidimensional, i.e. it includes sensory, physiological, affective, cognitive, behavioural and socio-cultural factors. Nociceptors are found throughout muscle, so that muscle can be a potential source of pain. Muscle nociceptors are sensitive to mechanical deformation and chemical irritation and thus can produce mechanical or chemical nociceptive pain. Chemical irritation may be due to inflammation, ischaemia or sympathetic nervous

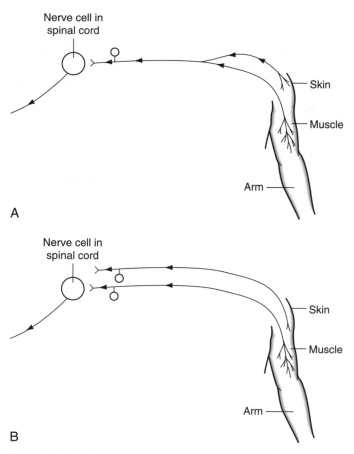

Figure 5.44 Referred pain due to convergence of afferents **A** in the periphery and **B** in the spinal cord (after Wells et al 1994, with permission).

system activity. Pain from muscle tends to be deep and localized over the muscle with some diffuse referred pain and tenderness to touch some distance away, possibly over the underlying joint, and may follow a segmental distribution.

Tendon injury and repair

Tendons can tear in the middle region, by avulsion of bone, and more rarely at the insertion site (Woo et al 1988). Repetitive strain of a tendon can produce micro- and macrotrauma of the tendon. The amount of strain needed to cause micro and macrotrauma is given in Figure 5.45. Repetitive strain may alter the collagenous structure of tendon with resultant inflammation, oedema and pain (Jozsa & Kannus 1997). Overuse injury occurs where this repetitive strain, causing tissue damage, is greater than the natural repair and healing process (Archambault et al 1995, Jozsa & Kannus 1997). Conditions include tendonitis, peritendinitis and tenosynovitis and this may lead, with further strain, to partial or complete rupture of the tendon. Often, these overuse injuries are seen in the upper extremity in occupations that require repetitive movement of the hands and forearms, and in the lower extremities in sport-related injuries.

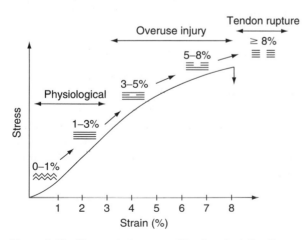

Figure 5.45 Stress–strain curve of tendon depicting the amount of stress involved in microtrauma (3–8%) and macrotrauma (<8%) (from Jozsa & Kannus 1997).

The aetiology of sports-related lower limb tendon injuries is thought to include vascularity of the tendon, malalignments, leg-length discrepancy, age and weight (Clement et al 1984, Jozsa et al 1989b, Jozsa & Kannus 1997), as well as extrinsic factors such as type of sport, training errors, environmental conditions, equipment and ineffective rules (Clement et al 1984, Jozsa & Kannus 1997).

Vascularity is thought to be an important aetiological factor because tendon injuries often occur where there is a relatively poor blood supply (Archambault et al 1995, Carr & Norris 1989, Clement et al 1984, Frey et al 1990, Reynolds & Worrell 1991). For example, the tendocalcaneus tendon has an avascular area 2–6 cm proximal to its distal attachment (Carr & Norris 1989), and it is in this region where the most severe tendon degeneration and spontaneous ruptures occur (Jozsa & Kannus 1997, Jozsa et al 1989b). The posterior tibial tendon has an area of poor vascularity posterior and distal to the medial malleolus, and it is in this region that it frequently ruptures (Frey et al 1990). The supraspinatus tendon has poor vascularity where it inserts onto the humerus (Chansky & Iannotti 1991, Lohr & Uhthoff 1990), and again, it is in this region where the tendon ruptures (Jozsa & Kannus 1997). Age-related degenerative changes within the tendon can cause narrowing or obliteration of blood vessels, further reducing the vascularity of the tendon (Kannus & Jozsa 1991).

In work-related upper-limb tendon injuries the strain placed on tendon may not be excessive, but the repetitive nature of the task may be sufficient to cause change in the tissue. It is proposed that, initially, in the first 5 days, there is ischaemia, metabolic disturbance and cell membrane damage leading to inflammation (Jozsa & Kannus 1997). The increase in tissue pressure further impairs the circulation and enhances the ischaemic changes. In the proliferation phase (5–21 days) there is fibrin clotting and proliferation of fibroblasts, synovial cells and capillaries. This is followed by the maturation phase (<21 days) in which adhesions and thickening of the tenosynovium and paratenon occur (Jozsa & Kannus 1997, Kvist & Kvist 1980).

Spontaneous tendon rupture is associated with degenerative changes (Jozsa et al 1989b). The diameter of collagen fibres decreases in degenerative tendon, suggesting an increase in weaker type III collagen fibres (Jozsa et al 1989a). Degenerative changes were found in 97% of ruptured tendons, which included the Achilles tendon, biceps brachii and extensor pollicis longus from nearly 900, compared to 35% in a control group (Kannus & Jozsa 1991).

Tendon repair

Healing of tendon is similar to that of other soft tissues and consists of three phases: lag or inflammation phase (1–7 days), regeneration or proliferation phase (7–21 days) and remodelling or maturation phase (21 days to 1 year) (Jozsa & Kannus 1997). Initially type III collagen is laid down which is replaced by type I collagen tissue during the late proliferation stage and maturation phase (Coombs et al 1980).

Muscle injury and repair

Muscle strain injury can occur with eccentric exercise, producing delayed muscle soreness (Friden et al 1983, Jones et al 1986). Pain, weakness and muscle stiffness are felt after unaccustomed eccentric exercise. There is disruption of the Z band, predominantly of type II fibres, with repair largely completed by 6 days (Friden et al 1983, Jones et al 1986). The reason for the delayed muscle soreness following eccentric contraction may be that eccentric contraction produces more force within the muscle than other types of muscle contraction (Katz 1939). The myotendinous region is the weakest part of the tendon–muscle unit and is the region most susceptible to strain injuries (Garrett 1990, Garrett et al 1989, Nikolaou et al 1987, Tidball 1991).

Muscle repair

Repair of muscle injury follows the typical healing process of all soft tissues: the lag phase, regeneration and remodelling.

There is initially the development of a necrotic zone at the site of damage and the adjacent uninjured myofibrils retract and begin the repair process, with activation of satellite cells (McComas 1996). The satellite cells migrate into the necrotic area and differentiate into myotubes, which begin to bridge the gap between the retracted uninjured myofibrils.

An experimental crush injury of the semitendinosus muscle of the rat reveals necrosis in the first 2 days, with new myotubes within the damaged area at 5 days and regeneration of muscle fibres bridging the necrotic area by 10 days, with full regeneration at 30 days (Stuart et al 1981). A controlled strain injury of the musculotendinous junction of tibialis anterior muscle was carried out on New Zealand White rabbits (Nikolaou et al 1987). Necrosis and infiltration of inflammatory cells, oedema and haemorrhage occurred after 1 day. After 2 days the damaged fibres had been broken down with proliferation of inflammatory cells, macrophages and fibroblasts. After 7 days inflammation was reduced and fibrocytes were evident (Nikolaou et al 1987). Clear evidence of muscle regeneration was evident after 4 days following an experimental strain injury of a rat tendon (Almekinders & Gilbert 1986).

Summary of muscle dysfunction

Common muscle dysfunctions seen clinically are reduced muscle strength, power and endurance, altered motor control, reduced muscle length and the production of symptoms. Muscle dysfunction does not exist in isolation; joint and nerve will also to some extent be involved. The next chapter discusses treatment of muscle dysfunction.

REFERENCES

Abrahams V C 1977 The physiology of neck muscles; their role in head movement and maintenance of posture. Canadian Journal of Physiology and Pharmacology 55:332–338

Abrahams V C 1981 Sensory and motor specialization in some muscles of the neck. Trends in Neuroscience 4:24–27

Adams M A, Bogduk N, Burton K, Dolan P 2002 The biomechanics of back pain. Churchill Livingstone, Edinburgh

Agre J C, Rodriquez A A 1989 Validity of manual muscle testing in post-polio subjects with good or normal strength. Archives of Physical Medicine and Rehabilitation 70(suppl):A17–A18

Ahles T A, Martin J B 1992 Cancer pain: a multidimensional perspective. In: Turk D C, Feldman C S (eds) Noninvasive approaches to pain management in the terminally ill. Haworth, New York, p 25–48

Akima H, Kano Y, Enomoto Y et al 2001 Muscle function in 164 men and women aged 20–84 yr. Medicine and Science in Sports and Exercise 33(2):220–226

Allen G M, Gandevia S C, McKenzie D K 1995 Reliability of measurements of muscle strength and voluntary activation using twitch interpolation. Muscle and Nerve 18:593–600

Allum J H J, Bloem B R, Carpenter M G et al 1998 Proprioceptive control of posture: a review of new concepts. Gait and Posture 8:214–242

Almekinders L C, Gilbert J A 1986 Healing of experimental muscle strains and the effects of nonsteroidal antiinflammatory medication. American Journal of Sports Medicine 14(4):303–308

Alter M J 1996 Science of flexibility, 2nd edn. Human Kinetics, Illinois

Antonutto G, Capelli C, Girardis M et al 1999 Effects of microgravity on maximal power of lower limbs during very short efforts in humans. Journal of Applied Physiology 86:85–92

Appell H-J 1990 Muscular atrophy following immobilisation, a review. Sports Medicine 10(1):42–58

Arangio G A, Chen C, Kalady M, Reed J F 1997 Thigh muscle size and strength after anterior cruciate ligament reconstruction and rehabilitation. Journal of Orthopaedics and Sports Physiotherapy 26(5):238–243

Archambault J M, Wiley J P, Bray R C 1995 Exercise loading of tendons and the development of overuse injuries, a review of current literature. Sports Medicine 20(2):77–89

Arvidsson I, Eriksson E, Knutsson E, Arner S 1986 Reduction of pain inhibition on voluntary muscle activation by epidural analgesia. Orthopaedics 9(10):1415–1419

Baratta R, Solomonow M, Zhou B H et al 1988 Muscular coactivation. The role of the antagonist musculature in maintaining knee stability. American Journal of Sports Medicine 16(2):113–122

Barker D 1974 The morphology of muscle receptors. In: Hunt C C (ed) Handbook of sensory physiology. Muscle receptors, vol 3 part 2. Springer-Verlag, Berlin, p 124

Barker D, Saito M 1981 Autonomic innervation of receptors and muscle fibres in cat skeletal muscle. Proceedings of the Royal Society Lond B Biological Science 212:317–332

Bastide G, Zadeh J, Lefebvre D 1989 Are the 'little muscles' what we think they are? Surgical and Radiological Anatomy 11:255–256

Beard D J, Soundarapandian R S, O'Connor J J, Dodd C A F 1996 Gait and electromyographic analysis of anterior cruciate ligament deficient subjects. Gait and Posture 4:83–88

Bennett J G, Stauber W T 1986 Evaluation and treatment of anterior knee pain using eccentric exercise. Medicine and Science in Sports and Exercise 18(5):526–530

Berberich P, Hoheisel U, Mense S 1988 Effects of a carrageenan-induced myositis on the discharge properties of group III and IV muscle receptors in the cat. Journal of Neurophysiology 59(5):1395–1409

Berchuck M, Andriacchi T P, Bach B R, Reider B 1990 Gait adaptations by patients who have a deficient anterior cruciate ligament. Journal of Bone and Joint Surgery 72A(6):871–877

Berg H E, Larsson L, Tesch P A 1997 Lower limb skeletal muscle function after 6 wk of bed rest. Journal of Applied Physiology 82:182–188

Bergmark A 1989 Stability of the lumbar spine. A study of mechanical engineering. Acta Orthopaedica Scandinavica 60(suppl 230):3–54

Bodine S C, Roy R R, Meadows D A et al 1982 Architectural, histochemical, and contractile characteristics of a unique biarticular muscle: the cat semitendinosus. Journal of Neurophysiology 48(1):192–201

Bogduk N 1997 Clinical anatomy of the lumbar spine and sacrum, 3rd edn. Churchill Livingstone, New York, ch 9, p 105

Bogduk N, MacIntosh J E 1984 The applied anatomy of the thoracolumbar fascia. Spine 9(2):164–170

Borg G A V 1982 Psychophysical bases of perceived exertion. Medicine and Science in Sport and Exercise 14(5):377–381

Bors E 1926 Uber das zahlenverhaltnis zwischen nerven und muskelfasern. Anatomy Anzeiger 60:415–420

Bouisset S, Zattara M 1981 A sequence of postural movements precedes voluntary movement. Neuroscience Letters 22:263–270

Boyd I A 1976 The mechanical properties of dynamic nuclear bag fibres, static nuclear bag fibres and nuclear chain fibres in isolated cat muscle spindles. Progress in Brain Research 44:33–50

Branch T P, Hunter R, Donath M 1989 Dynamic EMG analysis of anterior cruciate deficient legs with and without bracing during cutting. American Journal of Sports Medicine 17(1):35–41

Bredella M A, Tirman P F J, Fritz R C et al 1999 MR imaging findings of lateral ulnar collateral ligament abnormalities in patients with lateral epicondylitis. American Journal of Roentgenology 173:1379–1382

Brooke M H, Engel W K 1969 The histographic analysis of human muscle biopsies with regard to fibre types. 1. Adult male and female. Neurology 19:221–233

Brooks G A, Fahey T D 1987 Fundamentals of human performance. Macmillan, New York, ch 9 p 193–194

Brown M C, Hardman V J 1987 Plasticity of vertebrate motoneurones. In: Winlow W, McCrohan C R (eds)

Growth and plasticity of neural connections. Manchester University Press, Manchester, p 36–51

Buller A J, Eccles J C, Eccles R M 1960 Interactions between motoneurones and muscles in respect of the characteristic speeds of their responses. Journal of Physiology 150:417–439

Burkholder T J, Fingado B, Baron S, Lieber R L 1994 Relationship between muscle fiber types and sizes and muscle architectural properties in the mouse hindlimb. Journal of Morphology 221:177–190

Butler D S 2000 The sensitive nervous system. Noigroup, Adelaide

Carr A J, Norris S H 1989 The blood supply of the calcaneal tendon. Journal of Bone and Joint Surgery 71B(1):100–101

Chansky H A, Iannotti J P 1991 The vascularity of the rotator cuff. Clinics in Sports Medicine 10(4):807–822

Ciccotti M G, Kerlan R K, Perry J, Pink M 1994 An electromyographic analysis of the knee during functional activities. II. The anterior cruciate ligament-deficient and –reconstructed profiles. American Journal of Sports Medicine 22(5):651–658

Clark F J, Horch K W, Bach S M, Larson G F 1979 Contributions of cutaneous and joint receptors to static knee-position sense in man. Journal of Neurophysiology 42(3):877–888

Clement D B, Taunton J E, Smart G W 1984 Achilles tendonitis and peritendinitis: etiology and treatment. American Journal of Sports Medicine 12(3):179–184

Comerford M J, Mottram S L 2001a Functional stability re-training: principles and strategies for managing mechanical dysfunction. Manual Therapy 6(1):3–14

Comerford M J, Mottram S L 2001b Movement and stability dysfunction – contemporary developments. Manual Therapy 6(1):15–26

Coombs R R H, Klenerman L, Narcisi P et al 1980 Collagen typing in Achilles tendon rupture. Journal of Bone and Joint Surgery 62B(2):258

Cooper S, Daniel P M 1963 Muscles spindles in man; their morphology in the lumbricals and the deep muscles of the neck. Brain 86:563–592

Cooper R R, Misol S 1970 Tendon and ligament insertion: a light and electron microscopic study. Journal of Bone and Joint Surgery 52A(1):1–20

Cordo P J, Nashner L M 1982 Properties of postural adjustments associated with rapid arm movements. Journal of Neurophysiology 47(2):287–302

Corser T 1974 Temporal discrepancies in the electromyographic study of rapid movement. Ergonomics 17(3):389–400

Cousins M, Power I 1999 Acute and postoperative pain. In: Wall P D, Melzack R (eds) Textbook of pain, 4th edn. Churchill Livingstone, Edinburgh, ch 19, p 447–491

Cowan S M, Bennell K L, Crossley K M et al 2002 Physical therapy alters recruitment of the vasti in patellofemoral pain syndrome. Medicine and Science in Sports and Exercise 34(12):1879–1885

Cresswell A G 1993 Responses of intra-abdominal pressure and abdominal muscle activity during dynamic trunk loading in man. European Journal of Applied Physiology and Occupational Physiology 66:315–320

Cresswell A G, Grundstrom H, Thorstensson A 1992 Observations on intra-abdominal pressure and patterns of abdominal intra-muscular activity in man. Acta Physiologic Scandinavica 144:409–418

Cresswell A G, Thorstensson A 1994 Changes in intra-abdominal pressure, trunk muscle activation and force during isokinetic lifting and lowering. European Journal of Applied Physiology and Occupational Physiology 68:315–321

Crow J L, Haas B M 2001 The neural control of human movement. In: Trew M, Everett T (eds) Human Movement, an introductory text, 4th edn. Churchill Livingstone, Edinburgh, ch 4, p 69

David G, Magarey M E, Jones M A et al 2000 EMG and strength correlates of selected shoulder muscles during rotations of the glenohumeral joint. Clinical Biomechanics 15:95–102

deAndrade J R, Grant C, Dixon A St J 1965 Joint distension and reflex muscle inhibition in the knee. Journal of Bone and Joint Surgery 47A(2):313–322

Descartes R 1985 Discourse on method and the meditations. Penguin, Middlesex, 6th meditation p 150–169

DeVita P, Hortobagyi T, Barrier J et al 1997 Gait adaptations before and after anterior cruciate ligament reconstruction surgery. Medicine and Science in Sports and Exercise 29(7):853–859

De Vries H A, Housh T J 1994 Physiology of exercise for physical education, athletics and sports science, 5th edn. Brown & Benchmark, Madison, Wisconsin

Diehl B, Hoheisel U, Mense S 1988 Histological and neurophysiological changes induced by carrageenan in skeletal muscle of cat and rat. Agents and Actions 25(3/4):210–213

Edgerton V R, Zhou M-Y, Ohira Y et al 1995 Human fiber size and enzymatic properties after 5 and 11 days of spaceflight. Journal of Applied Physiology 78:1733–1739

Eisenberg B R, Milton R L 1984 Muscle fiber termination at the tendon in the frog's sartorius: a stereological study. American Journal of Anatomy 171:273–284

Elftman H 1966 Biomechanics of muscle. Journal of Bone and Joint Surgery 48A(2):363–377

Elliott D H 1965 Structure and function of mammalian tendon. Biological Review 40:392–421

Fahrer H, Rentsch H U, Gerber N J et al 1988 Knee effusion and reflex inhibition of the quadriceps – a bar to effective retraining. Journal of Bone and Joint Surgery 70B(4):635–638

Feinstein B, Langton J N K, Jameson R M, Schiller F 1954 Experiments on pain referred from deep somatic tissues. Journal of Bone and Joint Surgery 36A(5):981–997

Ferrell W R 1985 The response of slowly adapting mechanoreceptors in the cat knee joint to tetanic contraction of hind limb muscles. Quarterly Journal of Experimental Physiology 70:337–345

Fitts R H, Riley D R, Widrick J J 2000 Microgravity and skeletal muscle. Journal of Applied Physiology 89:823–839

Fitts R H, Riley D R, Widrick J J 2001 Functional and structural adaptations of skeletal muscle to microgravity. Journal of Experimental Biology 204:3201–3208

Foreman R D, Schmidt R F, Willis W D 1979 Effects of mechanical and chemical stimulation of fine muscle afferents upon primate spinothalamic tract cells. Journal of Physiology (Lond) 286:215–231

Frank C B, Loitz B, Bray R et al 1994 Abnormality of the contralateral ligament after injuries of the medial collateral ligament – an experimental study in rabbits. Journal of Bone and Joint Surgery 76A(3):403–412

Franz M, Mense S 1975 Muscle receptors with group IV afferent fibres responding to application of bradykinin. Brain Research 92:369–383

Freeman M A R, Wyke B 1967 Articular reflexes at the ankle joint: an electromyographic study of normal and abnormal influences of ankle joint mechanoreceptors upon reflex activity in the leg muscles. British Journal of Surgery 54(12):990–1001

Frey C, Shereff M, Greenidge N 1990 Vascularity of the posterior tibial tendon. Journal of Bone and Joint Surgery 72A(6):884–888

Friden J, Sjostrom M, Ekblom B 1983 Myofibrillar damage following intense eccentric exercise in man. International Journal of Sports Medicine 4:170–176

Friedli W G, Hallett M, Simon S R 1984 Postural adjustments associated with rapid voluntary arm movements 1. Electromyographic data. Journal of Neurology, Neurosurgery and Psychiatry 47:611–622

Fukunaga T, Ichinose Y, Ito M et al 1997 Determination of fascicle length and pennation in a contracting human muscle in vivo. Journal Applied Physiology 82(1):354–358

Fung Y C 1993 Biomechanics, biomechanical properties of living tissues, 2nd edn. Springer-Verlag, New York, p 260

Gajdosik R L, Linden D W V, Williams A K 1996 Influence of age on concentric isokinetic torque and passive extensibility variables of the calf muscles of women. European Journal of Applied Physiology 74:279–286

Gandevia S C, McClosky D I 1976 Joint sense, muscle sense, and their combination as position sense, measured at the distal interphalangeal joint of the middle finger. Journal of Physiology (Lond) 260:387–407

Gandevia S C, Hall L A, McCloskey D I, Potter E K 1983 Proprioceptive sensation at the terminal joint of the middle finger. Journal of Physiology (Lond) 335:507–517

Gandevia S C, Herbert R D, Leeper J B 1998 Voluntary activation of human elbow flexor muscles during maximal concentric contractions. Journal of Physiology 512(2):595–602

Garell P C, McGillis S L B, Greenspan J D 1996 Mechanical response properties of nociceptors innervating feline hairy skin. Journal of Neurophysiology 75(3):1177–1189

Garfin S R, Tipton C M, Mubarak S J et al 1981 Role of fascia in maintenance of muscle tension and pressure. Journal of Applied Physiology 51(2):317–320

Garrett W E 1990 Muscle strain injuries: clinical and basic aspects. Medicine and Science in Sports and Exercise 22(4):436–443

Garrett W E, Rich F R, Nikolaou P K, Vogler J B 1989 Computed tomography of hamstring muscle strains. Medicine and Science in Sports and Exercise 21(5):506–514

Ghez C 1991 Muscles: effectors of the motor systems. In: Kandel E R, Schwartz J H, Jessell T M (eds) Principles of neural science, 3rd edn. Elsevier, New York, ch 36, p 548–563

Gifford L 1998 Pain. In: Pitt-Brooke J, Reid H, Lockwood J, Kerr K (eds) Rehabilitation of movement, theoretical basis of clinical practice. W B Saunders, London, ch 5, p 196–232

Glousman R, Jobe F, Tibone J et al 1988 Dynamic electromyographic analysis of the throwing shoulder with glenohumeral instability. Journal of Bone and Joint Surgery 70A(2):220–226

Glousman R E, Barron J, Jobe F W et al 1992 An electromyographic analysis of the elbow in normal and injured pitchers with medial collateral ligament insufficiency. American Journal of Sports Medicine 20(3):311–317

Goldspink G 1976 The adaptation of muscle to a new functional length. In: Anderson D J & Matthews B (eds) Mastication. Wright, Bristol, ch 12, p 90–99

Goldspink G, Williams P E 1979 The nature of the increased passive resistance in muscle following immobilization of the mouse soleus muscle. Journal of Physiology 289: 55P (Proceedings of the Physiological Society December 15/16th 1978)

Gombrich E, Biancheri B, Thomas D et al 1989 Leonardo da Vinci. South Bank Centre, London

Goodwin G M, McCloskey D I, Matthews P B C 1972 The contribution of muscle afferents to kinaesthesia shown by vibration induced illusions of movement and by the effects of paralysing joint afferents. Brain 95:705–748

Granata K P, Marras W S 1995 The influence of trunk muscle coactivity on dynamic spinal loads. Spine 20(8):913–919

Granit R, Phillips C G, Skoglund S, Steg G 1957 Differentiation of tonic from phasic alpha ventral horn cells by stretch, pinna and crossed extensor reflexes. Journal of Neurophysiology 20(5):470–481

Greenleaf J E, Bulbulian R, Bernauer E M et al 1989 Exercise-training protocols for astronauts in microgravity. Journal of Applied Physiology 67:2191–2204

Grieve G P 1994 Referred pain and other clinical features. In Grieve's modern manual therapy, the vertebral column, 2nd edn. Boyling J D, Palastanga N (eds) Churchill Livingstone, Edinburgh, ch 19, p 271–292

Grigg P 1994 Peripheral neural mechanisms in proprioception. Journal of Sport Rehabilitation 3:2–17

Grimby G 1995 Muscle performance and structure in the elderly as studied cross-sectionally and longitudinally. Journal of Gerontology 50A(special issue):17–22

Gydikov A A 1976 Pattern of discharge of different types of alpha motoneurones and motor units during voluntary and reflex activities under normal physiological conditions. In: Komi P V (ed) Biomechanics V-A. University Park, Baltimore, p 45–57

Haggmark T, Jansson E, Eriksson E 1981 Fibre type area and metabolic potential of the thigh muscle in man after knee surgery and immobilization. International Journal of Sports Medicine 2:12–17

Hales J P, Gandevia S C 1988 Assessment of maximal voluntary contraction with twitch interpolation: an instrument to measure twitch responses. Journal of Neuroscience Methods 25:97–102

Harpuder K, Stein I D 1943 Studies on the nature of pain arising from an ischaemic limb. II. Biochemical studies. American Heart Journal 25(4):438–448

Hasan Z, Houk J C 1975 Transition in sensitivity of spindle receptors that occurs when muscle is stretched more than a fraction of a millimeter. Journal of Neurophysiology 38:673–689

Henneman E, Olson C B 1965 Relations between structure and function in the design of skeletal muscles. Journal of Neurophysiology 28:581–598

Henneman E, Somjen G, Carpenter D O 1965 Functional significance of cell size in spinal motoneurons. Journal of Neurophysiology 28:560–580

Herzog W 1999 Muscle. In: Nigg B M, Herzog W (eds) Biomechanics of the musculo-skeletal system, 2nd edn. John Wiley, Chichester, ch 2.7, p 148–188

Herzog W, Gal J 1999 Tendon. In: Nigg B M, Herzog W (eds) Biomechanics of the musculo-skeletal system, 2nd edn. John Wiley, Chichester, ch 2.6, p 127–147

Hess G P, Cappiello W L, Poole R M, Hunter S C 1989 Prevention and treatment of overuse tendon injuries. Sports Medicine 8(6):371–384

Heyley M V, Rees J, Newham D J 1998 Quadriceps function, proprioceptive acuity and functional performance in healthy young, middle-aged and elderly subjects. Age and Ageing 27(1):55–62

Hides J, Richardson C, Jull G, Davies S 1995 Ultrasound imaging in rehabilitation. Australian Journal of Physiotherapy 41(3):187–193

Hill A V 1938 The heat of shortening and the dynamic constants of muscle. Proceedings of The Royal Society of London (Biology) 126:136–195

Hirsch C 1974 Tensile properties during tendon healing. A comparative study of intact and sutured rabbit peroneus brevis tendons. Acta Orthopaedica Scandinavica 153(suppl):11

Hodges P W, Richardson C A 1996 Inefficient muscular stabilization of the lumbar spine associated with low back pain. A motor control evaluation of transversus abdominis. Spine 21(22):2640–2650

Hodges P W, Richardson C A 1997a Contraction of the abdominal muscles associated with movements of the lower limb. Physical Therapy 77(2):132–144

Hodges P W, Richardson C A 1997b Feedforward contraction of transversus abdominis in not influenced by the direction of arm movement. Experimental Brain Research 114:362–370

Hodges P W, Richardson C A 1997c Relationship between limb movement speed and associated contraction of the trunk muscles. Ergonomics 40(11):1220–1230

Horak F B, Esselman P, Anderson M E, Lynch M K 1984 The effects of movement velocity, mass displaced, and task certainty on associated postural adjustments made by normal and hemiplegic individuals. Journal of Neurology, Neurosurgery and Psychiatry 47:1020–1028

Hortobagyi T, DeVita P 2000 Muscle pre-and coactivity during downward stepping are associated with leg stiffness in aging. Journal of Electromyography and Kinesiology 10:117–126

Hortobagyi T, Zheng D, Weidner M et al 1995 The influence of aging on muscle strength and muscle fiber characteristics with special reference to eccentric strength. Journal of Gerontology 50A(6):B399-B406

Hortobagyi T, Dempsey L, Fraser D et al 2000 Changes in muscle strength, muscle fibre size and myofibrillar gene expression after immobilization and retraining in humans. Journal of Physiology 524(1):293–304

Horowits R, Maruyama K, Podolsky R J 1989 Elastic behavior of connectin filaments during thick filament movement in activated skeletal muscle. Journal of Cell Biology 109:2169–2176

Houk J, Henneman E 1967 Responses of golgi tendon organs to active contractions of the soleus muscle of the cat. Journal of Neurophysiology 30:466–481

Houk J C, Singer J J, Henneman E 1971 Adequate stimulus for tendon organs with observations on mechanics of ankle joint. Journal of Neurophysiology 34:1051–1065

Hughes V A, Frontera W R, Wood M et al 2001 Longitudinal muscle strength changes in older adults: influence of muscle mass, physical activity, and health. Journal of Gerontology 56A(5):B209-B217

Hughston J C, Walsh W M, Puddu G 1984 Patellar subluxation and dislocation, vol 5. W B Saunders, Philadelphia

Hukins D W L, Aspden R M, Hickey D S 1990 Thoracolumbar fascia can increase the efficiency of the erector spinae muscles. Clinical Biomechanics 5:30–34

Hunt C C 1990 Mammalian muscle spindle: peripheral mechanisms. Physiological Reviews 70(3):643–663

Hurley M V, Newham D J 1993 The influence of arthrogenous muscle inhibition on quadriceps rehabilitation of patients with early, unilateral osteoarthritic knees. British Journal of Rheumatology 32:127–131

Hurley M V, O'Flanagan S J, Newham D J 1991 Isokinetic and isometric muscle strength and inhibition after elbow arthroplasty. Journal of Orthopaedic Rheumatology 4:83–95

Hurley M V, Jones D W, Wilson D, Newham D J 1992 Rehabilitation of quadriceps inhibited due to isolated rupture of the anterior cruciate ligament. Journal of Orthopaedic Rheumatology 5:145–154

Hurley M V, Jones D W, Newham D J 1994 Arthrogenic quadriceps inhibition and rehabilitation of patients with extensive traumatic knee injuries. Clinical Sciences 86:305–310

Huxley A F 2000 Cross-bridge action: present views, prospects, and unknowns. In: Herzog W (ed) Skeletal muscle mechanics: from mechanisms to function. John Wiley, Chichester, ch 2, p 7–31

Iggo A 1961 Non-myelinated afferent fibres from mammalian skeletal muscle. Journal of Physiology 155:52P–53P

Iles J F, Stokes M, Young A 1990 Reflex actions of knee joint afferents during contraction of the human quadriceps. Clinical Physiology 10:489–500

Indahl A, Kaigle A, Reikeras O, Holm S 1995 Electromyographic response of the porcine multifidus musculature after nerve stimulation. Spine 20(24):2652–2658

Indahl A, Kaigle A, Reikeras O, Holm S 1997 Interaction between the porcine lumbar intervertebral disc, zygapophysial joints, and paraspinal muscles. Spine 22(24):2834–2840

Ingelmark BO E 1948 The structure of tendons at various ages and under different functional conditions II an electron-microscopic investigation of Achilles tendons from white rats. Acta Anatomy 6(3):193–225

Inman V T, Saunders J B DeC M 1944 Referred pain from skeletal structures. Journal of Nervous and Mental Disease 99:660–667

Jami L 1992 Golgi tendon organs in mammalian skeletal muscle: functional properties and central actions. Physiological Reviews 72(3):623–666

Janda V 1985 Pain in the locomotor system – a broad approach. In: Glasgow E F, Twomey L T, Scull E R, Kleynhans A M, Idczak R M (eds) Aspects of manipulative therapy. Churchill Livingstone, Melbourne, ch 22, p 148–151

Johns R J, Wright V 1962 Relative importance of various tissues in joint stiffness. Journal of Applied Physiology 17(5):824–828

Johnson M A, Polgar J, Weightman D, Appleton D 1973 Data on the distribution of fibre types in thirty-six human muscles: an autopsy study. Journal of the Neurological Sciences 18:111–129

Jones D A, Newham D J, Round J M, Tolfree S E J 1986 Experimental human muscle damage: morphological changes in relation to other indices of damage. Journal of Physiology 375:435–448

Jones D W, Jones D A, Newham D J 1987 Chronic knee effusion and aspiration: the effect on quadriceps inhibition. British Journal of Rheumatology 26:370–374

Jozsa L, Kannus P 1997 Human tendons: anatomy, physiology and pathology. Human Kinetics, Champaign, Illinois

Jozsa L, Kvist M, Kannus P, Jarvinen M 1988 The effect of tenotomy and immobilization on muscle spindles and tendon organs of the rat calf muscles. Acta Neurophathologica 76:465–470

Jozsa L, Lehto M, Kvist M et al 1989a Alterations in dry mass content of collagen fibers in degenerative tendinopathy and tendon-rupture. Matrix 9:140–146

Jozsa L, Kvist M, Balint B J et al 1989b The role of recreational sport activity in Achilles tendon rupture, a clinical, pathoanatomical, and sociological study of 292 cases. American Journal of Sports Medicine 17(3):338–343

Jozsa L, Kannus P, Balint J B, Reffy A 1991 Three-dimensional ultrastructure of human tendons. Acta Anatomica 142:306–312

Jozsa K, Kannus P, Jarvinen M et al 1992 Denervation and immobilization induced changes in the myotendinous junction. European Journal of Experimental Musculoskeletal Research 1:105–112

Kalund S, Sinkjaer T, Arendt-Nielsen L, Simonsen O 1990 Altered timing of hamstring muscle action in anterior cruciate ligament deficient patients. American Journal of Sports Medicine 18(3):245–248

Kannus P, Jozsa L 1991 Histopathological changes preceding spontaneous rupture of a tendon. Journal of Bone and Joint Surgery 73A(10):1507–1525

Kannus P, Jozsa L, Kvist M et al 1992 The effect of immobilization on myotendinous junction: an ultrastructural, histochemical and immunohistochemical study. Acta Physiologica Scandinavica 144:387–394

Kao F F 1963 An experimental study of the pathways involved in exercise hyperpnoea employing cross-circulation techniques. In: Cunningham D J C, Lloyd B B (eds) The regulation of human respiration, Blackwell, Oxford, p 461–502

Karpakka J, Vaananen K, Virtanen P et al 1990 The effects of remobilization and exercise on collagen biosynthesis in rat tendon. Acta Physiologica Scandinavica 139:139–145

Katz B 1939 The relation between force and speed in muscular contraction. Journal of Physiology 96:45–64

Kaufman M P, Iwamoto G A, Longhurst J C, Mitchell J H 1982 Effects of capsaicin and bradykinin on afferent fibers with endings in skeletal muscle. Circulatory Research 50:133–139

Kaufman M P, Longhurst J C, Rybicki K J et al 1983 Effects of static muscular contraction on impulse activity of groups III and IV afferents in cats. Journal of Applied Physiology 55:105–112

Kaufman M P, Waldrop T G, Rybicki K J et al 1984a Effects of static and rhythmic twitch contractions on the discharge of group III and IV muscle afferents. Cardiovascular Research 18:663–668

Kaufman M P, Rybicki K J, Waldrop T G, Ordway G A 1984b Effect of ischaemia on responses of group III and IV afferents to contraction. Journal of Applied Physiology 57:644–650

Kawakami Y, Ichinose Y, Fukunaga T 1998 Architectural and functional features of human triceps surae muscles during contraction. Journal of Applied Physiology 85(2):398–404

Keating J F, Crossan J F 1992 Evaluation of rotator cuff function following anterior dislocation of the shoulder. Journal of Orthopaedic Rheumatology 5:135–140

Kellgren J H 1938 Observations on referred pain arising from muscle. Clinical Science 3:175–190

Kellgren J H 1939 On the distribution of pain arising from deep somatic structures with charts of segmental pain areas. Clinical Science 4:35–46

Kennedy J C, Alexander I J, Hayes K C 1982 Nerve supply of the human knee and its functional importance. American Journal of Sports Medicine 10(6):329–335

Kent-Braun J A & Le Blanc R 1996 Quantification of central activation failure during maximal voluntary contractions in humans. Muscle and Nerve 19:861–869

Kerr K 1998 Exercise in rehabilitation. In: Pitt-Brooke J, Reid H, Lockwood J, Kerr K (eds) Rehabilitation of movement, theoretical basis of clinical practice. W B Saunders, London ch 12, p 423–457

Kidd G, Lawes N, Musa I 1992 Understanding neuromuscular plasticity a basis for clinical rehabilitation. Edward Arnold, London

Kieschke J, Mense S, Prabhakar N R 1988 Influence of adrenaline and hypoxia on rat muscle receptors in vitro. In: Hamann W, Iggo A (eds) Progress in Brain Research, Elsevier, Amsterdam, 74:91–97

Knatt T, Guanche C, Solomonow M et al 1995 The glenohumeral-biceps reflex in the feline. Clinical Orthopaedics and Related Research 314:247–252

Kniffki K-D, Mense S, Schmidt R F 1978 Responses of group IV afferent units from skeletal muscle to stretch, contraction and chemical stimulation. Experimental Brain Research 31:511–522

Kojima T 1991 Force-velocity relationship of human elbow flexors in voluntary isotonic contraction under heavy loads. International Journal of Sports Medicine 12:208–213

Krebs D E, Staples W H, Cuttita D, Zickel R E 1983 Knee joint angle: its relationship to quadriceps femoris activity in normal and postarthrotomy limbs. Archives of Physical Medicine and Rehabilitation 64:441–447

Kumazawa T, Mizumura K 1977 Thin-fibre receptors responding to mechanical, chemical, and thermal stimulation in the skeletal muscle of the dog. Journal of Physiology 273:179–194

Kvist H, Kvist M 1980 The operative treatment of chronic calcaneal paratenonitis. Journal of Bone and Joint Surgery 62B(3):353–357

Kvist M, Jozsa L, Kannus P et al 1991 Morphology and histochemistry of the myotendineal junction of the rat calf muscles. Histochemical, immunohistochemical and electron-microscopic study. Acta Anatomica 141:199–205

Kvist M, Hurme T, Kannus P et al 1995 Vascular density at the myotendinous junction of the rat gastrocnemius muscle after immobilization and remobilization. American Journal of Sports Medicine 23(3):359–364

Labarque V L, Eijnde B Op 't, Leemputte M Van 2002 Effect of immobilization and retraining on torque-velocity relationship of human knee flexor and extensor muscles. European Journal of Applied Physiology 86:251–257

Larsson L, Grimby G, Karlsson J 1979 Muscle strength and speed of movement in relation to age and muscle morphology. Journal of Applied Physiology 46(3):451–456

Laughlin M H, Korthuis R J 1987 Control of muscle blood flow during sustained physiological exercise. Canadian Journal of Sports Sciences 12(suppl):77S–83S

Levick J R 1983 Joint pressure–volume studies: their importance, design and interpretation. Journal of Rheumatology 10:353–357

Levine J D, Dardick S J, Basbaum A I, Scipio E 1985a Reflex neurogenic inflammation. 1. Contribution of the peripheral nervous system to spatially remote inflammatory responses following injury. Journal of Neuroscience 5(5):1380–1386

Levine J D, Moskowitz M A, Basbaum A I 1985b The contribution of neurogenic inflammation in experimental arthritis. Journal Immunology 135(2):843s–847s

Lewis C S 1998 The problem of pain. Fount, HarperCollins

Lieb F J, Perry J 1968 Quadriceps function. An anatomical and mechanical study using amputated limbs. Journal of Bone and Joint Surgery 50A(8):1535–1548

Lockwood J 1998 Musculoskeletal requirements for normal movement. In: Pitt-Brooke J, Reid H, Lockwood J, Kerr K (eds) Rehabilitation of movement, theoretical basis of clinical practice. W B Saunders, London, ch 2 p 107

Lohr J F, Uhthoff H K 1990 The microvascular pattern of the supraspinatus tendon. Clinical Orthopaedics and Related Research 254:35–38

Lomo T, Westgaard R H & Engebretsen L 1980 Different stimulation patterns affect contractile properties of denervated rat soleus muscles. In: Pette D (ed) Plasticity of muscle. Walter de Gruyter, Berlin

Louie J K, Mote C D 1987 Contribution of the musculature to rotatory laxity and torsional stiffness at the knee. Journal of Biomechanics 20(3):281–300

Louie J K, Kuo C Y, Gutierrez M D, Mote C D 1984 Surface EMG and torsion measurements during snow skiing: laboratory and field tests. Journal of Biomechanics 17(10):713–724

Lundborg G 1976 Experimental flexor tendon healing without adhesion formation – a new concept of tendon nutrition and intrinsic healing mechanisms. Hand 8(3):235–238

McArdle W D, Katch F I, Katch V L 2000 Essentials of exercise physiology 2nd edn. Lippincott Williams & Wilkins, Philadelphia, ch 15 p 417

McBryde A M, Anderson R B 1988 Sesamoid foot problems in the athlete. Clinics in Sports medicine 7(1):51–60

McCloskey D I, Mitchell J H 1972 Reflex cardiovascular and respiratory responses originating in exercising muscle. Journal of Physiology 224:173–186

McCloskey D I, Macefield G, Gandevia S C, Burke D 1987 Sensing position and movements of the fingers. News in Physiological Science 2:226–230

McComas A J 1996 Skeletal muscle: form and function. Human Kinetics, Champaign, Illinois

MacDougall J D 1986 Morphological changes in human skeletal muscle following strength training and immobilization. In: Jones N L, McCartney N, McComas A J (eds) Human muscle power. Human Kinetics, Champaign, ch 17, p 269–288

MacDougall J D, Elder G C B, Sale D G et al 1980 Effects of strength training and immobilisation on human muscle fibres. European Journal of Applied Physiology and Occupational Physiology 43:25–34

Macefield G, Gandevia S C, Burke D 1990 Perceptual responses to microstimulation of single afferents innervating joints, muscles and skin of the human hand. Journal of Physiology (Lond) 429:113–129

McGill S M, Norman R W 1986 Partitioning of the L4–L5 dynamic moment into disc, ligamentous, and muscular components during lifting. Spine 11(7):666–678

McGuire D B 1995 The multiple dimensions of cancer pain: a framework for assessment and management. In: McGuire D B, Yarbro C H, Ferrell B R (eds) Cancer pain management, 2nd edn. Jones and Bartlett, Boston, ch 1, p 1–17

McNair P J, Marshall R N, Maguire K 1994 Knee effusion and quadriceps muscle strength. Clinical Biomechanics 9(6):331–334

Maganaris C N, Baltzopoulos V, Sargeant A J 1998 In vivo measurements of the triceps surae complex architecture in man: implications for muscle function. Journal of Physiology 512(2):603–614

Maier A, Crockett J L, Simpson D R et al 1976 Properties of immobilized guinea pig hindlimb muscles. American Journal of Physiology 231(5):1520–1526

Matre D A, Sinkjaer T, Svensson P, Arendt-Nielsen L 1998 Experimental muscle pain increases the human stretch reflex. Pain 75:331–339

Matre D A, Sinkjaer T, Knardahl S et al 1999 The influence of experimental muscle pain on the human soleus stretch reflex during sitting and walking. Clinical Neurophysiology 110:2033–2043

Matthews P 1976 The fate of isolated segments of flexor tendons within the digital sheath – a study in synovial nutrition. British Journal of Plastic Surgery 29:216–224

Matthews P B C, Simmonds A 1974 Sensations of finger movement elicited by pulling upon flexor tendons in man. Journal of physiology (Lond) 239:27P–28P

Mense S 1981 Sensitization of group IV muscle receptors to bradykinin by 5-hyroxytryptamine and prostaglandin E₂. Brain Research 225:95–105

Mense S 1996 Group III and IV receptors in skeletal muscle: are they specific or polymodal? In: Kumazawa T, Kruger L, Mizumura K (eds) Progress in Brain Research 113, ch 5, p 83–100

Mense S, Meyer H 1985 Different types of slowly conducting afferent units in cat skeletal muscle and tendon. Journal of Physiology 363:403–417

Mense S, Stahnke M 1983 Responses in muscle afferent fibres of slow conduction velocity to contractions and ischaemia in the cat. Journal of Physiology 342:383–397

Merskey R, Albe-Fessard D G, Bonica J J et al 1979 Pain terms: a list with definitions and notes on usage. Pain 6:249–252

Milner-Brown H S, Stein R B, Yemm R 1973 The orderly recruitment of human motor units during voluntary isometric contractions. Journal of Physiology (Lond) 230:359–370

Mitchell F L 1993 Elements of muscle energy technique. In: Basmajian J V, Nyberg R (eds) Rational manual therapies. Williams & Wilkins, Baltimore, ch 12 p 297

Moberg E 1983 The role of cutaneous afferents in position sense, kinaesthesia, and motor function of the hand. Brain 106:1–19

Mooney V, Robertson J 1976 The facet syndrome. Clinical Orthopaedics and Related Research 115:149–156

Moore R M, Moore R E, Singleton A O 1934 Experiments on the chemical stimulation of pain-endings associated with small blood-vessels. American Journal of Physiology 107:594–602

Muller E A 1970 Influence of training and of inactivity on muscle strength. Archives of Physical Medicine and Rehabilitation 51:449–462

Myers T W 2001 Anatomy trains: myofascial meridians for manual and movement therapists. Churchill Livingstone, Edinburgh

Nakagawa Y, Totsuka M, Sato T et al 1989 Effect of disuse on the ultrastructure of the achilles tendon in rats. European Journal of Applied Physiology 59:239–242

Nakahara M 1971 The effect of a tourniquet on the kinin–kininogen system in blood and muscle. Thrombosis et Diathesis Haemorrhagia 26:264–274

Newham D J 1993 Eccentric muscle activity in theory and practice. In: Harms-Ringdahl K (ed) Muscle strength. Churchill Livingstone, Edinburgh, ch 5, p 63

Newham D J 2001 Strength, power and endurance. In: Trew M & Everett T (eds) Human Movement, 4th edn. Churchill Livingstone, Edinburgh, ch 6, p 105–128

Newham D J, Ainscough-Potts A-M 2001 Musculoskeletal basis for movement. In: Trew M & Everett T (eds) Human Movement, 4th edn. Churchill Livingstone, Edinburgh, ch 6, p 105–128

Newham D J, Hurley M V, Jones D W 1989 Ligamentous knee injuries and muscle inhibition. Journal of Orthopaedic Rheumatology 2:163–173

Newman P H 1968 The spine, the wood and the trees. Proceedings of the Royal Society of Medicine 61:35–41

Nicholls S P, Gathercole L J, Keller A, Shah J S 1983 Crimping in rat tail tendon collagen: morphology and transverse mechanical anisotrophy. International Journal of Biological Macromolecules 5:283–288

Nikolaou P K, MacDonald B L, Glisson R R et al 1987 Biomechanical and histological evaluation of muscle after controlled strain injury. American Journal of Sports Medicine 15(1):9–14

Nordin M, Frankel V H 1989 Basic biomechanics of the musculoskeletal system, 2nd edn. Lea & Febiger, Philadelphia

Norkin C C, Levangie P K 1992 Joint structure and function, a comprehensive analysis, 2nd edn. F A Davis, Philadelphia ch 3, p 101 and 115

Norman R W, Komi P V 1979 Electromechanical delay in skeletal muscle under normal movement conditions. Acta Physiologica Scandinavica 106:241–248

Osu R, Franklin D W, Kato H et al 2002 Short- and long-term changes in joint co-contraction associated with motor learning as revealed from surface EMG. Journal of Neurophysiology 88(8):991–1004

Paintal A S 1960 Functional analysis of group III afferent fibres of mammalian muscles. Journal of Physiology 152:250–270

Palastanga N, Field D, Soames R 2002 Anatomy and human movement – structure and function, 4th edn. Butterworth-Heinemann, Oxford

Panjabi M M 1992 The stabilizing system of the spine. Part 1. Function, dysfunction, adaptation, and enhancement. Journal of Spinal Disorders 5(4):383–389

Panjabi M M, White A A 2001 Biomechanics in the musculoskeletal system. Churchill Livingstone, New York

Panjabi M, Abumi K, Duranceau J, Oxland T 1989 Spinal stability and intersegmental muscle forces: a biomechanical model. Spine 14(2):194–200

Passatore M, Grassi C, Filippi G M 1985 Sympathetically-induced development of tension in jaw muscles: the possible contraction of intrafusal muscle fibres. Pflügers Archiv 405:297–304

Peacock E E 1959 A study of the circulation in normal tendons and healing grafts. Annals of Surgery 149(3):415–428

Peck D, Buxton D F, Nitz A 1984 A comparison of spindle concentrations in large and small muscles acting in parallel combinations. Journal of Morphology 180:243–252

Perry J, Antonelli D, Ford W 1975 Analysis of knee-joint forces during flexed-knee stance. Journal of Bone and Joint Surgery 57A(7):961–967

Pette D, Staron R S 1990 Cellular and molecular diversities of mammalian skeletal muscle fibres. Review of Physiology, Biochemistry and Pharmacology 116:1–76

Pette D, Peuker H, Staron R S 1999 The impact of biochemical methods for single muscle fibre analysis. Acta Physiologica Scandinavica 166:261–277

Petty R 2003 Evaluating muscle symptoms. Journal of Neurology, Neurosurgery & Psychiatry 74(suppl 11):ii38–ii42

Petty N J, Moore A P 2001 Neuromusculoskeletal examination and assessment, a handbook for therapists, 2nd edn. Churchill Livingstone, Edinburgh

Phillips D, Petrie S, Solomonow M et al 1997 Ligamentomuscular protective reflex in the elbow. Journal of Hand Surgery 22A(3):473–478

Pickering G W, Wayne E J 1933–1934 Observations on angina pectoris and intermittent claudication in anaemia. Clinical Science 1:305–325

Pope M H, Johnson R J, Brown D W, Tighe C 1979 The role of musculature in injuries to the medial collateral ligament. Journal of Bone and Joint Surgery 61A(3):398–402

Powers S K, Howley E T 1997 Exercise Physiology: theory and application to fitness and performance, 3rd edn. McGraw-Hill, Boston

Raja S N, Meyer R A, Ringkamp M, Campbell J N 1999 Peripheral neural mechanisms of nociception. In: Wall P D, Melzack R (eds) Textbook of pain, 4th edn. Churchill Livingstone, Edinburgh

Rantanen J, Rissanen A, Kalimo H 1994 Lumbar muscle fiber size and type distribution in normal subjects. European Spine Journal 3:331–335

Reinert A, Mense S 1992 Free nerve endings in the skeletal muscle of the rat exhibiting immunoreactivity to substance P and calcitonin gene-related peptide. Pflügers Archiv 420(suppl 1):R54

Reinert A, Vitek M, Mense S 1992 Effects of substance P on the activity of high- and low-threshold mechanosensitive receptors of the rat diaphragm in-vitro. Pflügers Archiv 420:R47

Renstrom P, Arms S W, Stanwyck T S 1986 Strain within the anterior cruciate ligament during hamstring and quadriceps activity. American Journal of Sports Medicine 14(1):83–87

Reynolds N L, Worrell T W 1991 Chronic achilles peritendinitis: etiology, pathophysiology, and treatment. Journal of Orthopaedic Sports Physical Therapy 13(4):171–176

Richardson C, Bullock M I 1986 Changes in muscle activity during fast, alternating flexion-extension movements of the knee. Scandinavian Journal of Rehabilitation Medicine 18:51–58

Richardson C, Jull G, Hodges P, Hides J 1999 Therapeutic exercise for spinal segmental stabilization in low back pain, scientific basis and clinical approach. Churchill Livingstone, Edinburgh

Rigby B J, Hirai N, Spikes J D, Eyring H 1959 The mechanical properties of rat tail tendon. Journal of General Physiology 43:265–283

Rowe R W D 1985 The structure of rat tail tendon fascicles. Connective Tissue Research 14:21–30

Royce J 1958 Isometric fatigue curves in human muscle with normal and occluded circulation. Research Quarterly 29(2):204–212

Rutherford O M, Jones D A, Newham D J 1986 Clinical and experimental application of the percutaneous twitch superimposition technique for the study of human muscle activation. Journal of Neurology, Neurosurgery and Psychiatry 49:1288–1291

Sacks R D, Roy R R 1982 Architecture of the hind limb muscles of cats: functional significance. Journal of Morphology 173:185–195

Saltin B, Henriksson J, Nygaard E, Andersen P 1977 Fiber types and metabolic potentials of skeletal muscles in sedentary man and endurance runners. Annals of New York Academy of Sciences 301:3–29

Sargeant A J, Davies C T M, Edwards R H T et al 1977 Functional and structural changes after disuse of human muscle. Clinical Science and Molecular Medicine 52:337–342

Schmid H, Spring H 1985 Muscular imbalance in skiers. Manual Medicine 2:23–26

Scott W, Stevens J, Binder-Macleod S A 2001 Human skeletal muscle fiber type classifications. Physical Therapy 81(11):1810–1816

Seki K, Taniguchi Y, Narusawa M 2001 Effects of joint immobilization on firing rate modulation of human motor units. Journal of Physiology 530(3):507–519

Shakespeare D, Stokes M, Sherman K P, Young A 1983 The effect of knee flexion on quadriceps inhibition after meniscectomy. Clinical Science 65:64P

Shakespeare D T, Stokes M, Sherman K P, Young A 1985 Reflex inhibition of the quadriceps after meniscectomy: lack of association with pain. Clinical Physiology 5:137–144

Shoemaker S C, Markolf K L 1982 In vivo rotary knee stability: ligamentous and muscular contributions. Journal of Bone and Joint Surgery 64A(2):208–216

Shumway-Cook A, Woollacott M H 1995 Motor control, theory and practical applications. Williams & Wilkins, Baltimore

Simone D A, Marchettini P, Caputi G, Ochoa J L 1994 Identification of muscle afferents subserving sensation of deep pain in humans. Journal of Neurophysiology 72(2):883–889

Simoneau J A, Lortie G, Boulay M R et al 1986 Inheritance of human skeletal muscle and anaerobic capacity adaptation

to high-intensity intermittent training. International Journal of Sports Medicine 7:167–171

Sirca A, Kostevc V 1985 The fibre type composition of thoracic and lumbar paravertebral muscles in man. Journal of Anatomy 141:131–137

Skinner H B, Barrack R L, Cook S D 1984 Age-related decline in proprioception. Clinical Orthopaedics and Related Research 184:208–211

Snyder-Mackler L, De Luca P F, Williams P R et al 1994 Reflex inhibition of the quadriceps femoris muscle after injury or reconstruction of the anterior cruciate ligament. Journal of Bone and Joint Surgery 76-A(4):555–560

Solomonow M, Guzzi A, Baratta R et al 1986 EMG-force model of the elbows antagonistic muscle pair: the effect of joint position, gravity and recruitment. American Journal Physical Medicine 65(5):223–244

Solomonow M, Baratta R, Zhou B H et al 1987 The synergistic action of the anterior cruciate ligament and thigh muscles in maintaining joint stability. American Journal of Sports Medicine 15(3):207–213

Solomonow M, Zhou B-H, Harris M et al 1998 The ligamento-muscular stabilizing system of the spine. Spine 23(23):2552–2562

Speers R A, Kuo A D, Horak F B 2002 Contributions of altered sensation and feedback responses to changes in coordination of postural control due to aging. Gait and Posture 16:20–30

Spencer J D, Hayes K C, Alexander I J 1984 Knee joint effusion and quadriceps reflex inhibition in man. Archives of Physical Medicine and Rehabilitation 65:171–177

Stacey M J 1969 Free nerve endings in skeletal muscle of the cat. Journal of Anatomy 105(2):231–254

Staron R S 1997 Human skeletal muscle fiber types: delineation, development, and distribution. Canadian Journal of Applied Physiology 22(4):307–327

Stauber W T 1989 Eccentric action of muscles: physiology, injury, and adaptation. Exercise and Sport Sciences Reviews 17:157–185

Stener B 1969 Reflex inhibition of the quadriceps elicited from a subperiosteal tumour of the femur. Acta Orthopaedica Scandinavica 40:86–91

Stener B, Petersen I 1963 Excitatory and inhibitory reflex motor effects from the partially ruptured medial collateral ligament of the knee joint. Acta Orthopaedica Scandinavica 33:359

Stokes M, Young A 1984 The contribution of reflex inhibition to arthrogenous muscle weakness. Clinical Science 67:7–14

Strasmann T, van der Wal J C, Halata Z, Drukker J 1990 Functional topography and ultrastructure of periarticular mechanoreceptors in the lateral elbow region of the rat. Acta Anatomica 138:1–14

Stratford P 1981 Electromyography of the quadriceps femoris muscles in subjects with normal knees and acutely effused knees. Physical Therapy 62(3):279–283

Stuart A, McComas A J, Goldspink G, Elder G 1981 Electrophysiologic features of muscle regeneration. Experimental Neurology 74:148–159

Suter E, Herzog W 1997 Extent of muscle inhibition as a function of knee angle. Journal of Electromyography and Kinesiology 7(2):123–130

Suter E, Herzog W 2000 Muscle inhibition and functional deficiencies associated with knee pathologies. In: Herzog W (ed) Skeletal Muscle Mechanics, from Mechanisms to Function. Wiley, Chichester, ch 21, p 365

Suter E, Herzog W, Huber A 1996 Extent of motor unit activation in the quadriceps muscles of healthy subjects. Muscle and Nerve 19:1046–1048

Suter E, Herzog W, Bray R C 1998a Quadriceps inhibition following arthroscopy in patients with anterior knee pain. Clinical Biomechanics 13:314–319

Suter E, Herzog W, De Souza K D, Bray R 1998b Inhibition of the quadriceps muscles in patients with anterior knee pain. Journal of Applied Biomechanics 14:360–373

Tabary J C, Tabary C, Tardieu C et al 1972 Physiological and structural changes in the cat's soleus muscle due to immobilization at different lengths by plaster casts. Journal of Physiology 224(1):231–244

Talishev F M, Fedina T I 1976 Influence of muscle viscoelastic characteristics on the accuracy of movement control. In: Komi P V (ed) Biomechanics V-A. University Park, Baltimore, p 124–128

Taylor D C, Dalton J D, Seaber A V, Garrett W E 1990 Viscoelastic properties of muscle–tendon units, the biomechanical effects of stretching. American Journal of Sports Medicine 18(3):300–309

Thelen D G, Shultz A B, Alexander N B, Ashton-Miller J A 1996 Effects of age on rapid ankle torque development. Journal Gerontology 51A(5):M226–M232

Thelen D G, Muriuki M, James J et al 2000 Muscle activities used by young and old adults when stepping to regain balance during a forward fall. Journal of Electromyography and Kinesiology 10:93–101

Threlkeld A J 1992 The effects of manual therapy on connective tissue. Physical Therapy 72(12):893–902

Tidball J G 1991 Myotendinous junction injury in relation to junction structure and molecular composition. Exercise and Sport Sciences Reviews 19:419–445

Torebjork H E, Ochoa J L, Schady W 1984 Referred pain from intraneural stimulation of muscle fascicles in the median nerve. Pain 18:145–156

Torry M R, Decker M J, Viola R W et al 2000 Intra-articular knee joint effusion induces quadriceps avoidance gait patterns. Clinical Biomechanics 15:147–159

Tracy B L, Enoka R M 2002 Older adults are less steady during submaximal isometric contractions with the knee extensor muscles. Journal of Applied Physiology 92:1004–1012

Trappe T A, Lindquist D M, Carrithers J A 2001 Muscle-specific atrophy of the quadriceps femoris with aging. Journal of Applied Physiology 90:2070–2074

Urbach D, Awiszus F 2002 Impaired ability of voluntary quadriceps activation bilaterally interferes with function testing after knee injuries. A twitch interpolation study. International Journal of Sports Medicine 23(4):231–236

van der Heide B, Allison G T, Zusman M 2001 Pain and muscular responses to a neural tissue provocation test in the upper limb. Manual Therapy 6(3):154–162

Vaughan V G 1989 Effects of upper limb immobilization on isometric muscle strength, movement time, and triphasic electromyographic characteristics. Physical Therapy 69(2):36–46

Vleeming A, Mooney V, Snijders C J et al 1997 Movement, stability and low back pain, the essential role of the pelvis. Churchill Livingstone, New York

Voight M L, Wieder D L 1991 Comparative reflex response times of vastus medialis obliquus and vastus lateralis in normal subjects and subjects with extensor mechanism dysfunction, an electromyographic study. American Journal of Sports Medicine 19(2):131–137

Wainwright S A, Biggs W D, Currey J D, Gosline J M 1982 Mechanical design in organisms. Princeton University Press, Princeton NJ, p 91

Wall P D, Melzack R 1999 Textbook of pain, 4th edn. Churchill Livingstone, Edinburgh

Walla D J, Albright J P, McAuley E et al 1985 Hamstring control and the unstable anterior cruciate ligament-deficient knee. American Journal of Sports Medicine 13(1):34–39

Watkins M P, Harris B A, Kozlowski B A 1984 Isokinetic testing in patients with hemiparesis. A pilot study. Physical Therapy 64:184–189

Watson D H 1994 Cervical headache: an investigation of natural head posture and upper cervical flexor muscle performance. In: Boyling J D, Palastanga N (eds) Grieve's modern manual therapy, the vertebral column, 2nd edn. Churchill Livingstone, Edinburgh, ch 24, p 349–360

Wells P E, Frampton V, Bowsher D 1994 Pain management by physiotherapy, 2nd edn. Butterworth-Heinemann, Oxford

Widrick J J, Romatowski J G, Norenberg K M et al 2001 Functional properties of slow and fast gastrocnemius muscle fibers after a 17-day spaceflight. Journal of Applied Physiology 90:2203–2211

Wilke H-J, Wolf S, Claes L E et al 1995 Stability increase of the lumbar spine with different muscle groups: a biomechanical in vitro study. Spine 20(2):192–198

Wilkie D R 1950 The relation between force and velocity in human muscle. Journal of Physiology 110:249–280

Williams P E 1988 Effect of intermittent stretch on immobilised muscle. Annals of the Rheumatic Diseases 47(12):1014–1016

Williams P E, Goldspink G 1973 The effect of immobilization on the longitudinal growth of striated muscle fibres. Journal of Anatomy 116(1):45–55

Williams P E, Goldspink G 1976 The effect of denervation and dystrophy on the adaptation of sarcomere number to the functional length of the muscle in young and adult mice. Journal of Anatomy 122(2):455–465

Williams P E, Goldspink G 1978 Changes in sarcomere length and physiological properties in immobilized muscle. Journal of Anatomy 127(3):459–468

Williams P E, Goldspink G 1984 Connective tissue changes in immobilized muscle. Journal of Anatomy 138(2):343–350

Williams P L, Bannister L H, Berry M M et al 1995 Gray's anatomy, 38th edn. Churchill Livingstone, New York

Witvrouw E, Sneyers C, Lysens R et al 1996 Reflex response times of vastus medialis oblique and vastus lateralis in normal subjects and in subjects with patellofemoral pain syndrome. Journal of Orthopaedic Sports Physical Therapy 24(3):160–165

Woo S, Maynard J, Butler D et al 1988 Ligament, tendon, and joint capsule insertions to bone. In: Woo S L-Y, Buckwalter J (eds) Injury and repair of the musculoskeletal soft tissues. American Academy of Orthopaedic Surgeons. Park Ridge, Illinois ch 4, p 133–166

Wood L, Ferrell W R, Baxendale R H 1988 Pressures in normal and acutely distended human knee joints and effects on quadriceps maximal voluntary contractions. Quarterly Journal of Experimental Physiology 73:305–314

Wood T O, Cooke P H, Goodship A E 1988 The effect of exercise and anabolic steroids on the mechanical properties and crimp morphology of the rat tendon. American Journal of Sports Medicine 16(2):153–158

Wuerker R B, McPhedran A M, Henneman E 1965 Properties of motor units in a heterogeneous pale muscle (M. Gastrocnemius) of the cat. Journal of Neurophysiology 28:85–99

Wyke B D, Polacek P 1975 Articular neurology: the present position. Journal of Bone and Joint Surgery 57B(3):401

Yamashita T, Minaki Y, Ozaktay A C et al 1996 A morphological study of the fibrous capsule of the human lumbar facet joint. Spine 21(5):538–543

Yoshihara K, Shirai Y, Nakayama Y, Uesaka S 2001 Histochemical changes in the multifidus muscle in patients with lumbar intervertebral disc herniation. Spine 26(6):622–626

Young A, Hughes I, Russell P et al 1980 Measurement of quadriceps muscle wasting by ultrasonography. Rheumatology and Rehabilitation 19(3):141–148

Young A, Stokes M, Crowe M 1982a The relationship between quadriceps size and strength in elderly women. Clinical Science 63(3):35P–36P

Young A, Hughes I, Round J M, Edwards R H T 1982b The effect of knee injury on the number of muscle fibres in the human quadriceps femoris. Clinical Science 62:227–234

Young A, Stokes M, Round J M, Edwards R H T 1983 The effect of high-resistance training on the strength and cross-sectional area of the human quadriceps. European Journal of Clinical Investigation 13:411–417

Young A, Stokes M, Iles J F 1987 Effects of joint pathology on muscle. Clinical Orthopaedics and Related Research 219:21–27

Zattara M, Bouisset S 1988 Posturo-kinetic organisation during the early phase of voluntary upper limb movement. 1. Normal subjects. Journal of Neurology, Neurosurgery and Psychiatry 51:956–965

Zhang L-Q, Nuber G, Butler J et al 1998 In vivo human knee joint dynamic properties as functions of muscle contraction and joint position. Journal of Biomechanics 31:71–76

Zhao W-P, Kawaguchi Y, Matsui H et al 2000 Histochemistry and morphology of the multifidus muscle in lumbar disc herniation comparative study between diseased and normal sides. Spine 25(17):2191–2199

6

Principles of muscle treatment

There is no pure treatment for muscle, that is, treatment cannot be isolated to muscle alone, it will always to a greater or lesser extent affect joint and/or nerve tissue. Some sort of classification system for treatment is needed in order to have meaningful communication between clinicians, and this text follows the traditional classification of muscle, joint and nerve treatment. In this text a 'muscle treatment' is defined as a 'treatment to effect a change in muscle'; that is, the intention of the clinician is to produce a change in muscle and therefore it is described as a muscle treatment. Similarly, where a technique is used to effect a change in a joint, it will be referred to as a 'joint treatment' and where a technique is used to effect a change in nerve, it will be referred to as a 'nerve treatment'. Thus, treatments are classified according to which tissue the clinician is predominantly attempting to affect. This relationship of treatment of muscle, joint and nerve is depicted in Figure 6.1.

An example may help to illustrate the impurity of a muscle treatment technique. With the patient sitting over the edge of the couch, the patient is asked to contract the knee extensors against the manual resistance of the clinician. After maximal contraction there is relaxation of the muscle and the clinician is able to move the knee into more flexion. This is a hold–relax technique for the knee extensors. Further analysis reveals that this technique is not purely a muscle treatment: it also involves joints and nerves. The quadriceps muscle contains the patella and so muscle contraction will cause movement of the patellofemoral joint and may cause some change to the tibiofemoral

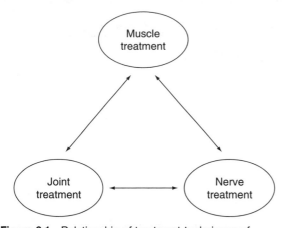

Figure 6.1 Relationship of treatment techniques of muscle, joint and nerve. Treatment of muscle will also affect joint and nerve.

joint. Following muscle relaxation, the clinician moves the knee joint further into flexion, which will affect the tibiofemoral joint and patellofemoral joint. Throughout this technique there will be neural activity in the form of afferent information from skin, joint and muscle, and efferent activity to muscle. In addition, the movement of the knee into further flexion will

lengthen the femoral nerve. It can be readily seen that a simple hold–relax technique, that might be described as a muscle treatment, also affects joint and nerve. For this reason the hold–relax technique could be used to effect a change in muscle, joint and/or nerve tissue. The therapeutic effect of the hold–relax technique is likely to be a combined effect on muscle, joint and nerve.

There are a variety of muscle treatments. Treatments are categorized in this text from the dysfunctions identified in the previous chapter, namely, reduced strength, power and endurance, altered motor control (muscle inhibition, increased muscle activation, delayed timing of onset, altered activation of agonist and antagonist), reduced length, and production of symptoms (Table 6.1). From this, a classification of muscle treatment can be identified: to increase muscle strength, power and endurance, alter motor control (increase muscle activation, reduce muscle activation, increase timing of onset, alter activation of agonist and antagonist), increase muscle length, and reduce muscle related symptoms. A variety of techniques to address each of these treatments is also given in Table 6.1.

Table 6.1 Muscle dysfunction, aims of muscle treatment and treatment techniques

Muscle dysfunction	Aims of muscle treatment	Treatment techniques
Reduced strength, power and endurance	Increase strength, power and endurance	Training regimes using free weights, springs, pulleys, theraband, dynamometers, PNF
Altered motor control: muscle inhibition	Increase muscle activation	Active assisted movements, rapid stretch mechanical vibration, PNF, touch, use of overflow, ice and taping
delayed timing of onset	Increase time of onset	Challenge posture and balance using for example sit fit, gym ball
increased muscle activation	Reduce muscle activation	Made aware of the unwanted muscle activity using a mirror, verbal feedback, touch, EMG feedback. Positioning, PNF, trigger points, deep inhibitory massage and taping
Reduced length	Increase length	Stretching: ballistic or static, passively by clinician or actively by patient PNF
Symptom production	Reduce symptoms	Soft-tissue mobilization: massage, connective tissue massage, specific soft tissue mobilizations, trigger points, frictions Joint mobilizations Taping Electrotherapy

PRINCIPLES OF INCREASING MUSCLE STRENGTH, POWER AND ENDURANCE

There are a variety of exercise regimes used to increase muscle strength, power and endurance and the reader is referred to the numerous exercise physiology textbooks for further details on these.

This text reviews the principles involved in increasing muscle strength, power and endurance. The principles are: overload, specificity, individuality, motivation, learning, reversibility and diminishing returns (Newham 2001); these principles are summarized in Box 6.1.

Overload

To improve the strength or endurance of a muscle it must be progressively overloaded (Bruton 2002). When strengthening a muscle, the resistance must be greater than that during everyday activities, and as the muscle gains strength the resistance must be progressively increased. When increasing muscle endurance, there must be a progressive increase in duration and frequency.

Specificity

This relates to the specific adaptation of muscle to the imposed demands (DiNubile 1991). The effect on muscle is specific to the nature of the exercise:

1. High resistance and low repetition will result in an increase in muscle strength (Hakkinen et al 1998, Staron et al 1994); there will

---

be little to no improvement in endurance (Newham 2001).

2. Low resistance and high repetition will result in an increase in muscle endurance; there will be little to no improvement in strength (Newham 2001).

3. Low resistance at high speed will increase muscle power, that is, an increase in the speed of contraction.

4. High resistance at slow speed will result in an increase in muscle strength (and will not improve the speed of contraction).

The implication of specificity is that the prescribed exercise needs to mirror the functional activity it aims to improve.

Individuality

Individuals will respond differently to the same exercise; this response is determined by genetics, cellular growth rates, metabolism and neural and endocrine regulation (Wilmore & Costill 1999).

Motivation

Only those motivated enough will make the physical and mental effort of following a training programme. The clinician can help to motivate the patient by the use of voice, explanation, enthusiasm etc.

Learning

The clinician educates the patient about the required exercise so that it is carried out effectively. Where the movement is unfamiliar, motor learning may need to occur. Motor learning is discussed in greater detail in Chapter 7.

Diminishing returns

An exercise regime will produce a greater improvement in people in poor physical condition than in those already in a good physical condition (Newham 2001).

Box 6.1 Principles of increasing muscle strength, power and endurance (Newham 2001)

- Overload
- Specificity
- Individuality
- Motivation
- Learning
- Reversibility
- Diminishing returns

Reversibility

This rather disappointing principle states that when training stops, any strength or endurance gains will be lost (Bruton 2002).

INCREASING MUSCLE STRENGTH

The above principles need to be applied when attempting to increase muscle strength. The resistance to a muscle contraction needed to strengthen a muscle can be provided by: gravity, the clinician, the patient, a wall or piece of furniture, free weights, pulleys, springs, theraband and dynamometers such as the Cybex machine (Cybex, Bay Shore, NY). Interestingly, an isotonic exercise programme using free weights has been found to be as effective in strengthening the quadricep femoris muscle as the more expensive Cybex machine (DeLateur et al 1972a).

Recommended strengthening regimes for healthy sedentary adults have been advocated by the American College of Sports Medicine (1998). This programme involves a minimum of 8–12 RM (repetition maximum) at least two times a week, where an eight-repetition maximum would be the maximum amount of weight that could be lifted eight times. This recommendation is supported by research findings. The majority of studies have found that one set is as effective as two or three sets of resisted exercises (Graves et al 1990, Pollock et al 1993, Starkey et al 1996, Westcott 1986, Westcott et al 1989). In one study, three sets was found to be the optimum number for strengthening muscle (Berger 1962).

The optimum frequency of exercise has also been investigated by a number of studies with varying results. An optimum frequency for strengthening the muscles around the chest, arms and legs has been found to be three or more times a week (Braith et al 1989, Gillam 1981), one, two or three times a week for spinal muscles (DeMichele et al 1997, Graves et al 1990, Leggett et al 1991, Pollock et al 1993), and trunk flexion and extension muscle strength has been found to increase following two or three sessions a week (Parkkola et al 1992). A reasonable guideline for frequency would be a minimum of twice a week (Feigenbaum & Pollock 1999).

A strengthening regime would normally start slowly with a low intensity of exercise (American College of Sports Medicine 1998, Feigenbaum & Pollock 1999). Following assessment of the 1 RM, the upper body should train at 30–40% of 1 RM and the lower body at 50–60%. Once the weight can be lifted well 12 times with a perceived exertion rating of 12–14 RPE, (Borg 1982), 5% can be added to the next training session (Fig. 6.2). Exercising to maximal effort, that is, to 19–20 RPE, will produce the greatest gains in strength (American College of Sports Medicine 1998), with progression of weight every 1–2 weeks.

It is recommended that, for the elderly, the intensity be reduced to one set of 10–15 RM, increasing the weight every 2–4 weeks (Feigenbaum & Pollock 1999). While muscle strength is less in the older person, the potential to strengthen muscle with a training programme is much the same as with a young person (Grimby 1995).

In conformity with the principle of specificity, the type of muscle contraction used in an exercise regime affects the change in muscle strength.

Eccentric muscle contraction appears to be more effective and efficient in increasing muscle strength. Eccentric exercises have been found to cause a greater increase in eccentric, isometric and concentric muscle strength than either con-

6	
7	Very very light
8	
9	Very light
10	
11	Fairly light
12	
13	Somewhat hard
14	
15	Hard
16	
17	Very hard
18	
19	Very very hard
20	

Figure 6.2 Fifteen-point scale for ratings of perceived exertion, the RPE scale. (Reproduced from Borg 1982, Psychophysical bases of perceived exertion. Medicine and Science in Sports and Exercise 14(5)377–381, with permission.)

centric exercises or a mixed exercise regime (Hortobagyi et al 2000). Eccentric exercises three times a week for 12 weeks have been found to increase eccentric strength three and a half times more than concentric exercises increase concentric strength (Hortobagyi et al 1996).

Isotonic exercise with free weights increases isotonic strength of quadriceps but not isometric strength, even after a few days of isometric exercises (DeLateur et al 1972b). Isometric exercises on the other hand, increase isometric strength and after 4 days of isotonic exercises produce a rapid increase in isotonic strength (DeLateur et al 1972b). The clinical implication of this is that if movement is not possible due to some pathological process or injury, isometric exercises will improve isometric strength and enhance isotonic strength gains when movement is allowed (DeLateur et al 1972b).

The value of isometric exercises is further highlighted in another study, exploring the optimal exercise regime to produce hypertrophy of multifidus in patients with chronic low back pain (Danneels et al 2001). General stabilization exercises, isometric contractions and concentric and eccentric muscle contractions at 70% of 1 RM (15–18 repetitions) three times a week for 10 weeks, resulted in hypertrophy of multifidus. However, the group of patients who carried out only general stabilization exercises, and the group of patients who carried out only general stabilization exercises and the concentric and eccentric exercises, failed to produce a significant hypertrophy of multifidus. It was therefore concluded that the isometric exercises were critical in producing hypertrophy of multifidus in patients with chronic low back pain. However, it is worth mentioning that isometric exercises produce strength gains only in the range within which the exercise is carried out.

The speed of isotonic muscle contractions can effect the strength changes in muscle. A high speed of contraction has been found to eliminate muscle inhibition, and so fast dynamic work may be the best form of strength training (Newham et al 1989).

Transcutaneous electrical stimulation for 10 to 15 minutes once a day for 5 weeks has been found to produce a significant increase ($P <0.001$) in quadriceps femoris torque and the improvement was similar to subjects who carried out isometric exercises (Laughman et al 1983).

The clinician can provide manual resistance to a concentric or isometric muscle contraction and this has been most fully explored with proprioceptive neuromuscular facilitation (PNF). PNF is thought to be useful when a muscle is very weak; once active contraction is possible equipment to provide resistance is more effective (Newham 2001). The advantages of PNF include a reduced need for equipment; PNF also allows tactile encouragement by the clinician and versatile movement patterns can be incorporated. The disadvantages of PNF are the time and effort required by the clinician and the imprecise measurement of the resistance applied and the muscle torque produced. Further information about PNF can be found elsewhere (Knott & Voss 1968, Waddington 1999).

Underlying effect of strengthening a muscle

A small number of repetitions against a high resistance will strengthen muscle (Hakkinen et al 1998, Staron et al 1994); the underlying effects are, first, a change in neural tissue, so that motor learning occurs, and second, a change in muscle tissue, so that there is muscle hypertrophy (Fig. 6.3). The stimulus for a strength change is the force of contraction, and this is reflected in the nature of the changes.

Motor learning

The first stage, which lasts for 6–8 weeks, is where motor learning occurs; performance improves but strength remains the same.

The changes include:

• increased neural activation to the muscle (Komi 1986, Moritani & DeVries 1979, Sale et al 1983). The amount of increase parallels the amount of increase in muscle strength.
• increased activation of prime movers (Sale 1988).
• improved coordination (Sale 1988).

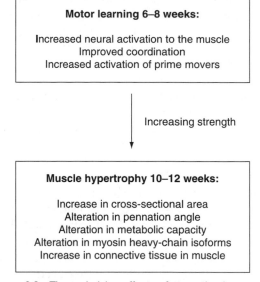

Motor learning 6–8 weeks:

Increased neural activation to the muscle
Improved coordination
Increased activation of prime movers

Increasing strength

Muscle hypertrophy 10–12 weeks:

Increase in cross-sectional area
Alteration in pennation angle
Alteration in metabolic capacity
Alteration in myosin heavy-chain isoforms
Increase in connective tissue in muscle

Figure 6.3 The underlying effects of strengthening muscle (Newham 2001).

It has been proposed that neural changes alone can produce an increase in muscle strength (Enoka 1988). During an 8-week training programme neural changes were responsible for almost all the strength gains in subjects with a mean age of 70 years. In subjects with a mean age of 22 years, neural changes were responsible for most of the strength changes in the first 4 weeks, with muscle hypertrophy after 4–6 weeks (Moritani & de Vries 1979). It appears from this study that the timing of the changes in nerve and muscle varies with age.

Neural activation may be responsible for improved muscle activation, strength and endurance beyond the suggested 6–8 weeks (Kaser et al 2001, Mannion et al 2001). Patients with chronic low back pain followed a 3-month back exercise programme (Mannion et al 2001), and while activation, strength and endurance improved this was not accompanied by any change in the size of the muscle fibres or proportion of muscle fibre type (Kaser et al 2001).

Muscle hypertrophy

The final stage after about 10–12 weeks is muscle hypertrophy where muscle increases in size and strength (Newham 2001). The changes are:

1. An increase in the cross-sectional area of the muscle, mainly at the proximal and distal parts of the muscle belly; this is visible after a few weeks of training (Housh et al 1992, Narici et al 1996). The increase in cross-sectional area of the muscle is due to hypertrophy of muscle fibres (see below) and an increase in the connective tissue in muscle (MacDougall 1986). In addition, where the strength training involves a group of muscles, the increase in cross-sectional area is not equal in each muscle (Housh et al 1992, Narici et al 1996). For example, with quadriceps strength training, greatest hypertrophy was seen in rectus femoris and least hypertrophy in vastus intermedius (Narici et al 1996).

2. An increase in the cross-sectional area of the muscle fibres (Andersen & Aagaard 2000, Hortobagyi et al 1996, MacDougall et al 1980, Melissa et al 1997). It is unclear whether fibre types respond differently to strength training; only two studies found an increase in cross-sectional area in type II fibres (Andersen & Aagaard 2000, Melissa et al 1997), and two studies found type II fibres increased in cross-sectional area at a faster rate than type I fibres (Hortobagyi et al 1996, MacDougall et al 1980). Yet another study found equal increases between type I and II fibres (Young et al 1983). Differences in methodology such as upper or lower limb muscle, exercise regime and type of muscle contraction may, in part, be responsible for the conflicting results. The most distinctive difference was found within one study which found that eccentric exercises produced a tenfold greater increase in type II cross-sectional area than concentric exercises (Hortobagyi et al 1996).

3. Alteration in muscle fibre types. Some studies have found no change in proportion of type I or type II fibres (Labarque et al 2002, Terrados et al 1990), while other studies have found an increase in the proportion of type IIa fibres and a decrease in type IIb fibres following strength training (Andersen & Aagaard 2000, Hortobagyi et al 1996).

4. An alteration in pennation angles has been demonstrated in hypertrophied muscle (Kawakami et al 1993, 1995).

5. An alteration in metabolic capacity of muscle has been demonstrated; this effect appears to be genetically determined (Simoneau et al 1986).

6. An alteration in myosin heavy-chain (MHC) isoforms (Andersen & Aagaard 2000, Gea 1997). The myosin head, which binds with actin during a muscle contraction, contains the myosin heavy-chain isoforms (Scott et al 2001).

7. There is an increase in the amount of connective tissue found in muscle structures proportional to muscle hypertrophy (MacDougall 1986).

INCREASING MUSCLE POWER

The principles of overload, specificity, individuality, motivation, learning, reversibility and diminishing returns (Newham 2001) need to be considered when attempting to increase muscle power. Because muscle power is a function of muscle force and velocity of contraction, improvement in either or both of these aspects will result in an increase in muscle power. Increasing muscle strength has been discussed in the previous section; increasing speed of contraction involves active contraction at speed. Repeated practice of the movement, or a component of the movement, at speed, is thought to produce an improvement in muscle power (deVries & Housh 1994). It is suggested that the whole movement, or a component of the movement, should be carried out as fast as possible against a resistance of 30% maximal isometric strength (Kerr 1998), although one study has found that exercises carried out at high speed only caused improvement in power at a high speed, whereas exercises at slow or intermediate speed increased power at slow, intermediate and high speed (Kanehisa & Miyashita 1983). In line with the principle of specificity, the speed at which the muscle needs to contract for a specific functional task is the ideal speed at which the exercises should be carried out.

INCREASING MUSCLE ENDURANCE

Muscle endurance can refer to the ability of a muscle to contract repetitively or to sustain a contraction for a period of time (Bruton 2002). The principles of overload, specificity, individuality, motivation, learning, reversibility and diminishing returns (Newham 2001) also need to be applied when attempting to increase muscle endurance.

The differing effect of exercise, between individuals, to improve endurance is beginning to emerge. The effect of exercises on muscle endurance training has been found to be related to an 'insertion' gene encoding angiotensin-converting enzyme which has been found in significantly (P <0.05) greater frequency in elite high-altitude mountaineers than in control subjects (Montgomery et al 1998). In addition, the same researchers found that subjects with 'insertion' allele had an eleven-fold greater improvement than those with 'deletion' allele following a 10-week endurance-training programme. The underlying mechanism is unclear but may affect the circulation system, hormone concentration and/or metabolism (Montgomery et al 1998).

To increase muscle endurance a muscle must contract at 30–50% of its maximum contraction, for 20–30 minutes three times a week (McArdle et al 1996) and 25–35 repetitions need to occur at each session (Berger 1982, Kerr 1998). Where endurance training incorporates general cardio-respiratory exercises, such as walking, running, swimming and cycling, the intensity of exercise should be sufficient to raise the heart rate to 60–90% of maximal, and it should be carried out for 15–60 minutes, three to five times each week (Newham 2001). Recommended maximal heart rates during training for different age groups are shown in Table 6.2 (Newham 2001).

Underlying effects of increasing muscle endurance

A high number of repetitions of muscle contractions against a low resistance will increase muscle endurance (Newham 2001) by effecting a change in muscle. The stimulus is the metabolic demand of the muscle and this is reflected in the nature of the changes (Box 6.2) and include an:

- increase in the number of type I and IIa fibres and a decrease in type IIb fibres (Demirel et al 1999, Ingjer 1979)

Table 6.2 The maximal heart rate recommended during training at different ages (Newham 2001)

Age (years)	Upper limit (beats per minute)
20–29	170
30–39	160
40–49	150
50–59	140
60 and over	130

- increase in the cross-sectional area of type I fibres (Ingjer 1979)
- increase in number of capillaries surrounding each muscle fibre (Hermansen & Wachtlova 1971, Ingjer 1979)
- increase in blood flow in muscle (Rohter et al 1963, Vanderhoof et al 1961)
- increase in myoglobin content, which increases oxidative power of muscle (Holloszy 1976)
- increase in oxidative power and enzyme activity of mitochondria. An endurance training programme resulted in a 40% increase in the mitochondrial oxidative power (Tonkonogi et al 2000)
- increase in oxidative enzymes (Fitts & Widrick 1996, Holloszy 1976)
- increase in glycogen and fat storage in muscle (Holloszy 1976)
- increase in activity of enzymes involved in beta-oxidation of fat (Holloszy 1976)
- a higher threshold level of lactate (Holloszy 1976)

Box 6.2 Underlying effect of increasing muscle endurance

- Increase in number of I and IIa fibres, and a decrease in type IIb fibres
- Increase in cross-sectional area of type I fibres
- Increase in number of capillaries
- Increase in myoglobin content
- Increase in oxidative power and enzyme activity of mitochondria
- Increase in oxidative enzymes
- Increased store of muscle glycogen and fat
- Increased activity of enzymes
- Higher threshold level of lactate
- Altered myosin heavy chain (MHC) isoforms

- alteration in myosin heavy chain (MHC) isoforms (Demirel et al 1999, O'Neill et al 1999).

ALTERING MOTOR CONTROL

Signs of altered motor control have been considered in the previous chapter as muscle inhibition, delayed timing of onset, increased muscle activation, and altered relative activation of agonist and antagonist. The aim of treatment, in this case, would therefore be to: increase muscle activation, increase the speed of onset of muscle contraction, reduce muscle activation or alter relative activation of agonist and antagonist. The common theme for each of these aims is to alter the pattern of muscle activation, which is to alter motor control. The principles of altering motor control are largely provided by the theory of motor learning and have been applied in patients with neurological problems and neuromusculoskeletal dysfunction; the underlying processes involved are thought to be similar (Carr & Shepherd 1998).

As in any learning environment, the learner – in this case the patient – is the key player. The patient comes with a unique set of abilities and past experience which can influence their ability to learn new motor patterns; these factors include: attitude to new experiences, body type, cultural background, emotional make-up, fitness level, dexterity, stamina, strength, learning style (visual, verbal or kinaesthetic), maturity, motivation, previous social and therapeutic experiences, prior movement experiences and stage of learning (Schmidt & Wrisberg 2000). These are summarized in Box 6.3. The motivation of the patient is critical and can be enhanced by fully involving the patient with the treatment by allowing them to set and evaluate their own goals of treatment. The patient needs to be motivated to practise because the improvement of performance is directly related to the amount of practice (Carr & Shepherd 1998).

Motor learning can be divided into three stages: verbal–cognitive, motor and autonomous (Schmidt & Wrisberg 2000); these stages are sum-

Box 6.3 Factors affecting the ability of a person to learn a new movement pattern (Schmidt & Wrisberg 2000)

- Attitude to new experiences
- Body type
- Cultural background
- Emotional makeup
- Fitness level
- Dexterity
- Stamina
- Strength
- Learning style (visual, verbal or kinaesthetic)
- Maturity
- Motivation
- Previous social and therapeutic experiences
- Prior movement experiences
- Stage of learning

marized in Figure 6.4. The verbal–cognitive stage is where the patient is being asked to do a new unfamiliar movement and is characterized by the patient thinking and perhaps talking about the movement they want to achieve. Any past experience of something similar will help the patient in this stage. Their ability to achieve the movement is likely to be jerky and uncertain.

The effects of mental practice compared to physical practice have been investigated in an interesting study on piano playing (Pascual-Leone et al 1995). One subject group undertook mental practice, and another group physical practice, for 2 hours a day over a 5-day period. Both groups demonstrated similar cortical changes in the motor system. The mental practice group were not as good as the physical practice group in performing the actual physical task; however,

they did become equivalent in their ability after just one 2-hour physical practice session. This suggests that mental practice can be used to minimize the time needed for physical practice and is of equal value to physical practice (Pascual-Leone et al 1995). The clinician can enhance learning by being aware of the learning style of the patient (Honey & Mumford 1986) and emphasizing their preferred cue, whether that be a visual, verbal or kinaesthetic cue. Thus, the clinician will explain, demonstrate, and use touch to help teach the patient a new movement strategy.

The motor stage is where the learner refines the movement pattern so that it is smoother and more certain. If the required movement or muscular control is slow, for example, challenging balance and posture, then the patient will focus on any internal or external feedback to improve motor control. If, on the other hand, the required movement is fast, the patient will focus on the movement itself. Whichever feedback is used, the patient can be encouraged to reflect on their performance, and any errors they may have made, as this has been found to promote development of skill (Liu & Wrisberg 1997). The patient may initially produce movement with co-contraction of agonist and antagonist and, as improvement occurs, there will be sequential contraction – producing an improved quality of movement (Moore & Marteniuk 1986). With improvement, the movement will be carried out more efficiently with less energy used (Sparrow & Irizarry-Lopez 1987), so that there will be less fatigue. This change can be measured by asking patients their rating of perceived effort using the Borg scale, shown in Figure 6.2 (Borg 1982). The clinician can enhance learning in this stage by providing the patient with specific and accurate feedback by the use of mirrors, palpation, verbal feedback, pressure biofeedback unit (PBU, Chatanooga, Australia), ultrasound imaging (Hides et al 1995), EMG biofeedback (Richardson et al 1999) and encouraging the patient to practise (McDonald et al 1989, Moore & Marteniuk 1986, Sparrow & Irizarry-Lopez 1987). If the movement is complex, then practice of individual components may help, but – as early as possible – the movement should be practised in its

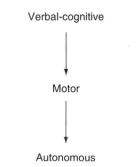

Verbal-cognitive

↓

Motor

↓

Autonomous

Figure 6.4 Stages in motor learning (Schmidt & Wrisberg 2000).

entirety and in its specific context (Carr & Shepherd 1998). This stage may last for several weeks or months.

The patient may then move to the autonomous stage in which a movement can be carried out without the patient having to concentrate on it and there is an increased ability to detect and correct error in their performance (McCullagh & Caird 1990). Learning in this stage can continue for months and even years (Crossman 1959). For example, in the manufacture of cigars workers perform a discrete motor task as quickly as possible. The speed of performance does not appreciably improve until it has been repeated some three million times over a 2-year period (Crossman 1959).

The nervous system is plastic, that is, it adapts and changes as the need arises (Carr & Shepherd 1998, Kandel 1991, Niemann et al 1991, Pascual-Leone et al 1995). The trigger for change within the central nervous system is an increased use of a body part or increased sensory feedback from it (Carr & Shepherd 1998, Jenkins et al 1990). An interesting study controlled the behaviour of the adult owl monkey's hand. The hand was trained to obtain food and repeated the task about 600 times each day for 10 days, equivalent to about 6000 repetitions. This learned motor task was accompanied by an expansion of the area of the brain's cortex concerned with the hand, demonstrating the cortical effects of motor learning (Jenkins et al 1990). Cortical changes have been found to occur in humans following limb amputation and spinal cord injury (Cohen et al 1991) and learning a complicated sequence of finger movements (Niemann et al 1991, Pascual-Leone et al 1995). Learning alters the pattern of interconnections between the involved sensory and motor systems (Kandel 1991). It appears that Brodmann's areas of mapping in the sensory cortex varies between individuals and depends on the dominant pathways in use (Kandel 1991). The underlying mechanisms of these changes have so far been identified as either the development of new neural connections or increased synaptic effectiveness (Kandel 1991, Kidd et al 1992). Proprioceptive neuromuscular facilitation (PNF), described by a number of workers

(Bobath 1990, Carr & Shepherd 1998, Knott & Voss 1968, Rood 1956, Waddington 1999), has provided treatments that encourage and guide normal movement patterns. Treatment aims to facilitate wanted movement and inhibit unwanted movement (Kidd et al 1992). The basis of these techniques is that, by producing normal movement patterns and repeating them, the central and peripheral nervous system will undergo plastic change such that it learns to initiate and reproduce this normal movement pattern (Carr & Shepherd 1998, Fletcher-Cook 1999).

Continual practice of normal movement patterns over a long period of time is often necessary to produce a change. The Peto Institute in Budapest provides an intensive (13 hours per day) residential teaching programme in motor learning for children and adults with motor disabilities, such as ataxia, hemiplegia etc. (Todd 1990). To alter normal functional movement patterns, treatment needs to use normal functional movement patterns (Carr & Shepherd 1998). This is reinforced by the principle of specificity of learning (Henry 1968) which, when applied to patients, means that the best practice of a movement is that which most closely mimics the functional movement required.

To increase muscle activation

Methods for increasing muscle activation, that is, for facilitating muscle contraction, include active assisted movements, rapid stretch mechanical vibration, PNF, touch, use of overflow, ice and taping (Box 6.4). Electrical stimulation of muscle is also available. With the muscle contracting and in a lengthened position, a rapid stretch is applied to the muscle; this stimulates the muscle

---

Box 6.4 Treatment to increase muscle activation

- Active assisted movements
- Rapid stretch
- PNF
- Touch
- Use of overflow
- Mechanical vibration
- Ice
- Taping

spindles to facilitate extrafusal muscle contraction (Newham 2001). Vibration similarly stimulates the muscle spindles. Proprioceptive neuromuscular facilitation (PNF) may also prove helpful in facilitating muscle contraction (Knott & Voss 1968, Waddington 1999). Touch can be used to facilitate muscle contraction; stimulation of the skin has been shown to enhance alpha and gamma motor neurone activity in the underlying muscles and cause inhibition of more distal muscles (Eldred & Hagbarth 1954). The principle of overflow may also be helpful in facilitating muscle activation, such that contraction of stronger muscles can lead to increased activation of the weak muscle (Kidd et al 1992). Quickly brushing ice over a muscle may facilitate its contraction (Rood 1956). Taping is thought to increase activation of the underlying muscle (Cowan et al 2002, Gilleard et al 1998).

Inhibition of an active voluntary contraction was eliminated with a fast velocity isotonic contraction (Newham et al 1989). This can be explained by the relationship of force and speed, where increased speed of concentric contraction reduces the force generated (Hill 1938).

The activation of a muscle during functional activities may need to be addressed in treatment. Contraction of the hamstring muscles can increase knee joint stiffness by 100–250% (Louie & Mote 1987) and reduce the strain on the ACL (Renstrom et al 1986). It may be helpful in treatment to increase the activation of the hamstring muscles to help stabilize the knee joint. It has been found that strengthening the knee flexors over a period of 2–3 weeks results in increased activity of the hamstrings during maximal active knee extension (Baratta et al 1988). It appears, then, that strengthening a muscle does not just affect its function as an agonist, it also facilitates its recruitment as an antagonist. Thus, hamstring strength training may be beneficial in patients with ACL injury, or after repair, to enhance knee joint stability (Baratta et al 1988). If this phenomenon occurs with other muscles, then the effect of strengthening a muscle increases its torque as an agonist and also increases its activation as an antagonist.

The plastic nature of muscle activation is highlighted by patients with ACL-deficient knees who have an increased EMG activity of biceps femoris, vastus lateralis, tibialis anterior during a range of functional activities, compared to a control group (Ciccotti et al 1994). This increased muscle activity is considered to be a protective mechanism which enhances the stability of the knee joint.

Measurement of muscle inhibition varies with joint angle (Suter & Herzog 1997). For this reason, standardization of the position of the joint is needed on each reassessment. Measurement of quadriceps inhibition, in the presence of a joint effusion, is best carried out at 30 degrees knee flexion, as intra-articular pressure is least at this angle (Jayson & Dixon 1970, Levick 1983). Measurement of quadriceps inhibition for patients with ACL reconstruction is best carried out beyond 60 degrees (Arms et al 1984) or 80 degrees (Hirokawa et al 1992) knee flexion because, at this angle, the tibia is translating posteriorly and will thus not strain the ACL.

Increase speed of onset

Using the principles of motor learning, it would seem reasonable to suggest that, to increase the speed of onset of muscle contraction, treatment needs to use normal functional activities that will produce a need for the muscle to contract. With delayed activation of transversus abdominis in patients with LBP (Hodges & Richardson 1996), treatment would include functional postures and movements that challenge postural stability and this would need to be continued repetitively over a period of time. The use of a gym ball and sit fit (Sissel UK Ltd, Halifax, UK) may help to facilitate speed of onset of muscle contraction (Richardson et al 1999). In patients with anterior knee pain, a combination of specific muscle exercise with biofeedback, muscle stretches, taping and patellofemoral accessory movements has been shown, over a 6-week period, to increase the timing of muscle onset of vastus medialis, when going up and down stairs (Cowan et al 2002, Gilleard et al 1998). The mechanism by which the tape increased the onset of vastus medialis is unclear. Cutaneous stimulation has been shown to alter recruitment threshold and recruitment order of motor units (Garnett & Stephens 1981, Jenner & Stephens 1982).

To reduce muscle activation

This may be needed where the clinician feels there is over-activity of muscles. For example, in the early stages of motor learning there is co-contraction of the agonist and antagonist when carrying out a movement (Moore & Marteniuk 1986). Similarly, there may be unwanted muscle activity as a patient attempts to produce a specific muscle contraction, for example, flexion of the lumbar spine, while trying to isolate contraction of the transversus abdominis and lumbar multifidus (Richardson et al 1999). The patient may have over-activity of muscles because of pain, which may be sufficient to produce muscle spasm. In all of these examples, the clinician may need to reduce the muscle activity. To do this the patient may need to be made aware of the unwanted muscle activity using a mirror, verbal feedback, touch, EMG feedback. Other methods for reducing muscle activation include positioning, PNF, trigger points, deep inhibitory massage, relaxation techniques and taping (Box 6.5). It has been speculated that tape to the posterior thigh inhibits overactive hamstring muscles (McConnell 2002) and some other studies would support this (Tobin & Robinson 2000). Tape across the belly of vastus lateralis in asymptomatic subjects has been found to reduce the EMG activity when coming down stairs (Tobin & Robinson 2000). Tape over the lower fibres of trapezius of asymptomatic subjects was found to inhibit the muscle by as much as 22% when measured using the H reflex (Alexander et al 2003). The underlying mecha-

nism is not known; it has been postulated that it could be due to an alteration in muscle length and/or stimulation of cutaneous afferents, leading to inhibition of the underlying muscle and/or leading to decrease in descending drive of the motor neurone pool (Alexander et al 2003).

Altered relative activation of agonist and antagonist

The above sections on increasing and reducing muscle activation address the relative activation of agonist and antagonist.

ALTERING MUSCLE LENGTH

Treatment may aim to decrease length or increase length. The reason a muscle may be considered long, and why treatment should be aimed at reducing its length, is likely to be associated with reduced muscle tone. Where the clinician identifies reduced tone, treatment would be directed at increasing the contraction of the muscle, which has been discussed above.

Increasing muscle length

When considering muscle stretching, it can be helpful to categorize muscle into the active contractile unit and the non-contractile connective tissue, within the muscle belly and tendon. Treatment can be classified according to which effect the clinician is attempting to have on the muscle. Increasing the length of a muscle can be achieved by passively lengthening the connective tissue such that there is a permanent increase in length, or by attempting to produce physiological relaxation of the active contractile unit of the muscle belly using, for example, proprioceptive neuromuscular facilitation (PNF). Clearly, the contractile and non-contractile elements are inseparable and what is not being said here is that treatment to lengthen the connective tissue affects the connective tissue alone and has no effect on the contractile unit, or vice versa. The classification of treatment is used simply to aid communication between clinicians and is not attempting to describe the effect of the treatment.

Box 6.5 Treatment to reduce muscle activity

- Mirror
- Verbal feedback
- Touch
- EMG feedback
- Positioning
- PNF
- Trigger points
- Deep inhibitory massage
- Taping

Muscle can be stretched passively, by the clinician or by the patient. The aim of treatment is to produce a permanent (plastic) lengthening of the connective tissue of muscle and tendon with minimal structural weakness.

Passive muscle stretching by the clinician

A passive stretch can be performed in much the same way as a passive stretch to a joint or a nerve, that is, the clinician applies a static or oscillatory force to lengthen the muscle. The dose of passive stretch incorporates a number of factors, and is outlined in Table 6.3.

Position.   This includes the general position of the patient, such as lying, sitting or standing, and the specific position of the body part, for example, the hip may be placed in medial rotation and then flexed. The choice of general and specific positioning will depend on a number of factors:

- the comfort and support of the patient
- the comfort of the clinician applying the technique
- accurate application of the technique
- the desired effect of the treatment
- whether weight-bearing or non-weight-bearing is desired
- to what extent the movement is to be functional
- to what extent symptoms are to be produced.

An effective passive stretch is produced when a force moves the proximal and distal muscle attachments further apart; often this involves fixing the proximal attachment while passively moving the distal attachment. Positioning can often be used to help fix the proximal attachment; for example, supine with one leg flexed onto the chest helps to fix the pelvis as the other hip is moved into extension to lengthen the iliopsoas muscle.

Direction of movement.   There is no single direction of movement that will stretch all parts of a muscle; the clinician needs to fully explore and treat all aspects of muscle length by combining movements (Hunter 1998). The muscle attachments, direction of its fibres, position of the muscle and the relationship of the muscle to other structures, enable the clinician to decide how to combine movements for any particular muscle. For example, to lengthen biceps femoris fully, a combination of hip flexion, medial rotation and adduction with knee extension and medial tibial rotation needs to be used. Similarly, to lengthen extensor carpi radialis brevis fully, elbow extension with forearm pronation, wrist flexion, ulna deviation and individual finger flexion need to be combined (Hunter 1998).

Magnitude of force.   When a muscle is stretched the force is distributed throughout the connective tissue framework of the muscle (Hill 1950). Whenever a permanent lengthening is achieved,

Table 6.3   Treatment dose for passive stretching by the clinician and active stretching by the patient

Factors	Passive stretching by the clinician	Active stretching by the patient
Patient's position	e.g. supine	e.g. sitting, standing with heel of foot on a stool with knee extended
Direction of movement	e.g. hip flexion	e.g. active knee extension
Magnitude of force applied	Related to therapist's perception of resistance: grades I to V	Related to patient's perception of stretch
Amplitude of oscillation	Static or small or large	Static or small or large
Speed	Slow or fast	Slow or fast (If fast may be referred to as ballistic)
Rhythm	Smooth or staccato	Smooth or staccato
Time	Of repetitions and number of repetitions	Of repetitions, number of repetitions
Temperature	Room temperature or heat with short-wave diathermy	Room temperature
Symptom response	Short of symptom production	Short of symptom production
	Point of onset or increase in resting symptom	Point of onset or increase in resting symptom
	Partial reproduction of symptom	Partial reproduction of symptom
	Full reproduction of symptom	Full reproduction of symptom

there is some degree of mechanical weakening (Rigby et al 1959, Warren et al 1971). Interestingly, the amount of weakening depends on the way the muscle has been lengthened, as well as how much it has been lengthened. A small force for a long duration will induce less weakening than a large force for a short duration (Sapega et al 1981, Taylor et al 1990, Warren et al 1971).

The force applied by the clinician may be described using grades of movement (Magarey 1985, 1986, Maitland et al 2001). Grades of movement were initially described for forces applied to joint movement, later for lengthening nerve, and in this text for lengthening muscle. As a joint is passively moved to lengthen a muscle, resistance will be felt by the clinician and this can be depicted on a movement diagram (Petty & Moore 2001). With physiological movements that lengthen muscle, there is often minimal resistance early in range of movement. For example, hip flexion will have little resistance in the early part of the range and the clinician may mark the onset of resistance (R_1) somewhere towards the end of the movement (Fig. 6.5). Grades of movement are then defined according to the resistance curve. The grades of movement defined in this text (Table 6.4) are a modification of Maitland et al (2001) and Magarey (1985, 1986). The modification allows every possible position in range to be described (cf. Magarey 1985, 1986), and each

Table 6.4 Grades of movement

Grade	Definition
I	Small-amplitude movement short of resistance
II	Large-amplitude movement short of resistance
III-	Large-amplitude movement in the first third of resistance
IV-	Small-amplitude movement in the first third of resistance
III	Large-amplitude movement in the middle third of resistance
IV	Small-amplitude movement in the middle third of resistance
III+	Large-amplitude movement in the last third of resistance
IV+	Small-amplitude movement in the last third of resistance

grade to be distinct from the others (cf. Maitland et al 2001). The choice of magnitude of force, like every other factor of treatment dose, depends on what the clinician is attempting to achieve.

Amplitude of oscillation. The movement can be a sustained or oscillatory force. If the force is oscillated, it is described as having a small or large amplitude. The amplitude is relative to the available range of any movement. The amplitude of oscillatory movement is described within the definition of a grade of movement: grades I and IV are small-amplitude movements, grades II and III are large-amplitude movements. It is impossible for a truly sustained force to be applied: there will always be some variation in the force, albeit very small. For this reason, it is sometimes referred to as a quasistatic force. Where a clinician applies a sustained force, it is suggested that the description would use grades I, IV−, IV, IV+, with the word 'sustained' written prior to the grade – for example, treatment notes would read 'sustained grade IV−'. What is important, however, is not the choice of notation but the full description of the treatment dose.

It can be seen that grades of movement describe the magnitude of the force and the amplitude of oscillation. The choice of grade of movement is determined by the relationship of pain (or other symptom) and resistance through the range of movement. Where resistance limits the range of movement and there is minimal pain, a grade III+ or IV+ would be appropriate

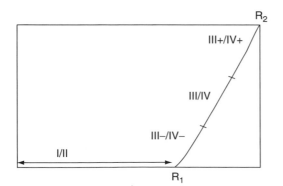

Figure 6.5 A movement diagram depicting grades of movement for a physiological movement. The onset of resistance (R_1) may be felt by the clinician somewhere towards the end of the movement, with R_2 depicting the end of range.

(Fig. 6.6A). Where pain limits the range of movement, and there is minimal resistance, a grade I or II may be appropriate, so that no pain is produced (Fig. 6.6B). A grade III– or IV– may be appropriate if the pain is non-severe and non-irritable and there is no caution related to the nature of the disorder. Where resistance limits the movement and there is a significant amount of pain, or where pain limits the movement and there is significant amount of resistance, the choice of grade will depend on the degree to which symptoms can be provoked (Fig. 6.6C and 6.6D). For example, in Figure 6.6C, if a grade IV is chosen at about 50% of resistance, this would, according to the movement diagram, provoke an intensity of pain of about 3 out of 10 (where A is 0 and C is 10). If a grade IV is chosen for 6.6D, this would provoke about 6 out of 10, which may or may not be acceptable to the patient.

Speed and rhythm of movement. The speed of the movement can be described as slow or fast, and the rhythm as smooth or staccato (jerky); of course, these terms will apply only to oscillatory forces. Speed and rhythm go hand in hand, and movements will tend to be slow and smooth, fast and smooth, or fast and staccato; it would be difficult to apply a slow staccato movement. The connective tissue in muscle is viscoelastic and is therefore sensitive to the speed of the applied force (Norkin & Levangie 1992). A force applied quickly will produce less movement, provoking a greater stiffness; that is, the gradient of the resistance curve will increase; a force applied more slowly, on the other hand, will cause more movement as the stiffness is relatively less (Norkin & Levangie 1992). If the intention of treatment is to maximize range of movement by lengthening connective tissue then a slow speed would seem preferable.

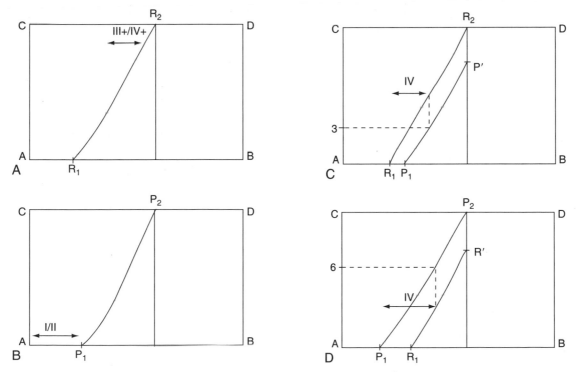

Figure 6.6 Grades of movement are determined by the relationship of pain and resistance through the range of movement; this is depicted on a movement diagram. A Resistance limiting movement. B Pain limiting movement. C Resistance limiting movement with a significant amount of pain. D Pain limiting movement with a significant amount of resistance.

Time. In terms of treatment dose, time relates to the amount of time a muscle is placed on a stretch, the number of times this is repeated, and the frequency of the appointments.

The required length of time to stretch a muscle is thought to be 6–12 seconds several times a day (Corbin & Noble 1980).

Hamstring muscle length has been found to be as effectively lengthened with daily static stretches using a 30-second stretch as with three repetitions of 1-minute stretches (Bandy et al 1997). Reassessment after each repetition enables the clinician to determine the effect of treatment on the patient's signs and symptoms. Depending on this change (better, same or worse), the clinician may alter the time and number of repetitions within a treatment session.

When a muscle is placed on a stretch, the time needed to lengthen the connective tissue a certain amount varies inversely with the magnitude of the force; that is, a low force will take longer to lengthen a set amount than a high force (Warren et al 1971). The proportion of lengthening that remains, once the force is removed, is greater following a long-duration, low force (Sapega et al 1981, Warren et al 1971). A permanent (plastic) lengthening of the connective tissue of muscle and tendon with minimal structural weakness is enhanced by a long-duration stretch (Sapega et al 1981).

Temperature. Temperature influences the mechanical behaviour of connective tissue under tensile load. As temperature rises to about 40–45°C, stiffness decreases and extensibility increases (LaBan 1962, Lehmann et al 1970, Rigby 1964, Rigby et al 1959). At about 40° C a change in the microstructure of collagen occurs which significantly enhances the extensibility and potential for a permanent (plastic) change in length (Rigby 1964, Rigby et al 1959). The viscoelastic properties can be increased by as much as 170% when muscle temperature is raised to 43° C (Talishev & Fedina 1976). A higher temperature will induce less weakening than a lower temperature (Sapega et al 1981, Warren et al 1971). Once the heat is removed, it has been found that maintaining the tension as the tissue cools enhances the plastic deformation (Lehmann et al 1970,

Sapega et al 1981). Increasing the temperature of a tissue depends on its depth; it will obviously be easier to heat more superficial muscles.

The ability of short-wave diathermy, hot-water baths and ultrasound to increase muscle and tendon temperature has been investigated. Twenty minutes of short-wave diathermy has been shown to raise muscle temperature by as much as 4° C (Millard 1961). If normal muscle temperature is assumed to be the same as normal body temperature, 37° C, then this would raise the temperature of muscle to 41° C, sufficient to enhance the effect of stretching. Twenty minutes immersion in a water bath at 42.5° C has been found to increase forearm muscle temperature to 39° C (Barcroft & Edholm 1943), which may be sufficient to enhance the effect of a stretch. Ultrasound at a frequency of 1 megacycle with a 12.5 cm^2 head at an intensity of 1 w/cm^2 for 7 minutes caused the muscle temperature (3.5 cm below the surface of the skin) to rise to 40° C (Lehmann et al 1966). This research suggests that heating muscle and tendon with short-wave diathermy, hot water or ultrasound will enhance the effect of muscle stretching.

Symptom response. The clinician decides which, and to what extent, each symptom is to be provoked during treatment. Choices include:

- no provocation
- provocation to the point of onset or increase in resting symptoms
- partial reproduction
- total reproduction.

The decision as to what extent symptoms are provoked during treatment depends on the severity and irritability of the symptom(s) and the nature of the condition. If the symptoms are severe, that is, the patient is unable to tolerate the symptom being produced, the clinician would choose not to provoke the symptoms. The clinician may also not choose to provoke symptoms if they are irritable, that is, once symptoms are provoked they take some time to ease. If, however, the symptoms are not severe and not irritable then the clinician is able to reproduce the patient's symptoms during treatment, and the extent to which symptoms are reproduced will depend on the tolerance of the patient. The nature of the condition may limit the extent to which symptoms are produced, such as a recent traumatic injury. Treatment is progressed or regressed by altering appropriate aspects of the treatment dose: patient position, movement, direction of force, magnitude of force, amplitude of oscillation, speed, rhythm, time or symptom response. Table 6.5 suggests the ways in which each aspect of the treatment dose can be progressed and regressed.

It is suggested that inexperienced clinicians alter only one aspect of treatment dose at an attendance so that they fully understand the value of the alteration; in this way they will quickly develop valuable clinical experience and clinical mileage which will contribute to growth in their clinical reasoning skills. The immediate and more long-term effect of the alteration can then be evaluated by reassessment of the subjective and physical asterisks. Table 6.6 provides an example of how a treatment dose for lengthening the upper fibres of trapezius may be progressed and regressed. An increase in time from 30 seconds to 1 minute provides a progression of the treatment dose, and a reduction in the amount of symptoms accounts for the regression. Other aspects of treatment dose which are closely linked are the length of time for each repetition and the number of repetitions; these, together, provide a dose of time and so each can be altered at the same time.

Passive muscle stretching by the patient

The patient can actively stretch a muscle. The factors defining the treatment dose are exactly the same as passive muscle stretching carried out by the clinician (Table 6.3). The only difference is that with passive stretching by the patient, the patient is in total control of the stretching movement and relies on their own perception of stretch and symptom production to determine the way the stretch is carried out. The patient needs to be fully informed as to how to carry out the stretch, that is, how forceful they need to be and to what extent they should reproduce the symptoms. The clinician in this case takes on a more educational and advisory role.

In sports medicine, two types of stretching are advocated: ballistic and static stretching. Ballistic stretching involves the person performing bouncing, rhythmic end-range movements. Alternatively, static stretching involves a simple hold at the end of range. Controversy exists over the effectiveness of each type of stretching in

Table 6.5 Progression and regression of treatment dose

Treatment dose	Progression	Regression
Position	Muscle towards end of available range	Muscle towards beginning of available range
Direction of force	More provocative	More provocative
Magnitude of force	Increase	Decrease
Amplitude of oscillation	Decreased	Increased
Rhythm	Staccato	Smoother
Time	Longer	Shorter
Speed	Slower or faster	Slower
Symptom response	Allowing more symptoms to be provoked	Allowing fewer symptoms to be provoked

Table 6.6 Example of how a treatment dose for increasing the passive length of the upper fibres of trapezius can be progressed and regressed

Regression	Dose	Progression
In full cervical flexion and 1/2 range contralateral flexion, static hold for 30 secs to partial reproduction of patient's neck pain	In full cervical flexion and 1/2 range contralateral flexion, static hold for 30 secs to full reproduction of patient's neck pain	In full cervical flexion and 1/2 range contralateral flexion, static hold for 1 min to full reproduction of patient's neck pain

producing an increase in muscle length. One study found that both methods were ineffective, only hold–relax produced an increase in muscle length (Sady et al 1982). The best method of stretching to cause a permanent increase in muscle length still remains unclear (Corbin & Noble 1980).

Summary of increasing muscle length

The important factors that affect a permanent increase in length of muscle following a passive stretch include the magnitude of force, time of force application and temperature of the muscle (Sapega et al 1981). From research to date, it appears that a permanent (plastic) lengthening of the connective tissue of muscle and tendon with minimal structural weakness will be enhanced by a relatively low force for a long-duration stretch (Sapega et al 1981, Warren et al 1971) at high temperatures (Rigby 1964, Rigby et al 1959, Sapega et al 1981, Talishev & Fedina 1976).

Increasing length via the contractile unit of muscle

The aim of this type of treatment is to cause a relaxation of the contractile unit of muscle in order to increase muscle length. Muscle energy techniques and positional release techniques can also be used to cause muscle relaxation (Chaitow 2001a, 2001b). Proprioceptive neuromuscular facilitation (PNF) is advocated to achieve this muscle relaxation (Knott & Voss 1968, Waddington 1999). These are rotational movement patterns through full range of movement, hold–relax, contract–relax and agonist–contract.

Rotational movement patterns. These patterns of movement take muscles from full outer range, where they are fully lengthened, to a fully shortened position. Specific patterns of movement for the head and neck, trunk and limbs have been described (Knott & Voss 1968).

Hold–relax. The muscle is positioned in its stretched position, either actively or passively. A strong isometric contraction of the muscle is achieved by the clinician providing manual resistance. The muscle contraction needs to be carefully controlled by the clinician. This is achieved by saying to the patient 'don't let me move you' or 'hold' and by slowly and smoothly increasing the manual resistance to maximum contraction. Following contraction the patient is asked to relax, the clinician gradually reduces the resistance, and time is allowed for muscle relaxation to occur. The clinician then moves further into range to increase the length of the muscle. The procedure of contraction followed by relaxation is then repeated until no further increase in muscle length can be achieved.

Contract–relax. This is the same as hold–relax except that, following the isometric contraction, the patient actively contracts to further lengthen the antagonistic muscle, rather than the clinician passively lengthening the muscle. For example, to lengthen quadriceps the patient isometrically contracts the quadriceps at, for example, 60 degrees flexion for 3–6 seconds. The patient is then asked to relax and actively to contract their hamstrings in an attempt to increase knee flexion and stretch the quadriceps muscle group. As in hold–relax, the procedure is repeated in the new range of movement and repeated until no further increase in muscle length is achieved.

Agonist–contract. The muscle is put in a position of stretch and a contraction of the agonist attempts to increase movement and thus increase stretch of the muscle. The clinician facilitates this movement by carefully applying a passive force. For example, to lengthen quadriceps the knee is positioned 60 degrees flexion. The patient actively contracts the hamstrings in an attempt to increase knee flexion and stretch the quadriceps muscle group. The clinician applies a force to the lower leg to enhance this movement.

Soft-tissue mobilization of muscle

Hunter (1998) has coined the phrase 'specific soft tissue mobilization' (SSTM). It is essentially the application of manual force to soft tissue, which can be considered to include muscle and tendon as well as skin, fascia, ligament and nerve.

There are essentially three types of treatment techniques: physiological SSTM, accessory

SSTM and combined SSTM (physiological and accessory).

1. Physiological SSTM involves full exploration of all anatomical regions of the muscle and tendon by a combination of physiological movements – in other words, putting a stretch on a muscle with a combination of movements. For example, to explore biceps femoris fully, hip flexion and knee extension need to be combined with medial rotation and adduction of the hip with medial rotation of the tibia (Hunter 1998).

2. Accessory SSTM involves applying manual force to muscle and tendon. For example, a horizontal force across the fibres of the tendocalcaneus could be applied. It is recommended that the force be applied in the plane of the muscle or tendon and at right angles to the site of dysfunction (Hunter 1998). In this regard it differs from transverse frictions (Fig. 6.7). Manual force can be applied with the muscle or tendon relaxed or with an isometric, concentric or eccentric muscle contraction.

3. Combined accessory and physiological SSTM involves the muscle and tendon in a lengthened position while an accessory force is applied. For example, the transverse glide across the tendocalcaneus could be carried out with the knee extended and the foot in dorsiflexion. It could also involve applying accessory movement with isometric, concentric or eccentric muscle contraction.

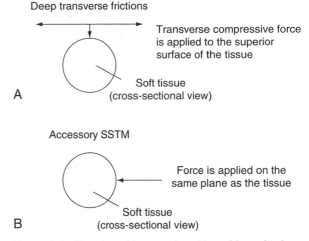

Figure 6.7 Direction of force and position of force for A deep transverse frictions and B accessory specific soft-tissue mobilization (from Hunter 1998, with permission).

Treatment dose. The decisions to be made by the clinician, in terms of treatment dose, include: the patient's position, movement, direction, magnitude of force applied, amplitude of oscillation, speed and rhythm of movement, time and symptom response. Table 6.7 provides a summary of the treatment options and is identical to the treatment dose for joint and nerve in Chapters 4 and 8 respectively.

The underlying effect of soft-tissue mobilization is not yet known. Soft-tissue mobilization is considered to be appropriate following soft-tissue

Table 6.7 Treatment dose for soft-tissue mobilization

Factors	Variables
Patient's position	e.g. prone, side lie, sitting
Movement	Physiological movement
	Accessory movement or a mixture of accessory and physiological
Direction of force applied	e.g. medial transverse, lateral transverse, AP, PA, caudad, cephalad
Magnitude of force applied	Related to therapist's perception of resistance: grades I to V
Amplitude of oscillation	None: sustained (quasistatic)
	Small: grades I and IV
	Large: grades II and III
Speed	Slow or fast
Rhythm	Smooth or staccato
Time	Of repetition and number of repetitions
Symptom response	Short of symptom production
	Point of onset or increase in resting symptom
	Partial reproduction of symptom
	Full reproduction of symptom

injury during the regeneration and remodelling phase of healing (Hunter 1998), details of which are given below with muscle injury. During the regeneration and remodelling phases soft-tissue mobilization is thought to enhance collagen synthesis and cross-linkage development, promote the orientation of collagen fibres along functional lines of stress, and promote 'normal' viscoelastic behaviour (Hunter 1998). SSTM is also proposed to be beneficial for degenerative lesions by stimulating an inflammatory response that initiates healing (Hunter 1998).

REDUCING SYMPTOMS

A useful premise for the clinician is to consider that the symptom is whatever the patient says it is, existing whenever they say it is (McCaffery 1979). This was originally used for pain, but can be widened to any symptom the patient feels.

The assumption in this text is that the cause of the muscle pain is some sort of injury to the muscle and/or tendon. In this situation, the pain will be a result of mechanical and/or chemical irritation of the muscle nociceptors. The subjective information from the patient, particularly the behaviour of symptoms and mechanism of injury, may enable the clinician to identify whether it is the contractile unit of muscle and/or connective tissue of muscle that is involved in the pain (Vicenzino et al 2002). For example, an overstretch injury may affect the connective tissue of muscle and require treatment to increase the muscle length and, by so doing, reduce pain.

Various palpatory techniques can be used to reduce symptoms emanating from muscle including: specific soft-tissue mobilization massage, connective tissue massage trigger points, frictions. Joint mobilizations, taping and electrotherapy can also be used. Specific soft-tissue mobilization has been described above. Electrotherapy is beyond the scope of this text; the reader is referred to other texts such as Low & Reed (1990) and an excellent review by Watson (2000).

Massage can be applied to muscle to reduce pain, using: stroking, effleurage, kneading, picking up, wringing and skin rolling (Thomson et al 1991). Additional effects are thought to include: an increase in the flow of the circulation, muscle relaxation, lengthening of tissues and an increased tissue drainage and pain relief (Thomson et al 1991). For further details see Thomson et al (1991).

Connective tissue massage (CTM) involves applying specific strokes to the skin and subcutaneous tissues from the lumbar spine to the upper limbs or from the lumbar spine to the lower limbs. It has been suggested that it affects the autonomic nervous system and, via this system, increases circulation which aids healing and eases pain (Thomson et al 1991). For further details see Thomson et al (1991).

A trigger point is defined as a focus of hyperirritability of a muscle and is thought to contribute to muscle tightness. On palpation of the muscle, an area of local tightness with tenderness, possible muscle twitch and referral of pain in a typical pattern, is found. Having identified this, treatment involves applying manual pressure over the area. The reader is referred to the textbook by Travell & Simons (1983, 1992) for further information. The underlying cause of the phenomenon of trigger points has been proposed as secondary hyperalgesia originating from peripheral nerves (Quintner & Cohen 1994).

Frictions are small-amplitude deep pressures applied to tissue such as muscle and tendon. The clinician's finger or thumb moves with the patient's skin across the tissue. The tissue is often positioned such that it is in a lengthened position. It has been proposed that frictions cause hyperaemia, break down adhesions, and stimulate mechanoreceptors (Cyriax 1984). In an experimental study on New Zealand white rabbits, 10 minutes of frictions caused mechanical trauma to muscle tissue, which, after 6 days, had largely healed (Gregory et al 2003). Whether this traumatic effect may be therapeutic in the presence of a muscle injury remains unknown, but it certainly highlights the mechanical effects of force on muscle.

Joint mobilizations may be used to reduce pain and change muscle. For example, anterior knee pain often involves the dysfunction of the quadriceps muscle group and the patellofemoral joint. Treatment to the muscle will affect the joint, and similarly, treatment to the joint will affect the muscle. Accessory movements applied to the patellofemoral joint, with or without concentric, eccentric or isometric quadriceps contraction, may be useful. Similarly, with lateral elbow pain there may be dysfunction of the extensor muscles of the forearm as well as a radiohumeral joint dysfunction. Again, accessory movements may be applied to the joint with or without concentric, eccentric or isometric contraction of the wrist and finger extensor muscles. For example, a lateral glide combined with the patient performing an isometric grip with the hand, has been found in a randomized double-blind placebo-controlled study to increase by approximately 10% the pressure pain threshold and increase by almost 60% the pain-free grip strength (Vicenzino et al 2001). In another study, spinal accessory movements have been found to reduce pain and improve muscle activation in the cervical spine (Sterling et al 2001). Further information on accessory movements combined with active muscle contractions can be found elsewhere (Mulligan 1995, Vicenzino 2003). The mechanism by which joint accessory movements reduce pain and cause a change in muscle activity is discussed in Chapter 4.

Tape may be used to relieve muscle pain. A useful principle is to apply the tape in such a way that it replicates the direction of the pain-relieving force applied by the clinician during treatment. For details of methods of taping the reader is referred to other texts (Macdonald 1994, Vicenzino 2003).

The mechanism by which pain is relieved with each of these manual techniques is still unclear. Large-diameter type III afferents are distributed throughout muscle tissue and are stimulated by pressure, mechanical force caused by lengthening muscle or by muscle contraction (Mense & Meyer 1985). It is possible that the manual techniques described above may stimulate the type III afferents and cause a reflex inhibition of the type IV muscle nociceptors according to the pain gate theory (Melzack & Wall 1965). Clearly, large-diameter afferents in the skin and joint may also contribute to this

pain inhibition. The pain may also be reduced via a descending inhibitory system explained below and expanded rather more in Chapter 8 on nerve treatment.

Descending inhibition of pain

The periaqueductal grey (PAG) area has been found to be important in the control of nociception. PAG projects to the dorsal horn and has a descending control of nociception (Fig. 6.8). It also projects upwards to the medial thalamus, orbital frontal cortex, and so may have an ascending control of nociception (Fields & Basbaum 1999). The PAG has two distinct regions, the dorsolateral PAG (dPAG) and the ventrolateral PAG (vPAG).

dPAG

The dorsolateral PAG (dPAG) runs to the dorsolateral pons and ventrolateral medulla, which is involved in autonomic control (Fields & Basbaum 1999). In the rat, stimulation of the dPAG causes analgesia, increased blood pressure, increased heart rate, vasodilation of the hind limb muscles, increased rate and depth of respiration, and coordinated hind limb, jaw and tail movements, suggesting increased activity of the sympathetic nervous system (SNS), and alpha motor neurones (Lovick 1991). The neurotransmitter from dPAG is noradrenaline (norepinephrine), and the analgesic effect appears to mediate morphine analgesia of mechanical nociceptor stimuli (Kuraishi et al 1983). At the spinal cord level, dPAG causes inhibition of substance P from peripheral noxious mechanical stimulation (Kuraishi 1990).

vPAG

The ventrolateral PAG (vPAG) runs mainly to the nucleus raphe magnus. In the rat, stimulation of vPAG causes analgesia with decreased blood pressure, decreased heart rate, vasodilation of the hind limb muscles and reduced hind limb, jaw and tail movements, suggesting inhibition of the SNS and inhibition of alpha motor neurones

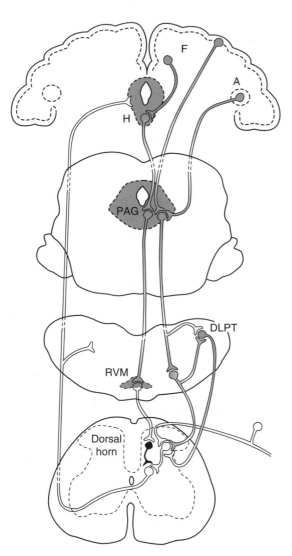

Figure 6.8 Pain modulating pathway. PAG receives input from the frontal lobe (F), the amygdala (A) and the hypothalamus (H). Afferents from PAG travel to the rostral ventromedial medulla (RVM) and the dorsolateral pontomesencephalic tegmentum (DLPT) and on to the dorsal horn. The RVM has bidirectional control of nociceptive transmission. There are inhibitory (filled) and excitatory (unfilled) interneurones. (From Fields & Basbaum 1999, with permission.)

somatostatin, produced by peripheral noxious thermal stimulation (Kuraishi 1990). These mechanisms have been linked to the behaviour of an animal under threat, which initially acts with a defensive flight-or-fight response, followed by recuperation (Fanselow 1991, Lovick 1991); this is summarized in Figure 6.9.

Noxious stimuli can cause activation of the descending control system (Fields & Basbaum 1999, Yaksh & Elde 1981), which may reduce nociceptive transmission. Noxious stimulation has been found to cause release of enkephalins at the supraspinal and spinal levels (Yaksh & Elde 1981). It has also been found that stimulation of the spinothalamic tract, transmitting nociceptive information from one foot, can be inhibited by

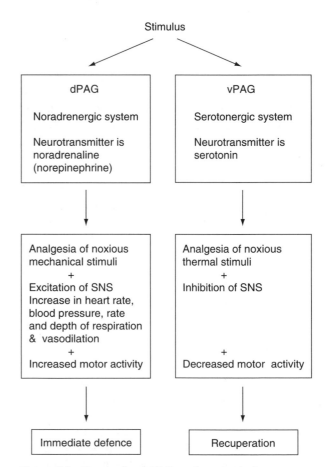

Figure 6.9 Descending inhibition of mechanical nociception from dPAG (noradrenergic system) and thermal nociception from vPAG (serotonergic system).

(Lovick 1991). The neurotransmitter used in vPAG is serotonin, and the analgesic effect appears to mediate morphine analgesia of thermal nociceptive stimuli (Kuraishi et al 1983). At the dorsal horn vPAG inhibits the release of

noxious input from the contralateral foot, hand, face or trunk (Gerhart et al 1981). It has been suggested that this may explain the relief of pain with acupuncture, and pain behaviours such as 'biting your lip and banging your head against a wall'(!) (Melzack 1975). Painful treatment of muscle may also activate the descending control system.

Addressing the biopsychosocial aspects of symptoms

Injury, or the perception of injury, produces anxiety and fear (Craig 1999). Who has ever injured themselves, however minimally, and not experienced an emotional reaction? The psychological aspects of pain sometimes focus on 'emotional individuals', or on chronic pain patients. However, all of us will have a cognitive and emotional response to injury, because injury interrupts our lives. There is never a right time for an injury: it will always be, to a greater or lesser degree, a nuisance to us. That 'nuisance' will drive our emotional reactions. It seems reasonable to suggest, therefore, that all patients with neuromusculoskeletal dysfunction will have thoughts and feelings about their problem, and it would be an oversight on the part of the clinician not to enquire about these. This enquiry involves the clinician understanding the patient's thoughts and feelings. This is no easy task, and to do it well requires a high level of skill in active listening. Active listening involves putting our own thoughts, beliefs and feelings to one side and choosing, instead, to hear what the patient has to say. It involves trying to understand the patient and their world, through their eyes, and avoiding the all-too-easy error of re-interpreting through our eyes. It requires the clinician to listen with compassion, patience and without judgement. It involves the clinician using words carefully and meaningfully and using open-ended questions to search for information, until understanding is reached. It involves sensitive verbal and non-verbal communication, encouraging safe and open communication. This is a tall order, but the benefits of truly being able to come alongside the patient will far outweigh the effort of developing these skills.

The use of 'yellow flags' was devised specifically for acute low-back pain to identify beliefs, emotions and behaviours that may contribute to long-term disability (Watson & Kendall 2000). Screening questionnaires (e.g. Main & Waddell 1999) have been devised; these, like all questionnaires, have major limitations. Questions provide a superficial, and sometimes false, understanding of the problem – as anyone who has filled in any questionnaire knows only too well. For example, while a question may ask 'how much have you been bothered by feeling depressed in the last week' and the recipient answers on a 0 to 10 scale from 'not at all' to 'extremely', little information is gleamed from this – there may be a wide variety of factors underlying the given score. For this reason, if a questionnaire is used, a discussion with the patient will also be necessary to understand the problems the patient faces (Watson & Kendall 2000). The questionnaire can be useful for providing the clinician with aspects to discuss with the patient; however, there is a danger that it becomes a mechanistic form-filling exercise. It is worth remembering that the clinical management of patients is fundamentally based on human relationships which are not normally enriched by form filling!

Following the enquiry of the patient, as to their thoughts and feelings, two further steps are recommended: education and exposure (Vlaeyen & Crombez 1999). Education involves the clinician carefully facilitating the patient's understanding of their problem. The way this is carried out with patients will vary according to a number of factors, including the patient's prior knowledge, thoughts and beliefs, and how they feel about the problem. All the listening skills discussed above will be imperative in this process. The ability of the clinician to be honest is important. The clinician needs to explain the problem to the patient in a careful way. There is a world of difference between 'the pain in your back is from the disc' and 'I think the pain in your back could be coming from the disc'. The former explanation suggests that you know that the pain is coming from the disc, and yet there is overwhelming evidence that you cannot make such claims; it has been estimated that a definite diagnosis of the pathology can be made in about only 15% of cases (Waddell 1999). Furthermore, there is a long-term problem with being so confident as the patient may, in the future, have a recurrence of the same pain and may see another clinician who may say 'the pain in your back is from your sacroiliac joint'. The patient is aware that this is a repeat episode and now, quite rightly, begins to have doubts about the ability of these two clinicians. This will be a familiar story to experienced clinicians who will have come across patients who may have received three, four or even more, confident 'diagnoses' of the same problem, and who come to you depressed, cynical and disillusioned with the medical profession.

The final aspect is exposure, which involves careful and graded exposure to the movements or postures that provoke pain (Vlaeyen & Crombez 1999). While this is designed for chronic pain patients who learn to avoid movements and posture through fear (Waddell & Main 1999), it may also be an important part of the treatment of acute tissue damage. Using movements and postures in a careful, controlled and graded way may help to avoid long-term movement dysfunctions.

MUSCLE INJURY AND REPAIR

Muscle can be damaged by a direct injury, such as a laceration or contusion, or indirectly by a sudden forceful contraction causing a muscle or tendon tear; damage may also be due to a chronic overuse injury (Kellett 1986). Whatever the mechanism of injury, the effect on muscle tissue is similar (Hurme et al 1991) and can be considered in three phases: inflammatory or lag phase, regeneration phase, and remodelling phase (Jarvinen & Lehto 1993).

The inflammatory or lag phase is characterized by haematoma formation, tissue necrosis and an inflammatory reaction. Necrosis of muscle tissue occurs with retraction of the muscle fibres on either side of the necrotic zone. It is generally accepted that treatment for the first 48 to 72 hours of a muscle injury is summarized by RICE, that is, rest, ice, compression and elevation (Evans 1980, Kellett 1986).

During the regeneration phase there is phagocytosis of damaged tissue, production of connective scar tissue. Capillary growth satellite cells migrate into the necrotic area. Muscle fibres regenerate by differentiation into myoblasts and then into myotubes, which link the two stumps on either side of the necrotic region (McComas 1996). The connective tissue within muscle is also damaged and undergoes healing with subsequent scar formation (Jarvinen & Lehto 1993). Following a short period of immobilization – more than 3–5 days for rats (Jarvinen & Lehto 1993) – it is considered beneficial to mobilize the muscle, within the limits of symptoms. Early mobilization is thought to enhance tensile strength, orientation of the regenerating muscle fibres, resorption of connective scar tissue and blood flow to the damaged area and to avoid atrophy brought about by immobilization (Jarvinen & Lehto 1993). The tensile strength of a tendon has been found to increase as a result of 60 repetitions per day of manual wrist and finger flexion/extension following a primary repair (Takai et al 1991).

The remodelling phase is characterized by the maturation of regenerated muscle (Jarvinen & Lehto 1993). There is contraction and reorganization of scar tissue and a gradual recovery of the functional capacity of the muscle.

An experimental crush injury of the semitendinosus muscle of the rat reveals necrosis of muscle tissue in the first 2 days, with new myotubes within the damaged area at 5 days and regeneration of muscle fibres bridging the necrotic area by 10 days, with full regeneration at 30 days (Stuart et al 1981). A controlled strain injury of the musculotendinous junction of tibialis anterior muscle was carried out on New Zealand white rabbits (Nikolaou et al 1987). Necrosis and infiltration of inflammatory cells, oedema and haemorrhage occurred after 1 day. After 2 days the damaged fibres had been broken down with proliferation of inflammatory cells, macrophages and fibroblasts. After 7 days inflammation was reduced and fibrocytes were evident (Nikolaou et al 1987). Clear evidence of muscle regeneration was evident after 4 days following an experimental strain injury of a rat tendon (Almekinders & Gilbert 1986).

Treatment of a muscle injury may include soft-tissue mobilization, frictions, controlled exercises, lengthening, tape and electrotherapy. The reader is directed to relevant texts for further information.

It is worth mentioning here that a patient presenting with classical signs of a hamstring tear may, in fact, have a neurodynamic component to their problem. In Australian-rules football, players with signs of a hamstring tear had a positive slump test and when this was addressed in treatment there was a better result than more traditional muscle treatment techniques (Kornberg & Lew 1989). This highlights the need for a full and comprehensive examination of a patient.

Delayed muscle soreness

Muscle strain injury occurs with eccentric exercise, producing delayed muscle soreness (Friden et al 1983, Jones et al 1986). Pain, weakness and muscle stiffness are felt after unaccustomed eccentric exercise. There is breakdown of collagen (Brown et al 1997) and disruption of the Z band, predominantly in type II fibres, with repair largely completed by 6 days (Friden et al 1983, Jones et al 1986). The reason for the delayed muscle soreness following eccentric contraction may be that eccentric contraction produces more force within the muscle than other types of muscle contraction (Katz 1939).

TENDON INJURY AND REPAIR

Tendons can tear in the middle region, by avulsion of bone and, more rarely, at the insertion site (Woo et al 1988). The myotendinous region is the weakest part of the tendon–muscle unit and is the region most susceptible to strain injuries (Garrett 1990, Garrett et al 1989, Nikolaou et al 1987, Tidball 1991). Healing of tendon is similar to that of other soft tissues and consists of three phases: lag or inflammation phase (1–7 days), regeneration or proliferation phase (7–21 days) and remodelling or

maturation phase (21 days to 1 year) (Jozsa & Kannus 1997).

Repetitive strain may alter the collagenous structure of tendon with resultant inflammation, oedema and pain (Jozsa & Kannus 1997). Overuse injury occurs where this repetitive strain causing tissue damage is greater than the natural repair and healing process (Archambault et al 1995, Jozsa & Kannus 1997). Conditions include tendonitis, peritendinitis and tenosynovitis, and this may lead, with further strain, to partial or complete rupture of the tendon. Eccentric pain-free exercises have been advocated for chronic achilles peritendinitis (Reynolds & Worrell 1991).

In work-related upper-limb tendon injuries, the repetitive nature of the task may be sufficient to cause change in the tissue. It is proposed that, initially, in the first 5 days, there is ischaemia, metabolic disturbance and cell membrane damage leading to inflammation (Jozsa & Kannus 1997). The increase in tissue pressure further impairs the circulation and enhances the ischaemic changes. In the proliferation phase (5–21 days) there is fibrin clotting, and fibroblast, synovial cell and capillary proliferation followed by the maturation phase (<21 days) in which adhesions and thickening of the tenosynovium and paratenon occur (Jozsa & Kannus 1997, Kvist & Kvist 1980).

Treatment of a tendon injury may include soft-tissue mobilization, frictions, controlled exercises, lengthening, tape and electrotherapy. The reader is directed to relevant texts for further information.

CHOICE OF MUSCLE TREATMENT

The choice of treatment depends on the assessment of the patient, whether the patient has a dysfunction of muscle and, if so, what that dysfunction is. Treatment may be to increase muscle strength, power and/or endurance, increase muscle length, alter motor control (increase muscle activation, reduce muscle activation, increase time of onset) and reduce symptoms. The overall aim of treatment is to normalize a dysfunction, that is, to eradicate the abnormal signs and symptoms.

There is a wide variety of treatment techniques, and it is not the intention of this textbook to reproduce what is already well described in other texts. Rather, this text aims to provide a broad overview of the principles behind the broad range of treatments to enable clinicians to solve the problem of what might be best for a particular patient at a particular time.

The best treatment is the one that improves the patient's signs and symptoms in the shortest period of time. The clinician monitors the patient's signs and symptoms within and between treatment sessions in order to identify the effectiveness of the treatment choice. Any change in signs and symptoms is considered in the light of the prognosis and treatment goals, following the examination and assessment on day one. In this way, the clinician can be creative and imaginative in considering all the possible treatment choices, while constantly monitoring the effectiveness of treatment. If the treatment is proved to be ineffective, then the clinician can alter the treatment; if it proves to be effective, and the patient is improving at the expected rate, then the treatment can be continued or progressed.

Any physical test which reproduces/eases the patient's symptoms can be converted to a treatment technique by applying the components of a treatment dose. Converting positive physical testing procedures to treatment techniques would seem the most logical approach to choosing treatment, as the clinician can be confident that the treatment is somehow or other affecting the structure at fault. Reproduction of the patient's symptoms is a vital anchor from which to decide aspects of treatment dose. Only when symptoms are produced can the clinician be sure that they are affecting, somehow or other, the structure(s) at fault. For example, the classic test of the length of the upper fibres of trapezius is contralateral lateral flexion and flexion of the cervical spine with the shoulder girdle depressed. If a patient's symptoms are brought on only when this test is accompanied by slight ipsilateral rotation, then it seems reasonable to ignore the classical test and follow the movement that reproduces the patient's symptoms. It may be that this particular patient has some sort of anatomical variation that requires the rotation movement.

MODIFICATION, PROGRESSION AND REGRESSION OF TREATMENT

The continuous monitoring of the patient's subjective and physical asterisks guides the entire treatment and management programme of the patient. The clinician judges the degree of change with treatment and relates this to the expected rate of change from the prognosis, and decides whether or not a treatment needs to be altered in some way. The nature of this alteration can be to modify the technique in some way, to progress or regress the treatment. Regardless of which alteration is made, the clinician makes every effort to determine what effect this alteration has on the patient's subjective and physical asterisks. In order to do this, the clinician alters one aspect of treatment at a time, and reassesses immediately to determine the value of the alteration.

Modification of treatment

The clinician may modify the treatment given to a patient by altering an existing treatment, adding a new treatment, or stopping a treatment. At all times the treatment should have the functional goals of the patient in mind. Altering an existing treatment involves altering some aspect of the treatment dose (outlined earlier). The immediate and more long-term effect of the alteration is then evaluated by reassessment of the subjective and physical asterisks; this process is outlined in Figure 6.10. The clinician then decides whether, overall, the patient is better, the same or worse, relating this to the prognosis. For instance, if a quick improvement was expected but only some improvement occurred, the clinician may progress treatment. If the patient is worse after treatment, the dose may be regressed in some way, and if the treatment made no difference at all then a more substantial modification may made be. Before discarding a treatment it is worth making sure that it has been fully utilized, as it may be that a much stronger or much weaker treatment dose may be effective.

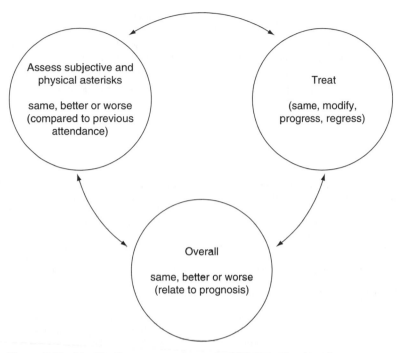

Figure 6.10 Modification, progression and regression of treatment.

Progression and regression of treatment

A treatment is progressed or regressed by altering appropriate aspects of the treatment dose in such a way that more treatment, or less treatment, is applied to the tissues.

PROGNOSIS

A full discussion on muscle and tendon injuries and their prognosis is beyond the scope of this text. Muscle rehabilitation following an anterior cruciate ligament tear is briefly outlined to highlight the difficulties in obtaining a restoration of muscle function. There is often incomplete recovery of muscle function following joint injury, despite a rehabilitation programme (Ciccotti et al 1994, Suter & Herzog 2000). A deficit in motor performance (Pfeifer & Banzer 1999), altered EMG activity (Ciccotti et al 1994), quadriceps strength (Hurley et al 1994) and muscle power (DeVita et al 1998) have been found during the first year following an injury or reconstruction of the anterior cruciate ligament of the knee. Patients who had greater muscle inhibition at the beginning of treatment had a poorer outcome by the end of the year (Hurley et al 1994). A deficit in muscle strength of up to 20% may continue for 4–9 years (Arangio et al 1997, Natri et al 1996, Seto et al 1988) owing to muscle atrophy (Arangio et al 1997) and incomplete muscle activation (Suter & Herzog 2000). The consequences of these deficits is unclear; it has been suggested that alterations in muscle activity may alter joint loading and this may, in the long term, lead to osteoarthritis in the joint (Brandt 1997, Felson & Zhang 1998). This is partly supported by the prediction that 50–70% of patients with a rupture of the anterior cruciate ligament will develop radiographical signs of osteoarthritis 15 to 20 years post-injury (Gillquist & Messner 1999). Osteoarthritic changes have been found 14 years (McDaniel & Dameron 1983) and between 2 and 27 years (Walla et al 1985) after an untreated anterior cruciate ligament rupture and were found to be associated with varus deformity and medial meniscectomy (McDaniel & Dameron 1983). This evidence suggests that joint injury will have profound effects on muscles, and restoration of muscle function may take a considerable length of time, and even then, may be incomplete.

Summary

This chapter has outlined the principles of muscle treatment. Treatment is only a part of the overall management of a patient; the reader is therefore encouraged to go now to Chapter 9 where the principles of management are discussed.

REFERENCES

Alexander C M, Stynes S, Thomas A et al 2003 Does tape facilitate or inhibit the lower fibres of trapezius? Manual Therapy 8(1):37–41

Almekinders L C, Gilbert J A 1986 Healing of experimental muscle strains and the effects of nonsteroidal antiinflammatory medication. American Journal of Sports Medicine 14(4):303–308

American College of Sports Medicine (ACSM) 1998 Resource Manual for Guidelines for Exercise Testing and Prescription, 3rd edn. Williams & Wilkins, Baltimore

Andersen J L, Aagaard P 2000 Myosin heavy chain IIX overshoot in human skeletal muscle. Muscle and Nerve 23(7):1095–1104

Arangio G A, Chen C, Kalady M, Reed J F 1997 Thigh muscle size and strength after anterior cruciate ligament reconstruction and rehabilitation. Journal of Orthopaedics and Sports Physiotherapy 26(5):238–243

Archambault J M, Wiley J P, Bray R C 1995 Exercise loading of tendons and the development of overuse injuries, a review of current literature. Sports Medicine 20(2):77–89

Arms S W, Pope M H, Johnson R J et al 1984 The biomechanics of anterior cruciate ligament rehabilitation and reconstruction. American Journal of Sports Medicine 12(1):8–18

Bandy W D, Irion J M, Briggler M 1997 The effect of time and frequency of static stretching on flexibility of the hamstring muscles. Physical Therapy 77(10): 1090–1096

Baratta R, Solomonow M, Zhou B H et al 1988 Muscular coactivation: the role of the antagonist musculature in maintaining knee stability. American Journal of Sports Medicine 16(2):113–122

Barcroft H, Edholm O G 1943 The effect of temperature on blood flow and deep temperature in the human forearm. Journal of Physiology 102:5–20

Berger R 1962 Effect of varied weight training programs on strength. Research Quarterly 33(2):168–181

Berger R A 1982 Applied exercise physiology. Lea & Febiger, Philadelphia, ch 1, p 33

Bobath B 1990 Adult hemiplegia: evaluation and treatment, 3rd edn. Butterworth-Heinemann, Oxford

Borg G A V 1982 Psychophysical bases of perceived exertion. Medicine and Science in Sports and Exercise 14(5):377–381

Braith R W, Graves J E, Pollock M L et al 1989 Comparison of 2 vs 3 days/week of variable resistance training during 10- and 18-week programs. International Journal of Sports Medicine 10:450–454

Brandt K D 1997 Putting some muscle into osteoarthritis. Annals of Internal Medicine 127(2):154–156

Brown S J, Child R B, Day S H, Donnelly A E 1997 Indices of skeletal muscle damage and connective tissue breakdown following eccentric muscle contractions. European Journal of Applied Physiology 75:369–374

Bruton A 2002 Muscle plasticity: response to training and detraining. Physiotherapy 88(7):398–408

Carr J H, Shepherd R B 1998 Neurological rehabilitation, optimizing motor function. Butterworth-Heinemann, Oxford

Chaitow L 2001a Muscle energy techniques, 2nd edn. Churchill Livingstone, Edinburgh

Chaitow L 2001b Positional release techniques, 2nd edn. Churchill Livingstone, Edinburgh

Ciccotti M G, Kerlan R K, Perry J, Pink M 1994 An electromyographic analysis of the knee during functional activities. II. The anterior cruciate ligament-deficient and –reconstructed profiles. American Journal of Sports Medicine 22(5):651–658

Cohen L G, Roth B J, Wassermann E M et al 1991 Magnetic stimulation of the human cerebral cortex, an indicator of reorganization in motor pathways in certain pathological conditions. Journal of Clinical Neurophysiology 8(1):56–65

Corbin C B, Noble L 1980 Flexibility: a major component of physical fitness. Journal of Physical Education and Recreation 51(6):23–24, 57–60

Cowan S M, Bennell K L, Crossley K M et al 2002 Physical therapy alters recruitment of the vasti in patellofemoral pain syndrome. Medicine and Science in Sports and Exercise 34(12):1879–1885

Craig K D 1999 Emotions and psychobiology. In: Wall P D, Melzack R (eds) Textbook of pain, 4th edn. Churchill Livingstone, Edinburgh, ch 12, p 331–343

Crossman E R F W 1959 A theory of the acquisition of speed-skill. Ergonomics 2:153–166

Cyriax J 1984 Textbook of orthopaedic medicine, vol 2 treatment by manipulation, massage and injection. Baillière Tindall, London

Danneels L A, Vanderstraeten G G, Cambier D C et al 2001 Effects of three different training modalities on the cross sectional area of the lumbar multifidus muscle in patients with chronic low back pain. British Journal of Sports Medicine 35:186–191

DeLateur B, Lehmann J F, Warren C G, et al 1972a Comparison of effectiveness of isokinetic and isotonic exercise in quadriceps strengthening. Archives of Physical Medicine and Rehabilitation 53:60–64

DeLateur B, Lehmann J, Stonebridge J, Warren C G 1972b Isotonic versus isometric exercise: a double-shift transfer-of-training study. Archives of Physical Medicine and Rehabilitation 53:212–216

Demirel H A, Powers S K, Naito H et al 1999 Exercise-induced alterations in skeletal muscle myosin heavy chain phenotype: dose-response relationship. Journal of Applied Physiology 86:1002–1008

DeMichele P L, Pollock M L, Graves J E et al 1997 Isometric torso rotation strength: effect of training frequency on its development. Archives of Physical Medicine and Rehabilitation 78:64–69

DeVita P, Hortobagyi T, Barrier J 1998 Gait biomechanics are not normal after anterior cruciate ligament reconstruction and accelerated rehabilitation. Medicine and Science in Sports and Exercise 30(10):1481–1488

deVries H A, Housh T J 1994 Physiology of exercise for physical education, athletics and exercise science, 5th edn. Brown & Benchmark, Madison, Wisconsin

DiNubile N A 1991 Strength training. Clinics in Sports Medicine 10(1):33–62

Eldred E, Hagbarth K-E 1954 Facilitation and inhibition of gamma efferents by stimulation of certain skin areas. Journal of Neurophysiology 17:59–65

Enoka R M 1988 Muscle strength and its development: new perspectives. Sports Medicine 6:146–168

Evans P 1980 The healing process at cellular level: a review. Physiotherapy 66(8):256–259

Fanselow M S 1991 The midbrain periaqueductal gray as a coordinator of action in response to fear and anxiety. In: Depaulis A, Bandler R (eds) The midbrain periaqueductal gray matter. Plenum Press, New York, p 151–173

Feigenbaum M S, Pollock M L 1999 Prescription of resistance training for health and disease. Medicine and Science in Sports and Exercise 31(1):38–45

Felson D T, Zhang Y 1998 An update on the epidemiology of knee and hip osteoarthritis with a view to prevention. Arthritis and Rheumatism 41(8):1343–1355

Fields H L, Basbaum A I 1999 Central nervous system mechanisms of pain modulation. In: Wall P D, Melzack R (eds) Textbook of pain, 4th edn. Churchill Livingstone, Edinburgh, ch 11, p 309–329

Fitts R H, Widrick J J 1996 Muscle mechanics: adaptations with exercise-training. Exercise and Sports Sciences Reviews 24:427–473

Fletcher-Cook P 1999 Neurophysiology of movement. In: Hollis M, Fletcher-Cook P (eds) Practical exercise therapy, 4th edn. Blackwell Science, Oxford, ch 18, p 189–201

Friden J, Sjostrom M, Ekblom B 1983 Myofibrillar damage following intense eccentric exercise in man. International Journal of Sports Medicine 4:170–176

Garnett R, Stephens J A 1981 Changes in the recruitment threshold of motor units produced by cutaneous stimulation in man. Journal of Physiology (Lond) 311:463–473

Garrett W E 1990 Muscle strain injuries: clinical and basic aspects. Medicine and Science in Sports and Exercise 22(4):436–443

Garrett W E, Rich F R, Nikolaou P K, Vogler J B 1989 Computed tomography of hamstring muscle strains. Medicine and Science in Sports and Exercise 21(5):506–514

Gea J G 1997 Myosin gene expression in the respiratory muscles. European Respiratory Journal 10:2404–2410

Gerhart K D, Yezierski R P, Giesler G J, Willis W D 1981 Inhibitory receptive fields of primate spinothalamic tract cells. Journal of Neurophysiology 46(6):1309–1325

Gillam G M 1981 Effects of frequency of weight training on muscle strength enhancement. Journal of Sports Medicine 21:432–436

Gilleard W, McConnell J, Parsons D 1998 The effect of patellar taping on the onset of vastus medialis obliquus and vastus lateralis muscle activity in persons with patellofemoral pain. Physical Therapy 78(1):25–32

Gillquist J, Messner K 1999 Anterior cruciate ligament reconstruction and the long term incidence of gonarthrosis. Sports Medicine 27(3):143–156

Graves J E, Pollock M L, Foster D et al 1990 Effect of training frequency and specificity on isometric lumbar extension strength. Spine 15(6):504–509

Gregory M A, Deane M N, Mars M 2003 Ultrastructural changes in untraumatised rabbit skeletal muscle treated with deep transverse friction. Physiotherapy 89(7):408–416

Grimby G 1995 Muscle performance and structure in the elderly as studied cross-sectionally and longitudinally. Journal of Gerontology 50A(special issue):17–22

Hakkinen K, Newton R U, Gordon S E et al 1998 Changes in muscle morphology, electromyographic activity, and force production characteristics during progressive strength training in young and older men. Journal of Gerontology 53A(6):B415–423

Henry F M 1968 Specificity vs. generality in learning motor skill. In: Brown R C, Kenyon G S (eds) Classical studies on physical activity. Prentice Hall, New Jersey, ch 5, p 328–331

Hermansen L, Wachtlova M 1971 Capillary density of skeletal muscle in well-trained and untrained men. Journal of Applied Physiology 30(6):860–863

Hides J, Richardson C, Jull G, Davies S 1995 Ultrasound imaging in rehabilitation. Australian Journal of Physiotherapy 41(3):187–193

Hill A V 1938 The heat of shortening and the dynamic constants of muscle. Proceedings of The Royal Society of London (Biology) 126:136–195

Hill A V 1950 The series elastic component of muscle. Proceedings of the Royal Society B137:273–280

Hirokawa S, Solomonow M, Lu Y et al 1992 Anterior-posterior and rotational displacement of the tibia elicited by quadriceps contraction. American Journal of Sports Medicine 20(3):299–306

Hodges P W, Richardson C A 1996 Inefficient muscular stabilization of the lumbar spine associated with low back pain. A motor control evaluation of transversus abdominis. Spine 21(22):2640–2650

Holloszy J O 1976 Adaptations of muscular tissue to training. Progress in Cardiovascular Diseases 18(6):445–458

Honey P, Mumford A 1986 The manual of learning styles. Printique, London

Hortobagyi T, Hill J P, Houmard J A et al 1996 Adaptive responses to muscle lengthening and shortening in humans. Journal of Applied Physiology 80(3):765–772

Hortobagyi T, Dempsey L, Fraser D et al 2000 Changes in muscle strength, muscle fibre size and myofibrillar gene expression after immobilization and retraining in humans. Journal of Physiology 524(1):293–304

Housh D J, Housh T J, Johnson G O, Wei-kom C 1992 Hypertrophic response to unilateral concentric isokinetic resistance training. Journal of Applied Physiology 73:65–70

Hunter G 1998 Specific soft tissue mobilization in the management of soft tissue dysfunction. Manual Therapy 3(1):2–11

Hurley M V, Jones D W, Newham D J 1994 Arthrogenic quadriceps inhibition and rehabilitation of patients with

extensive traumatic knee injuries. Clinical Sciences
86:305–310

Hurme T, Kalimo H, Lehto M, Jarvinen M 1991 Healing of
skeletal muscle injury: an ultrastructural and
immunohistochemical study. Medicine and Science in
Sports and Exercise 23(7):801–810

Ingjer F 1979 Capillary supply and mitochondrial content
of different skeletal muscle fiber types in untrained and
endurance-trained men. A histochemical and
ultrastructural study. European Journal of
Applied Physiology and Occupational Physiology
40:197–209

Jarvinen M J, Lehto M U K 1993 The effects of early
mobilisation and immobilisation on the healing
process following muscle injuries. Sports Medicine
15(2):78–89

Jayson M I V, Dixon A St J 1970 Intra-articular pressure in
rheumatoid arthritis of the knee. III. Pressure changes
during joint use. Annals of the Rheumatic Diseases
29:401–408

Jenkins W M, Merzenich M M, Ochs M T et al 1990
Functional reorganization of primary somatosensory
cortex in adult owl monkeys after behaviorally controlled
tactile stimulation. Journal of Neurophysiology
63(1):82–104

Jenner J R, Stephens J A 1982 Cutaneous reflex responses
and their central nervous system pathways studied in
man. Journal of Physiology (Lond) 333:405–419

Jones D A, Newham D J, Round J M, Tolfree S E J 1986
Experimental human muscle damage: morphological
changes in relation to other indices of damage. Journal of
Physiology 375:435–448

Jozsa L, Kannus P 1997 Human tendons: anatomy,
physiology and pathology. Human Kinetics, Champaign,
Illinois

Kandel E R 1991 Cellular mechanisms of learning and the
biological basis of individuality. In: Kandel E R, Schwartz
J H, Jessell T M (eds) Principles of neural science, 3rd edn.
Elsevier, New York

Kanehisa H, Miyashita M 1983 Specificity of velocity in
strength training. European Journal of Applied
Physiology 52:104–106

Kaser L, Mannion A F, Rhyner A et al 2001 Active Therapy
for chronic low back pain part 2 effects on paraspinal
muscle cross-sectional area, fiber type size, and
distribution. Spine 26(8):909–919

Katz B 1939 The relation between force and speed in
muscular contraction. Journal of Physiology 96:45–64

Kawakami Y, Abe T, Fukunaga T 1993 Muscle-fiber
pennation angles are greater in hypertrophied than in
normal muscles. Journal of Applied Physiology
74(6):2740–2744

Kawakami Y, Abe T, Kuno S-Y, Fukunaga T 1995 Training-
induced changes in muscle architecture and specific
tension. European Journal of Applied Physiology
72:37–43

Kellett J 1986 Acute soft tissue injuries – a review of the
literature. Medicine and Science in Sports and Exercise
18(5):489–500

Kerr K 1998 Exercise in rehabilitation. In: Pitt-Brooke J, Reid
H, Lockwood J, Kerr K (eds) Rehabilitation of movement,
theoretical basis of clinical practice. W B Saunders,
London, ch 12, p 423–457

Kidd G, Lawes N, Musa I 1992 Understanding
neuromuscular plasticity a basis for clinical rehabilitation.
Edward Arnold, London

Knott M, Voss D E 1968 Proprioceptive neuromuscular
facilitation. Harper Row, New York

Komi P V 1986 Training of muscle strength and power:
interaction of neuromotoric, hypertrophic, and mechanical
factors. International Journal of Sports Medicine 7:10–15
Supplement

Kornberg C, Lew P 1989 The effect of stretching neural
structures on grade one hamstring injuries. Journal
of Orthopaedic and Sports Physical Therapy
6:481–487

Kuraishi Y 1990 Neuropeptide-mediated transmission of
nociceptive information and its regulation. Novel
mechanisms of analgesics. Yakugaku Zasshi
110(10):711–726

Kuraishi Y, Harada Y, Aratani S et al 1983 Separate
involvement of the spinal noradrenergic and serotonergic
systems in morphine analgesia: the differences in
mechanical and thermal algesic tests. Brain Research
273:245–252

Kvist H, Kvist M 1980 The operative treatment of chronic
calcaneal paratenonitis. Journal of Bone and Joint Surgery
62B(3):353–357

LaBan M M 1962 Collagen tissue: implications of its
response to stress in vitro. Archives of Physical Medicine
and Rehabilitation 43(9):461–466

Labarque V L, Eijnde B Op 't, Leemputte M Van 2002 Effect
of immobilization and retraining on torque-velocity
relationship of human knee flexor and extensor
muscles. European Journal of Applied Physiology
86:251–257

Laughman R K, Youdas J W, Garrett T R, Chao E Y S 1983
Strength changes in the normal quadriceps femoris
muscle as a result of electrical stimulation. Physical
Therapy 63(4):494–499

Leggett S H, Graves J E, Pollock M L et al 1991 Quantitative
assessment and training of isometric cervical extension
strength. American Journal of Sports Medicine
19(6):653–659

Lehmann J F, DeLateur B J, Silverman D R 1966 Selective
heating effects of ultrasound in human beings.
Archives of Physical Medicine and Rehabilitation
47:331–339

Lehmann J F, Masock A J, Warren C G, Koblanski J N 1970
Effect of therapeutic temperature on tendon extensibility.
Archives of Physical Medicine and Rehabilitation
51(8):481–487

Levick J R 1983 Joint pressure–volume studies: their
importance, design and interpretation. Journal of
Rheumatology 10:353–357

Liu J, Wrisberg C A 1997 The effect of knowledge of results
delay and the subjective estimation of movement form
on the acquisition and retention of a motor skill.
Research Quarterly for Exercise and Sport 68(2):
145–151

Louie J K, Mote C D 1987 Contribution of the musculature
to rotatory laxity and torsional stiffness at the knee.
Journal of Biomechanics 20(3):281–300

Lovick T 1991 Interactions between descending pathways
from the dorsal and ventrolateral periaqueductal gray
matter in the rat. In: Depaulis A, Bandler R (eds) The

midbrain periaqueductal gray matter. Plenum Press, New York, p 101–120

Low J, Reed A 1990 Electrotherapy explained, principles and practice. Butterworth-Heinemann, London

McArdle W D, Katch F I, Katch V L 1996 Exercise physiology: energy, nutrition and human performance, 4th edn. Williams & Wilkins, Baltimore

McCaffery M 1979 Nursing the patient in pain. Harper & Row, London

McComas A J 1996 Skeletal muscle: form and function. Human Kinetics, Champaign, Illinois

McConnell J 2002 Recalcitrant chronic low back and leg pain – a new theory and different approach to management. Manual Therapy 7(4):183–192

McCullagh P, Caird J K 1990 Correct and learning models and the use of model knowledge of results in the acquisition and retention of a motor skill. Journal of Human Movement Studies 18:107–116

McDaniel W J, Dameron T B 1983 The untreated anterior cruciate ligament rupture. Clinical Orthopaedics and Related Research 172:158–163

Macdonald R 1994 Taping techniques. Butterworth-Heinemann, Oxford

McDonald P V, van Emmerick R E A, Newell K M 1989 The effects of practice on limb kinematics in a throwing task. Journal of Motor Behavior 21(3):245–264

MacDougall J D 1986 Morphological changes in human skeletal muscle following strength training and immobilization. In: Jones N L, McCartney N, McComas A J (eds) Human muscle power, Human Kinetics, Champaign, Illinois, ch 17, p 269–288

MacDougall J D, Elder G C B, Sale D G et al 1980 Effects of strength training and immobilization on human muscle fibres. European Journal of Applied Physiology 43:25–34

Magarey M E 1985 Selection of passive treatment techniques. In: Proceedings of 4th Biennial Conference of the Manipulative Therapists' Association of Australia, Brisbane, p 298–320

Magarey M E 1986 Examination and assessment in spinal joint dysfunction. In: Grieve G P (ed.) Modern manual therapy of the vertebral column. Churchill Livingstone, Edinburgh, ch 44, p 481–497

Main C J, Waddell G 1999 Psychological distress. In: Waddell G (ed) The back pain revolution. Churchill Livingstone, Edinburgh, ch 11 p 173–186

Maitland G D, Banks K, English K, Hengeveld E 2001 Maitland's vertebral manipulation, 6th edn. Butterworth-Heinemann, Oxford

Mannion A F, Taimela S, Muntener M, Dvorak J 2001 Active therapy for chronic low back pain part I effects on back muscle activation, fatigability, and strength. Spine 26(8):897–908

Melissa L, MacDougall J D, Tarnopolsky M A et al 1997 Skeletal muscle adaptations to training under normobaric hypoxic versus normoxic conditions. Medicine and Science in Sports and Exercise 29(2):238–243

Melzack R 1975 Prolonged relief of pain by brief, intense transcutaneous somatic stimulation. Pain 1:357–373

Melzack R, Wall P D 1965 Pain mechanisms: a new theory. Science 150:971–979

Mense S, Meyer H 1985 Different types of slowly conducting afferent units in cat skeletal muscle and tendon. Journal of Physiology 363:403–417

Millard J B 1961 Effect of high-frequency currents and infrared rays on the circulation of the lower limb in man. Annals of Physical Medicine 6(2):45–66

Montgomery H E, Marshall R, Hemingway H et al 1998 Human gene for physical performance. Nature 393:221–222

Moore S P, Marteniuk R G 1986 Kinematic and electromyographic changes that occur as a function of learning a time-constrained aiming task. Journal of Motor Behavior 18(4):397–426

Moritani T, DeVries H A 1979 Neural factors versus hypertrophy in the time course of muscle strength gain. American Journal of Physical Medicine 58(3):115–130

Mulligan B R 1995 Manual therapy 'nags', 'snags', 'MWM' etc, 3rd edn. Plane View Services, New Zealand

Narici M V, Hoppeler H, Kayser B et al 1996 Human quadriceps cross-sectional area, torque and neural activation during 6 months strength training. Acta Physiologica Scandinavica 157:175–186

Natri A, Jarvinen M, Latvala K, Kannus P 1996 Isokinetic muscle performance after anterior cruciate ligament surgery. International Journal of Sports Medicine 17:223–228

Newham D J 2001 Strength, power and endurance. In: Trew M & Everett T (eds) Human Movement, 4th edn. Churchill Livingstone, Edinburgh, ch 6 p 105–128

Newham D J, Hurley M V, Jones D W 1989 Ligamentous knee injuries and muscle inhibition. Journal of Orthopaedic Rheumatology 2:163–173

Niemann J, Winker T, Gerling J et al 1991 Changes of slow cortical negative DC-potentials during the acquisition of a complex finger motor task. Experimental Brain Research 85:417–422

Nikolaou P K, MacDonald B L, Glisson R R et al 1987 Biomechanical and histological evaluation of muscle after controlled strain injury. American Journal of Sports Medicine 15(1):9–14

Norkin C C, Levangie P K 1992 Joint structure and function, a comprehensive analysis, 2nd edn. F A Davis, Philadelphia

O'Neill D S, Zheng D, Anderson W K et al 1999 Effect of endurance exercise on myosin heavy chain gene regulation in human skeletal muscle. American Journal of Physiology 276:R414-R419

Parkkola R, Kujala U, Rytokoski U 1992 Response of the trunk muscles to training assessed by magnetic resonance imaging and muscle strength. European Journal of Applied Physiology and Occupational Physiology 65:383–387

Pascual-Leone A, Dang N, Cohen L G et al 1995 Modulation of muscle responses evoked by transcranial magnetic stimulation during the acquisition of new fine motor skills. Journal of Neurophysiology 74(3):1037–1045

Petty N J, Moore A P 2001 Neuromusculoskeletal examination and assessment, a handbook for therapists, 2nd edn. Churchill Livingstone, Edinburgh

Pfeifer K, Banzer W 1999 Motor performance in different dynamic tests in knee rehabilitation. Scandinavian Journal of Medicine and Science in Sports 9:19–27

Pollock M L, Graves J E, Bamman M M et al 1993 Frequency and volume of resistance training: effect on cervical extension strength. Archives of Physical Medicine and Rehabilitation 74:1080–1086

Quintner J L, Cohen M L 1994 Referred pain of peripheral nerve origin: an alternative to the 'myofascial pain' construct. Clinical Journal of Pain 10(3):243–251

Renstrom P, Arms S W, Stanwyck T S 1986 Strain within the anterior cruciate ligament during hamstring and quadriceps activity. American Journal of Sports Medicine 14(1):83–87

Reynolds N L, Worrell T W 1991 Chronic achilles peritendinitis: etiology, pathophysiology, and treatment. Journal of Orthopaedic Sports Physical Therapy 13(4):171–176

Richardson C, Jull G, Hodges P, Hides J 1999 Therapeutic exercise for spinal segmental stabilization in low back pain, scientific basis and clinical approach. Churchill Livingstone, Edinburgh

Rigby B J 1964 The effect of mechanical extension upon the thermal stability of collagen. Biochimica et Biophysica Acta 79 (SC 43008):634–636

Rigby B J, Hirai N, Spikes J D, Eyring H 1959 The mechanical properties of rat tail tendon. Journal of General Physiology 43:265–283

Rohter F D, Rochelle R H, Hyman C 1963 Exercise blood flow changes in the human forearm during physical training. Journal of Applied Physiology 18(4):789–793

Rood M S 1956 Neurophysiological mechanisms utilized in the treatment of neuromuscular dysfunction. American Journal of Occupational Therapy 10(4):220–224

Sady S P, Wortman M, Blanke D 1982 Flexibility training: ballistic, static or proprioceptive neuromuscular facilitation? Archives of Physical Medicine and Rehabilitation 63(6):261–263

Sale D G 1988 Neural adaptation to resistance training. Medicine and Science in Sports and Exercise 20(5):S135–S145

Sale D G, MacDougall J D, Upton A R M, McComas A J 1983 Effect of strength training upon motor neurone excitability in man. Medicine and Science in Sports and Exercise 15(1):57–62

Sapega A A, Quedenfield T C, Moyer R A, Butler R A 1981 Biophysical factors in range-of-motion exercise. Physician and Sportsmedicine 9(12):57–65

Schmidt R A, Wrisberg C A 2000 Motor learning and performance, a problem-based learning approach, 2nd edn. Human Kinetics, Champaign, Illinois

Scott W, Stevens J, Binder-Macleod S A 2001 Human skeletal muscle fiber type classifications. Physical Therapy 81(11):1810–1816

Seto J L, Orofino A S, Morrissey M C et al 1988 Assessment of quadriceps/hamstring strength, knee ligament stability, functional and sports activity levels five years after anterior cruciate ligament reconstruction. American Journal of Sports Medicine 16(2):170–180

Simoneau J A, Lortie G, Boulay M R et al 1986 Inheritance of human skeletal muscle and anaerobic capacity adaptation to high-intensity intermittent training. International Journal of Sports Medicine 7:167–171

Sparrow W A, Irizarry-Lopez V M 1987 Mechanical efficiency and metabolic cost as measures of learning a novel gross motor task. Journal of Motor Behavior 19(2):240–264

Starkey D B, Pollock M L, Ishida Y et al 1996 Effect of resistance training volume on strength and muscle thickness. Medicine and Science in Sports and Exercise 28:1311–1320

Staron R S, Karapondo D L, Kraemer W J et al 1994 Skeletal muscle adaptations during early phase of heavy-resistance training in men and women. Journal of Applied Physiology 76:1247–1255

Sterling M, Jull F, Wright A 2001 Cervical mobilisation: concurrent effects on pain, sympathetic nervous system activity and motor activity. Manual Therapy 6(2):72–81

Stuart A, McComas A J, Goldspink G, Elder G 1981 Electrophysiologic features of muscle regeneration. Experimental Neurology 74:148–159

Suter E, Herzog W 1997 Extent of muscle inhibition as a function of knee angle. Journal of Electromyography and Kinesiology 7(2):123–130

Suter E, Herzog W 2000 Muscle inhibition and functional deficiencies associated with knee pathologies. In: Herzog W (ed) Skeletal muscle mechanics, from mechanisms to function. John Wiley, Chichester, ch 21, p 365–376

Takai S, Woo S L-Y, Horibe S et al 1991 The effects of frequency and duration of controlled passive mobilization on tendon healing. Journal of Orthopaedic Research 9:705–713

Talishev F M, Fedina T I 1976 Influence of muscle viscoelastic characteristics on the accuracy of movement control. In: Komi P V (ed) Biomechanics V-A. University Park, Baltimore, p 124–128

Taylor D C, Dalton J D, Seaber A V, Garrett W E 1990 Viscoelastic properties of muscle-tendon units the biomechanical effects of stretching. American Journal of Sports Medicine 18(3):300–309

Terrados N, Jansson E, Sylven C, Kaijser L 1990 Is hypoxia a stimulus for synthesis of oxidative enzymes and myoglobin. Journal of Applied Physiology 68:2369–2372

Thomson A, Skinner A, Piercy J 1991 Tidy's Physiotherapy, 12th edn. Butterworth-Heinemann, Oxford

Tidball J G 1991 Myotendinous junction injury in relation to junction structure and molecular composition. Exercise and Sport Sciences Reviews 19:419–445

Tobin S, Robinson G 2000 The effect of McConnell's vastus lateralis inhibition taping technique on vastus lateralis and vastus medialis obliquus activity. Physiotherapy 86(4):173–183

Todd J E 1990 Conductive education: the continuing challenge. Physiotherapy 76(1):13–16

Tonkonogi M, Walsh B, Svensson M, Sahlin K 2000 Mitochondrial function and antioxidative defence in human muscle: effects of endurance training and oxidative stress. Journal of Physiology 528(2):379–388

Travell J G, Simons D G 1983 Myofascial pain and dysfunction: the trigger point manual, the upper extremities, vol 1. Williams & Wilkins, Baltimore

Travell J G, Simons D G 1992 Myofascial pain and dysfunction: the trigger point manual: the lower extremities, vol 2. Williams & Wilkins, Baltimore

Vanderhoof E R, Imig C J, Hines H M 1961 Effect of muscle strength and endurance development on blood flow. Journal of Applied Physiology 16(5):873–877

Vicenzino B 2003 Lateral epicondylalgia: a musculoskeletal physiotherapy perspective. Manual Therapy 8(2):66–79

Vicenzino B, Paungmali A, Buratowski S, Wright A 2001 Specific manipulative therapy treatment for chronic lateral epicondylalgia produces uniquely characteristic hypoalgesia. Manual Therapy 6(4):205–212

Vicenzino B, Souvlis T, Wright A 2002 Musculoskeletal pain. In: Strong J, Unruh A M, Wright A, Baxter G D (eds) Pain: a textbook for therapists. Churchill Livingstone, Edinburgh, ch 17 p 327–349

Vlaeyen J W S, Crombez G 1999 Fear of movement/(re)injury, avoidance and pain disability in chronic low back pain patients. Manual Therapy 4(4):187–195

Waddell G 1999 Diagnostic triage. In: Waddell G (ed) The back pain revolution. Churchill Livingstone, Edinburgh, ch 2 p 9

Waddell G, Main C J 1999 Beliefs about back pain. In: Waddell G (ed) The back pain revolution. Churchill Livingstone, Edinburgh, ch 12 p 187–202

Waddington P J 1999 In: Hollis M & Fletcher-Cook P (ed) Practical exercise therapy. Blackwell Scientific, Oxford

Walla D J, Albright J P, McAuley E et al 1985 Hamstring control and the unstable anterior cruciate ligament-deficient knee. American Journal of Sports Medicine 13(1):34–39

Warren C G, Lehmann J F, Koblanski J N 1971 Elongation of rat tail tendon: effect of load and temperature. Archives of Physical Medicine and Rehabilitation 52:465–474

Watson T 2000 The role of electrotherapy in contemporary physiotherapy practice. Manual Therapy 5(3):132–141

Watson P, Kendall N 2000 Assessing psychological yellow flags. In: Gifford L (ed) Topical issues in pain 2, biopsychosocial assessment and management relationships and pain. CNS, Kestral, ch 3, p 111–129

Westcott W L 1986 Four key factors in building a strength program. Scholastic Coach 55:104–105,123

Westcott W L, Greenberger K, Milius D 1989 Strength-training research: sets and repetitions. Scholastic Coach 58:98,100

Wilmore J H, Costill D L 1999 Physiology of Sport and Exercise, 2nd edn. Human Kinetics, Illinois, p 17

Woo S, Maynard J, Butler D et al 1988 Ligament, tendon, and joint capsule insertions to bone. In: Woo S L-Y, Buckwalter J (eds) Injury and repair of the musculoskeletal soft tissues. American Academy of Orthopaedic Surgeons. Park Ridge, Illinois ch 4, p 133–166

Yaksh T L, Elde R P 1981 Factors governing release of methionine enkephalin-like immunoreactivity from mesencephalon and spinal cord of the cat in vivo. Journal of Neurophysiology 46(5):1056–1075

Young A, Stokes M, Round J M, Edwards R H T 1983 The effect of high-resistance training on the strength and cross-sectional area of the human quadriceps. European Journal of Clinical Investigation 13:411–417

7

Function and dysfunction of nerve

The function of the neuromusculoskeletal system is to produce movement and this is dependent on optimal functions of nerves, joints and muscles. This interrelationship is depicted in Figure 7.1, which was originally devised to describe the stability of the spine (Panjabi 1992) but is applicable to the function of the whole neuromusculoskeletal system. So while this chapter is concerned with the function of nerves, it is important to stress that nerves do not function in isolation but in a highly interdependent way with joints and muscles. For a nerve to function optimally there must be normal functioning of the relevant joints and muscles.

Some examples of how nerves, joints and muscles function together may help to highlight this close relationship. Anatomically nervous tissues are clearly related to joint and muscle. Sensory nerve endings lie within ligamentous tissue, in extrafusal muscle fibres and in musculotendinous junctions. Peripheral nerves also lie close to muscle and joint; for example, the median nerve at the elbow runs under a fibrous arch of flexor digitorum superficialis, the sciatic nerve sometimes pierces through piriformis, and the common peroneal nerve runs around the superior tibiofibular joint. There is thus a very close anatomical relationship between nerve, joint and muscle.

Passive dorsiflexion of an anaesthetized cat ankle joint activates mechanoreceptors in the posterior joint capsule. This produces a reflex facilitation of gastrocnemius motor neurones and inhibition of tibialis anterior. Similarly, passive plantarflexion causes activation of mechanoreceptors in the anterior joint capsule which produces facilitation of tibialis anterior and inhibition of

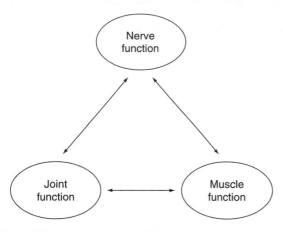

Figure 7.1 Interdependence of the function of nerve, joint and muscle for normal movement (after Panjabi 1992, with permission). Normal function of the neuromusculoskeletal system requires normal functioning of nerve, joint and muscle.

gastrocnemius (Freeman & Wyke 1967). In the same way, in the human lumbar spine the supraspinous ligament (Solomonow et al 1998) facet joint capsule and intervertebral disc (Indahl et al 1995, 1997) contain mechanoreceptors which, when stimulated, cause a reflex contraction of multifidus muscle; this reflex is thought to improve spinal stability (Solomonow et al 1998). These examples clearly link nerve function with joint movement and muscle activation.

Proprioception also highlights the interdependent relationship of nerve, joint and muscle. Evidence suggests that the brain uses information collectively from joint, muscle and skin afferents and that isolated information from one of these tissues provides limited information (Gandevia et al 1983, McCloskey et al 1987, Macefield et al 1990, Moberg 1983). Clearly, the nerves are the means by which this information is relayed to the central nervous system.

Normal control of movement occurs as a result of incoming sensory information and is integrated at all levels of the nervous system. Automatic and simple reflex movements occur in the spinal cord, postural and balance reactions occur at the level of the brain stem and basal ganglia, and more complicated movements are initiated and controlled at the motor/sensory cortices, while the cerebellum controls and coor-

dinates movement (Crow & Haas 2001). This clearly links nerves with muscles and joints.

Summary

These examples have sought to highlight the complex interdependent nature of nerve with joint and muscle. It seems clear that normal joint and muscle functions are prerequisites for normal nerve function.

NERVE FUNCTION

This chapter is limited to aspects of nerve function that underpin nerve examination and treatment in patients with neuromusculoskeletal dysfunction. It is anticipated that readers will need to refer to anatomy and physiology textbooks for further information.

The nervous system can be broadly divided into the central nervous system (brain and spinal cord), autonomic nervous system (which will be discussed under nerve movement) and peripheral nervous system (cranial nerves and spinal nerves with their branches).

The following aspects of nerve function will be considered:

- gross anatomy of the spinal cord
- anatomy and physiology of peripheral nerves
- biomechanics of peripheral nerves
- blood supply of peripheral nerves
- nerve supply of peripheral nerves
- movement of the nervous system.

Gross anatomy of the spinal cord

There are ascending and descending tracts in the spinal cord, some of which are demonstrated in Figures 7.2 and 7.3.

There are six major tracts transmitting sensory information from the periphery to the brain. These are briefly outlined below:

- dorsal columns: conveying light touch, pressure, vibration and limb and joint position to the sensory cortex. A few nociceptor fibres run in these columns. Fasciculus cuneatus runs as far as the mid-thoracic region and conveys sensation

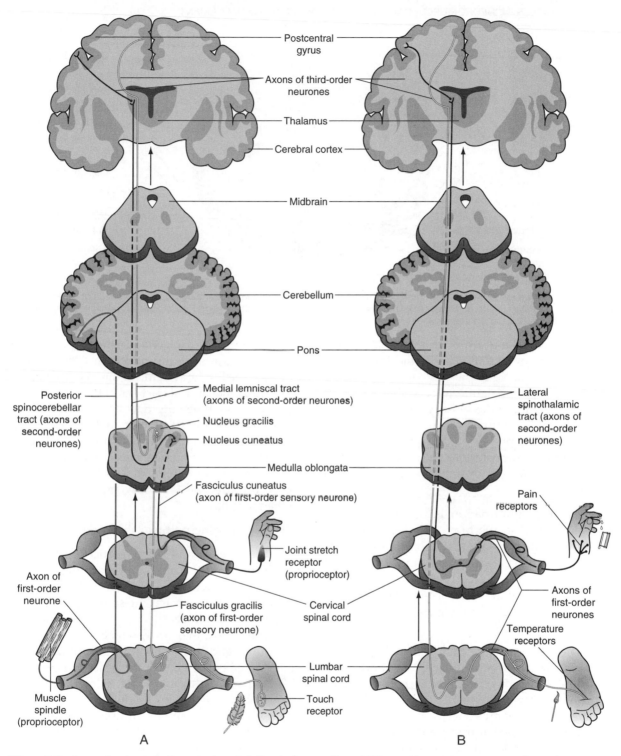

Figure 7.2 Ascending tracts in the spinal cord. **A** Fasciculus gracilis and cuneatus for touch, pressure and proprioception. **B** Lateral spinothalamic tract for pain, temperature, deep pressure and crude touch. (From Human Anatomy and Physiology, 3rd ed by Elaine N Marieb. Copyright © 1995 by The Benjamin/Cummings Publishing Company, Inc. Reprinted by permission of Pearson Education, Inc.)

The following labels appear in the figure:

Postcentral gyrus
Axons of third-order neurones
Thalamus
Cerebral cortex
Midbrain
Cerebellum
Pons
Posterior spinocerebellar tract (axons of second-order neurones)
Medial lemniscal tract (axons of second-order neurones)
Nucleus gracilis
Nucleus cuneatus
Lateral spinothalamic tract (axons of second-order neurones)
Medulla oblongata
Fasciculus cuneatus (axon of first-order sensory neurone)
Pain receptors
Joint stretch receptor (proprioceptor)
Axon of first-order neurone
Fasciculus gracilis (axon of first-order sensory neurone)
Cervical spinal cord
Axons of first-order neurones
Temperature receptors
Lumbar spinal cord
Muscle spindle (proprioceptor)
Touch receptor

A   B

Ascending tracts

Fasciculus gracilis

Fasciculus cuneatus

Posterior spinocerebellar tract

Anterior spinocerebellar tract

Lateral spinothalamic tract

Anterior spinothalamic tract

Descending tracts

Lateral corticospinal tract

Lateral reticulospinal tract

Rubrospinal tract

Anterior reticulospinal tract

Olivospinal tract

Tectospinal tract

Vestibulospinal tract

Anterior corticospinal tract

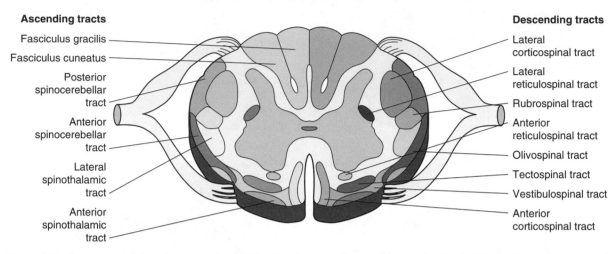

Figure 7.3 Transverse section of the spinal cord showing the ascending and descending tracts. (From Human Anatomy and Physiology, 3rd ed by Elaine N Marieb. Copyright © 1995 by The Benjamin/Cummings Publishing Company, Inc. Reprinted by permission of Pearson Education, Inc.)

from the upper limb, trunk and neck; fasciculus gracilis conveys sensation from the lower limb and lower trunk.

• lateral spinothalamic tract: conveying pain and temperature to the sensory cortex.

• anterior spinothalamic tract: transmitting crude touch and pressure to the sensory cortex.

• anterior and posterior spinocerebellar tracts transmitting muscle or tendon stretch to the cerebellum.

Nociceptive information is transmitted from the spinal cord to the brain via five pathways: the spinothalamic, spinoreticular, spinomesencephalic, spinocervical tracts and the dorsal columns (Jessell & Kelly 1991). The spinothalamic, spinoreticular and spinomesencephalic pathways are shown in Figure 7.4. These are briefly outlined below:

1. The spinothalamic tract transmits nociceptive information from laminar I, V, VI and VII of the dorsal horn. It contains nociceptive-specific neurones and wide-dynamic neurones that terminate at the thalamus.

2. The spinoreticular tract transmits nociceptive information from lamina VII and VIII and travels to the reticular formation and the thalamus.

3. The spinomesencephalic tract transmits nociceptive information from lamina I and lamina V to the mesencephalic reticular formation,

the lateral part of the periaqueductal grey region (PAG) and parts of the midbrain. The PAG is linked to the limbic system via the hypothalamus.

4. The spinocervical tract lies in the upper cervical spine and transmits nociceptive information from lamina III and IV running to the lateral cervical nucleus and on to the mid-brain and thalamus.

5. The dorsal columns transmits nociceptive information from lamina III and IV, in the fasciculus cuneatus and fasciculus gracilis and travel to the medulla.

The descending pathways include:

1. The anterior and lateral corticospinal tracts, which run from the motor cortex to the anterior horn cells and activate skeletal muscles (Figs. 7.3 and 7.5). These two tracts are sometimes referred to as pyramidal tracts.

2. The tectospinal tract, which runs from the mid-brain and transmits motor impulses for coordinated movement of the head and eyes.

3. The vestibulospinal tract, which runs from the vestibular nuclei in the medulla to the anterior horn cells; it maintains muscle tone and activates limb and trunk extensor muscles, thus aiding posture and balance.

4. The rubrospinal tract, which runs from the red nucleus in the mid-brain to the anterior horn and maintains muscle tone of mostly distal flexor muscles in the limbs.

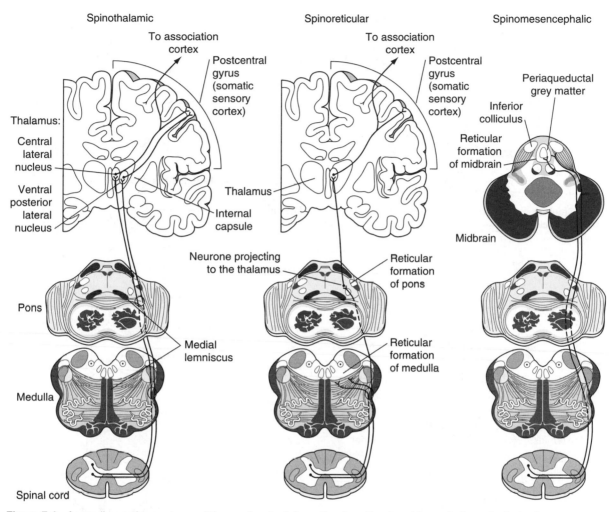

Figure 7.4 Ascending pathways transmitting nociceptor information from the dorsal horn via the spinothalamic, spinoreticular and spinomesencephalic pathways (from Jessell & Kelly 1991).

5. The reticulospinal tract, which runs from the reticular formation in the brain stem to the anterior horn and maintains muscle tone and visceral motor function.

Anatomy and physiology of the peripheral nerves

Sensory and motor fibres

Each spinal nerve is connected to the spinal cord via a dorsal root containing sensory fibres and a ventral root containing motor fibres (Fig. 7.6).

The spinal nerve roots descend the spinal canal by varying amounts and then exit the intervertebral foramina, as shown in Figure 7.7. The spinal nerve divide into two branches, the dorsal and ventral rami. The dorsal rami supply the zygapophyseal joints, muscles and skin overlying the head, neck and spine. The ventral rami supply the anterior and lateral trunk, and the upper and lower limbs. The ventral rami join in the cervical region to form the cervical and brachial plexi and in the lumbar and sacral regions to form the lumbar, lumbosacral and sacral plexi (Fig. 7.8).

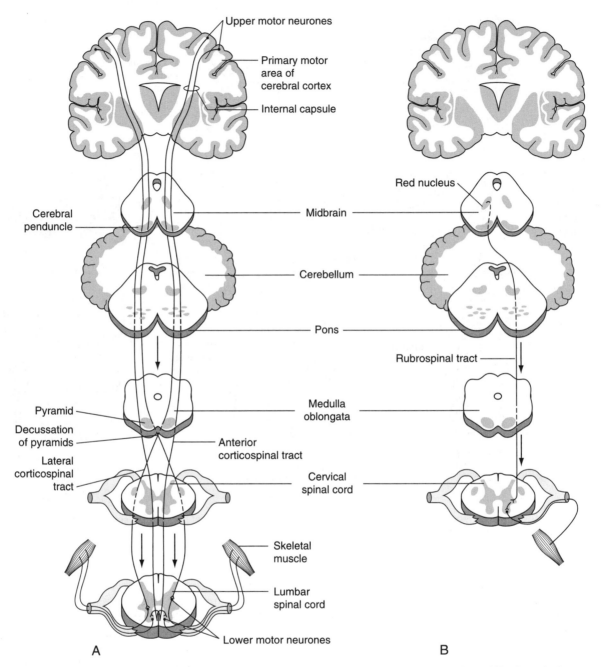

Figure 7.5 Descending tracts: **A** lateral and anterior corticospinal tracts activate skeletal muscle, and **B** rubrospinal tract involved in maintaining muscle tone. (From Human Anatomy and Physiology, 3rd ed by Elaine N Marieb. Copyright © 1995 by The Benjamin/Cummings Publishing Company, Inc. Reprinted by permission of Pearson Education, Inc.)

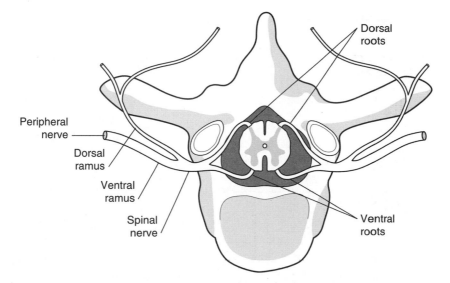

Figure 7.6 A horizontal cross section of the spinal cord demonstrating branches of a spinal nerve (after Palastanga et al 2002, with permission).

Peripheral nerves typically consist of sensory and motor nerve fibres surrounded by connective tissue. A typical sensory nerve fibre consists of dendrites at its distal end, (peripheral axon), a cell body lying in the dorsal root ganglion in the intervertebral foramen, and a central axon to the dorsal horn in the spinal cord (Fig. 7.9A). A typical motor nerve fibre consists of dendrites, a cell body in the ventral horn of the spinal cord and an axon (Fig. 7.9B). Each sensory or motor nerve fibre is a single, extremely elongated, cell which may run from the spinal cord as far as the toe or finger.

The fascicles (nerve fibres enclosed by the endoneurium, see later in this chapter) do not have a straight course along a nerve; rather, they repeatedly join and divide to form a complex plexus (Fig. 7.10). The number of fascicles seen on cross section of a nerve increases where a nerve crosses a joint, increasing its tensile strength (Sunderland 1990).

Most axons are myelinated, that is, they are surrounded by a myelin sheath; some, however, do not have this covering and are said to be unmyelinated. The myelin sheath is formed by Schwann cells wrapped a number of times around part of an axon (Fig. 7.11A).

Longitudinally along the axon, gaps occur between the Schwann cells, and these are known as nodes of Ranvier. Impulses travel along the nerve and 'jump' from one node of Ranvier to the next, a process known as saltatory conduction, which increases the speed of nerve conduction (Rydevik et al 1989). Unmyelinated nerve fibres are also covered in Schwann cells but they have no myelin sheath (Fig. 7.11B). Impulses travel in a continuous manner along an unmyelinated nerve fibre; there is no 'jumping', which reduces the speed of conduction. Large myelinated nerve fibres conduct the sense of touch, pressure, sense of position, temperature and sharp pain, while the small unmyelinated nerve fibres conduct dull diffuse pain (Rydevik et al 1989).

Peripheral nerve fibres (sensory, motor and autonomic) are classified according to their conduction velocities (Table 7.1). Afferent fibres can be classified in a variety of ways (Palastanga et al 2002). In this text the following terms only are used:

A α, which is the same as group I afferent
A β, which is the same as group II afferent
A δ, which is the same as group III afferent
C fibres, which are the same as group IV fibres.

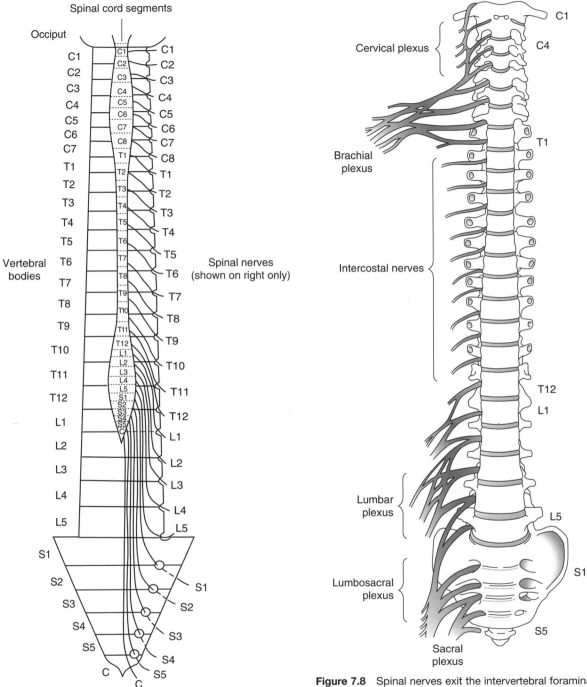

Figure 7.7 The relationship of exiting nerves with vertebral levels. It can be seen, for example, that the T9 nerve root exits between the T9 and T10 vertebra. (From Oliver & Middleditch 1991, with permission.)

Figure 7.8 Spinal nerves exit the intervertebral foramina to form the cervical, brachial, lumbar, lumbosacral and sacral plexi (from Palastanga et al 2002, with permission).

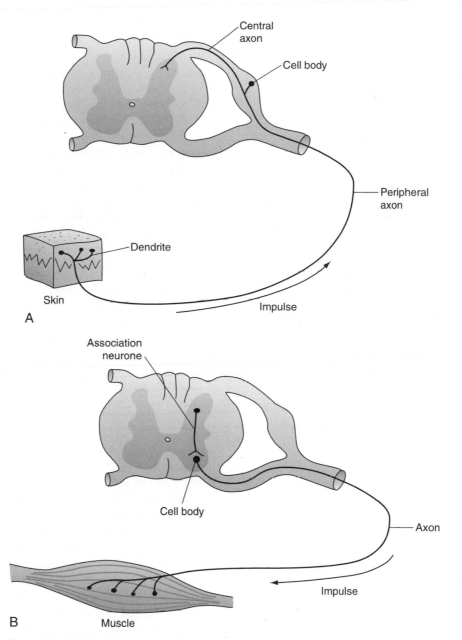

Figure 7.9 Typical **A** sensory and **B** motor nerve fibres. (After Human Anatomy and Physiology, 3rd ed by Elaine N Marieb. Copyright © 1995 by The Benjamin/Cummings Publishing Company, Inc. Reprinted by permission of Pearson Education, Inc.)

Efferent fibres, that is, motor fibres supplying muscle, can be broadly classified as A α and A γ (or fusimotor) fibres, both of which are fast-conducting myelinated fibres (Palastanga et al 2002).

The sensory nerves end distally in various types of receptor in almost all the tissues of the body. The sensory receptors in joint and muscle have been covered in the relevant chapters on joint and muscle. What remains to be clarified here are the receptors found in skin, which will clearly have relevance for all types of nerve, muscle and joint treatments.

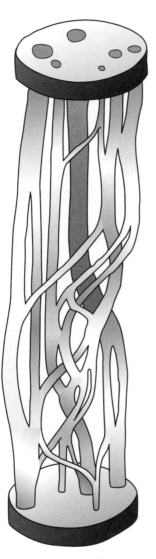

Figure 7.10 Fascicular plexus within a nerve (from Sunderland 1990, with permission).

Cutaneous sensory receptors

There is a variety of sensory receptors in the skin (Fig. 7.12); these are briefly outlined below:

1. Free nerve endings. These lie in the dermis and at the root of hair follicles. They respond to low-threshold mechanical stimuli such as touch, pressure and temperature, and high-threshold noxious mechanical stimuli; they thus act as nociceptors.

2. Merkel's discs. These lie in the epidermis in hairless skin, particularly the finger tips and are low-threshold mechanical receptors providing the sense of touch.

3. Meissner's corpuscles. These are surrounded by a fibrous capsule and lie in the dermis. They respond to touch.

4. Krause end bulbs. These are also surrounded by a fibrous capsule and lie in the dermis. They are low-threshold mechanical receptors, and so respond to touch.

5. Ruffini corpuscles. These lie within a covering of collagen fibres and lie in the dermis. They respond to pressure.

6. Pacinian corpuscles. These are covered in layers of modified Schwann cells encased in a fibrous capsule. They lie in the dermis and respond to pressure.

Free nerve endings responding to noxious mechanical and thermal stimuli are supplied by fast myelinated A delta and slow unmyelinated C fibres (Palastanga et al 2002). All the other skin receptors are supplied by fast-conducting myelinated A beta fibres (Palastanga et al 2002).

Normal, age-related change in nerve function occurs by approximately the seventh decade (Schaumburg et al 1983). The clinical tests manifesting reduced nerve function reflect both anatomical and physiological changes. There are degenerative changes in both myelinated and unmyelinated afferent fibres and their receptors, and efferent fibres and their motor endings, as well as a thickening of the connective tissue in the perineurium and endoneurium (Schaumburg et al 1983). These alterations are reflected in a reduction in sensitivity to touch, two-point discrimination, and vibration in the lower limbs, and a slightly elevated pain threshold (Schaumburg et al 1983). Motor changes include a reduction in tendon reflexes and a reduction in nerve conduction velocity (Kimura 1983). There is also a reduced function of the autonomic nervous system with increasing age (Schaumburg et al 1983).

Axoplasmic flow

Nerve cells contain axoplasm (synonymous with cytoplasm) which, as in all cells, plays a vital role in cell function. Nerve cells (cell body and axon)

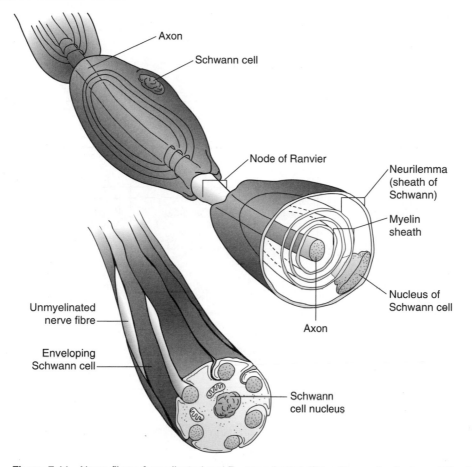

Figure 7.11 Nerve fibres **A** myelinated and **B** unmyelinated. (From Human Anatomy and Physiology, 3rd ed by Elaine N Marieb. Copyright © 1995 by The Benjamin/Cummings Publishing Company, Inc. Reprinted by permission of Pearson Education, Inc.)

can be extremely elongated structures, running, for example, from the lumbar spine to the toe, or from the cervical spine to the finger. Because of these long distances, a special method is required to transport substances from the cell body to the end of the axon and back. This method of transportation is known as axoplasmic flow (Schwartz 1991). Substances transported include: proteins, membranous vesicles, neurotransmitters, lipids, mitochondria and RNA (Grafstein & Forman 1980). There are three methods of axonal transport: fast anterograde (forward moving to the end of the axon, to the periphery), fast retrograde (backward moving towards the cell body), and slow anterograde axoplasmic flow (Schwartz 1991).

1. Fast anterograde axoplasmic flow transports synaptic vesicles to the terminal of the nerve where they take part in the release of transmitter substances. Axoplasmic flow occurs at a rate of approximately 400 mm/day (Dahlin & Lundborg 1990).

2. Fast retrograde axoplasmic flow transports materials from the end of the axon to the cell body. These materials can be degraded or recycled, or inform the cell body about events at the end of the axon (Bisby 1982, Dahlin & Lundborg 1990). For example, where nerve growth factor is released to stimulate growth of neurones, this is transported back to inform the cell body (Schwartz 1991). The rate of flow is about 200–260 mm/day.

Table 7.1 Classification of peripheral nerve fibres (Williams & Warwick 1980)

Characteristics of fibre / Type of sheath	Myelinated					Non-myelinated
Fibre diameter	22 μm				1.5 μm	2.0–0.1 μm
Conduction speed (metres/second)	120	60	50	30	4	0.5
Classification 1. Erlanger and Gasser *All fibres*	A			B		C
Subclasses: Efferent	Aα Skeletomotor	Aβ Fusimotor collaterals of A fibres	Aγ Fusimotor	B Preganglionic autonomic		C Postganglionic autonomic
Afferent	Aα and smaller. Muscle and tendon; cutaneous			Aδ Cutaneous, muscle visceral, etc.		C Cutaneous, muscle visceral, etc.
2. Lloyd Afferent – skeletal muscle and articular	I *a* primary spindle ending *b* tendon ending	II Secondary spindle ending		III Free ending (nociceptor, etc.) paciniform ending?		IV Free ending (nociceptor, etc.)

It should be noted that the scale for conduction velocities is not arithmetical.

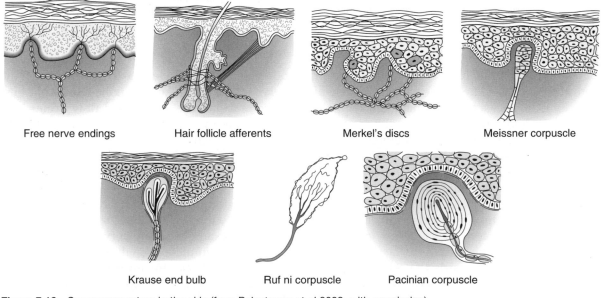

Free nerve endings   Hair follicle afferents   Merkel's discs   Meissner corpuscle

Krause end bulb   Ruf ni corpuscle   Pacinian corpuscle

Figure 7.12 Sensory receptors in the skin (from Palastanga et al 2002, with permission).

3. Slow anterograde axoplasmic flow is the method by which the majority of axoplasm moves. Fibrous and soluble proteins, and enzymes, are transported slowly along the axon at either a rate of 0.2–2.5 mm/day or at a slightly faster rate of 0.4–5 mm/day.

Connective tissue covering of peripheral nerves

Nerve fibres are organized into a bundle (or fascicle) by a layer of connective tissue called the endoneurium; this makes up the functional unit of a nerve. The endoneurium surrounding individual nerve fibres is made up of collagen and fibroblasts. The pressure within the endoneurium is slightly more than in the tissues surrounding a nerve (Rydevik et al 1989). A number of fascicles are surrounded by another layer of connective tissue called the perineurium. The perineurium acts as a diffusion barrier between the adjacent tissues (Rydevik & Lundborg 1977, Sunderland 1990) and is considered by Sunderland (1990) to be mostly responsible for providing nerve with tensile strength and elasticity. The outermost layer of connective tissue of a peripheral nerve is called the epineurium (Fig. 7.13). The epineurium consists of loose connective tissue which helps to protect the nerve during movement. The epineurium rather than the perineurium is considered by Haftek (1970) to be mostly responsible for providing nerve with tensile strength and elasticity.

Biomechanics of peripheral nerves

Because peripheral nerves lie on either side of joints they must shorten and lengthen with movement. The connective tissue surrounding nerves contain elastin; this therefore enables nerves to return to a shortened position following lengthening; for example, the median nerve has to shorten by about 15% on elbow flexion (Zoech et al l991).

When lengthening occurs, tensile (longitudinal) force is transmitted along the length of a nerve. Nerves have considerable tensile strength to withstand this tensile force. For example, the maximum load that can be sustained by the median nerve ranges from 71 to 218 N, the ulnar nerve from 63 to 152 N, the medial popliteal nerve from 202 to 329 N, and the lateral popliteal nerve from 116 to 210 N (Sunderland & Bradley 1961). The tensile properties of nerve roots, compared to bone, cartilage, ligament, muscle and tendon is given in Table 7.2 (Panjabi & White 2001).

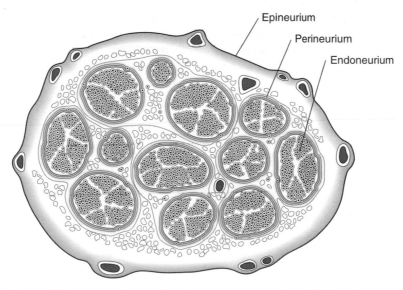

Figure 7.13 Layers of connective tissue around nerve fibres (after Lundborg et al 1987, with permission).

Table 7.2 Tensile properties of nerve roots compared to bone, cartilage, ligament, muscle and tendon (Panjabi & White 2001)

Tissue	Stress at failure (MPa)	Strain at failure (%)
Nerve roots	15	19
Cortical bone	100–200	1–3
Cancellous bone	10	5–7
Cartilage	10–15	80–120
Ligament	10–40	30–45
Muscle (passive)	0.17	60
Tendon	55	9–10

Peripheral nerve is viscoelastic and, as such, has a force–displacement (or stress–strain) curve similar to that of other tissues (Sunderland & Bradley 1961). The load–displacement curve is dependent on the rate of lengthening (Sunderland 1990): the faster the lengthening the greater the resistance. A typical force–displacement curve of a rabbit tibial nerve demonstrates an early toe region (Fig. 7.14) where a small force causes a relatively large displacement (Haftek 1970). During the toe region, the undulation of the nerve is straightened out (Haftek 1970), accounting for about 75% of the total change in length (Zoech et al 1991). Resistance then increases to produce the linear part of the curve until the limit of elasticity is reached. During this phase, all of the nerve, but particularly the epineurium and perineurium, resists the movement until, at the limit of elasticity, the epineurium ruptures (Haftek 1970). Generally this occurs at about 20% elongation, although it can occur as low

as 8% (Sunderland & Bradley 1961). Resistance then decreases as elongation continues. Complete rupture generally occurs at about 30% of elongation, although there is a wide variation between nerves (Sunderland & Bradley 1961).

A stress–strain graph of human median nerve from cadavers is shown in Figure 7.15 (Zoech et al 1991). It can be seen that there is an increase in stress at quite low strain values. On the graph, the stress is not sufficient to identify the limit of elasticity.

Like all viscoelastic materials, nerve undergoes stress relaxation. A 6% strain held for 1 hour causes a 57% reduction in tension (Wall et al 1992), an 8% strain held for 30 minutes causes a 50% reduction in tension (Clark et al 1992), while a 12% strain held for 1 hour causes a 50% reduction in tension (Wall et al 1992) and a 15% strain held for 30 minutes causes a 40% reduction in tension (Clark et al 1992). There is no structural damage to the nerve after a 12% strain held for 1 hour (Wall et al 1992), although there could be a change in function if the blood supply to the nerve is affected.

Lengthening a nerve will cause a number of changes: there will be a reduction in the cross-sectional area, increased tension within the nerve, compression of the nerve fibres and a reduction in the microcirculation of nerve (Sunderland 1990).

Whether the resistance to lengthening a nerve is provided mainly by the perineurium (Sunderland 1990) or by the epineurium (Haftek

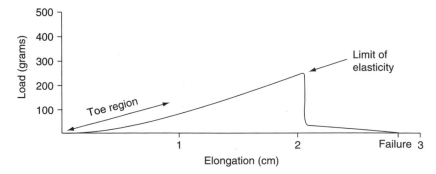

Figure 7.14 Force–displacement of the tibial nerve of the albino rabbit (after Haftek 1970, with permission).

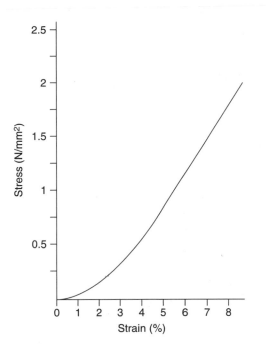

Figure 7.15 Stress–strain curve of the median nerve at the cubital fossa during elbow extension (after Zoech et al 1991, with permission).

1970), it seems clear that it is the connective tissue in nerve that resists the lengthening, and not the nerve fibres (Fig. 7.16). It can be seen that, under normal physiological lengthening, the

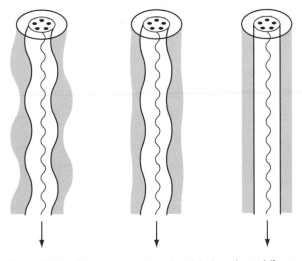

Figure 7.16 Changes to nerve when it is lengthened (from Sunderland 1990, with permission).

nerve fibres remain undulated and thus protected (Sunderland 1990).

The thickness of the epineurium varies between different nerves, and at different parts of the same nerve. Where a nerve requires greater protection there is an increase in the thickness of the epineurium (Sunderland 1978). So, for example, the cross-sectional area of the epineurium of the median nerve in the forearm is about 39% but at the elbow and wrist it is about 60% (Sunderland 1978). The epineurium around the sciatic nerve in the gluteal region is as much as 70–80% (Sunderland 1990). The percentage of epineurium that makes up the cross-sectional area of a nerve varies between 30 and 70% (Sunderland 1990). Nerve roots, on the other hand, exiting from the spinal cord, lack an epineurium and perineurium and are less protected from a traction or compression injury (Sunderland 1990).

Blood supply of peripheral nerves

Peripheral nerves are well vascularized (Fig. 7.17). Blood vessels running alongside nerves send regional feeding vessels to the epineurium which then divide and supply the deep and superficial layers of the epineurium, perineurium and endoneurium (Lundborg et al 1987). The blood vessels are coiled, which allows a certain amount of lengthening to occur without affecting blood flow (Fig. 7.18). Vessels lie obliquely in the perineurium, and it is thought that increased endoneurial pressure will therefore close these vessels (Lundborg 1975). This is supported by the fact that a small increase in endoneurial pressure results in a reduction in blood flow within the endoneurium (Lundborg et al 1983). For example, if a nerve is elongated by more than 8%, the intraneural blood flow is reduced, and at 15% the vessels are completely occluded, causing nerve ischaemia (Lundborg & Rydevik 1973).

Nerve supply of peripheral nerve

The connective tissue sheaths surrounding peripheral nerves are innervated by the nervi nervorum (Fig. 7.19) (Bove & Light 1995,

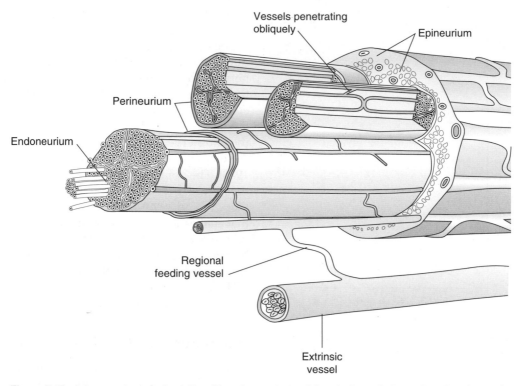

Figure 7.17 Intraneural microcirculation. Vessels penetrate obliquely through the perineurium (arrows). (After Lundborg et al 1987, with permission.)

Hromada 1963). The epineurium, perineurium and endoneurium contain both free nerve endings and encapsulated endings, and the afferent fibres are mostly unmyelinated C fibres with some thinly myelinated fibres (Hromada 1963). The nerve supply originates from the axons within the sheath and from the blood vessels that supply the nerve (Bahns et al 1986, Bove & Light 1995, Hromada 1963). The nerve endings respond to high-threshold mechanical stimuli as well as chemical stimuli (capsaicin, bradykinin, hypertonic sodium chloride or potassium chloride) and thermal stimuli, and are therefore considered to have a nociceptive function (Bahns et al 1986, Bove & Light 1995). The connective tissue of nerve can therefore be a direct source of pain, by mechanical deformation or chemicals released with inflammation.

The epineurium covering the ventral and dorsal roots is also innervated, as are the spinal and sympathetic ganglia (Hromada 1963).

Movement of the nervous system

During normal functional movements the nervous system moves as a continuum, as one whole system. For descriptive purposes here, movement of the brain, spinal cord and peripheral nerves will be considered separately.

Movement of the brain

Three layers of connective tissue, collectively known as the meninges, surround the brain and spinal cord; they are the dura mater, arachnoid mater and pia mater. The dura mater covering the brain is referred to as cerebral dura mater, and that around the spinal cord as spinal dura mater.

The cerebral dura mater is the outermost layer and is attached to the inner aspect of the cranium (Fig. 7.20). Large folds are reflected into the centre of the cranial cavity (Fig. 7.21), the largest

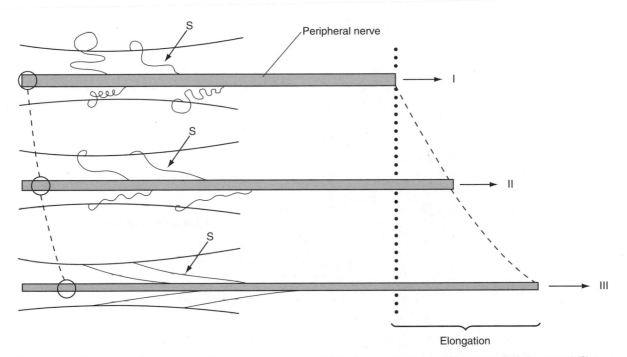

Figure 7.18 Effect of stretching on the blood supply to the rabbit tibial nerve. Stage I is where the coiled segmental (S) blood vessels are unaffected by nerve lengthening. Stage II is where further increase in nerve lengthening begins to stretch the blood vessels and impair flow. Stage III is where the cross-sectional area of the nerve (circled) is reduced which further impairs blood flow. (From Rydevik et al 1989, with permission.)

being the falx cerebri and the tentorium cerebelli (Palastanga et al 2002). The arachnoid layer contains the subarachnoid space filled with cerebrospinal fluid, which absorbs forces. The pia mater is adherent to the outside of the brain. The dura mater, arachnoid and pia mater in the cranium are all innervated and therefore can be a source of symptoms.

The cranial nerves are covered in connective tissue and lie close to the cerebral dura mater (Williams et al 1995). Movements of the head are thought to cause sliding, elongation, and compression of the dura mater, falx cerebri, tentorium cerebelli and the cranial nerves (Breig 1978, von Piekartz & Bryden 2001). Upper cervical flexion and contralateral lateral flexion have been found to cause 5–7 mm of movement in the trigeminal, hypoglossal, facial and accessory cranial nerves (Breig 1978). Figure 7.22 demonstrates the effect of cervical flexion on the spinal cord and branches of the mandibular nerve.

Movement of the spinal cord

The spinal cord is covered in dura mater, arachnoid mater and pia mater (Fig.7.23). The pia mater is a thin transparent membrane covering the spinal cord; caudally it attaches to the coccyx. The arachnoid contains the subarachnoid space, which is filled with cerebrospinal fluid. Dorsal ligaments link the inner surface of the arachnoid with the spinal cord. The outermost layer of spinal dura mater forms a tube known as the dural theca which contains the spinal cord. Twenty-one pairs of fibrous denticulate ligaments (or ligamentum denticulatum) lie between the level of the foramen magnum and T12/L1 level and attach to the pia mater and the dural sac (Fig. 7.24). They keep the spinal cord central in the dural theca, and they deform and move during spinal movements (Epstein 1966).

The dura mater is made up of longitudinally arranged collagen and a few elastic fibres, and

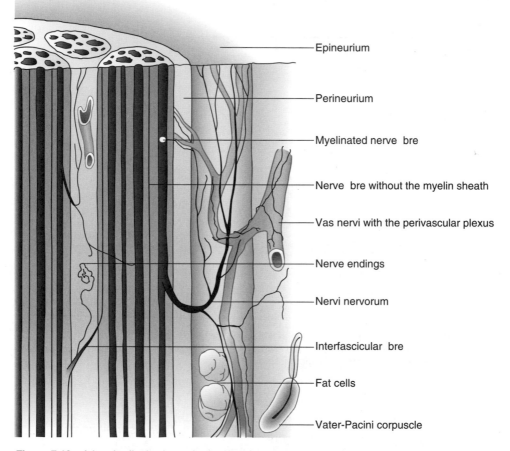

- Epineurium
- Perineurium
- Myelinated nerve bre
- Nerve bre without the myelin sheath
- Vas nervi with the perivascular plexus
- Nerve endings
- Nervi nervorum
- Interfascicular bre
- Fat cells
- Vater-Pacini corpuscle

Figure 7.19 A longitudinal schematic drawing demonstrating the nervi nervorum and nerve endings within the connective tissue sheath of a peripheral nerve. (After Hromada 1963, Acta Anatomica 55:343–351, with permission from the publisher, S. Karger AG, Basel.)

has great tensile strength. The dura mater is innervated anteriorly by the sinuvertebral nerve, but not posteriorly. The anterior innervation of the dura seems a useful defence mechanism. It lies adjacent to the posterior longitudinal ligament of the spine, which is also innervated, and these two structures form a protective wall between the intervertebral disc and the spinal cord (Fig. 7.25). The pia mater and arachnoid are also innervated (Williams et al 1995). Thus the dura mater, arachnoid and pia mater may transmit nociception and thus be a source of pain.

The autonomic nervous system must also adapt with movement, and of particular interest is the sympathetic trunk that is closely related to

the vertebral column (Fig 7.26). It can be seen that the trunk lies anterior to the axis of movement in the cervical region and posterior to the axis in the thoracic and lumbar regions. Consequently, the trunk will be lengthened when the cervical spine is extended and when the thoracic and lumbar regions are flexed. From the anterior view of the vertebral column it can be seen that the trunk lies to one side and will therefore be lengthened on contralateral lateral flexion, that is, the left side of the trunk will be lengthened when the spine laterally flexes to the right. It is perhaps also worth highlighting the close position of the sympathetic trunk to the costotransverse joints; movement at this joint

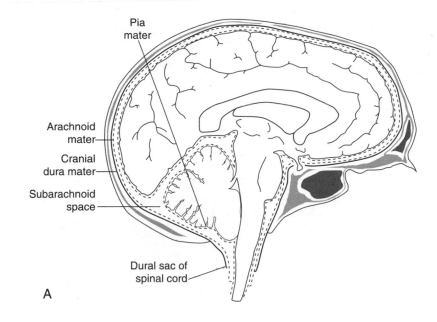

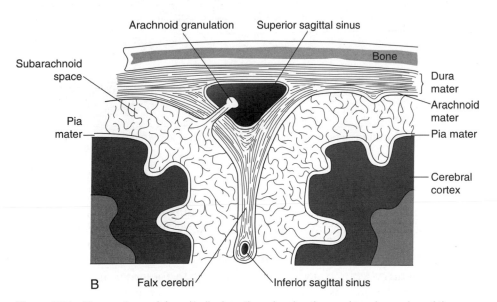

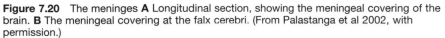

Figure 7.20 The meninges **A** Longitudinal section, showing the meningeal covering of the brain. **B** The meningeal covering at the falx cerebri. (From Palastanga et al 2002, with permission.)

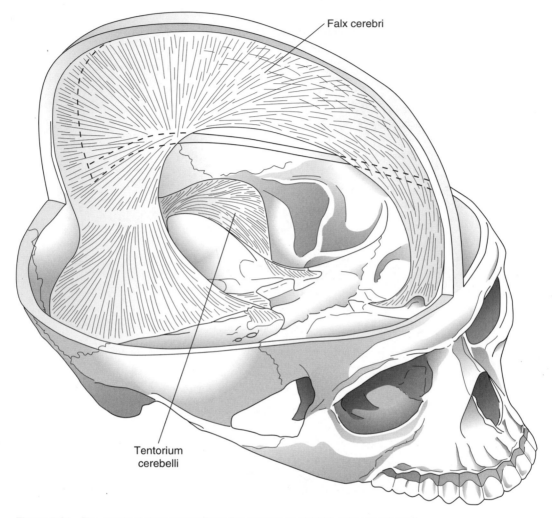

Falx cerebri

Tentorium
cerebelli

Figure 7.21 The cerebral dura mater (from Palastanga et al 2002, with permission).

will cause movement of the trunk. The close anatomical arrangement of the pre- and postganglionic axons of the grey and white rami communicans (Fig. 7.27) also demonstrates that movements that affect the spinal nerve roots will also affect the sympathetic nervous system.

Cervical flexion in isolation has also been shown to move and tension the spinal dura in the cervical spine in particular, but also in the thoracic and lumbar regions (Breig & Marions 1963, Tencer et al 1985).

With whole-spine movements, from full extension to full flexion, the spinal canal lengthens by about 5–9 cm (Breig 1978, Inman & Saunders 1942, Louis 1981). The axis of flexion and extension movements lie in the vertebral bodies, which is anterior to the spinal canal. For this reason, during flexion, the posterior wall lengthens more than the anterior wall. During flexion the neuroaxis (all the nervous tissue and meninges in the skull and vertebral canal) elongates and moves anteriorly in the spinal canal (Breig 1978). The movement, however, is not even throughout: little movement occurs at C6, T6 and L4 (Louis 1981). Butler (1991) refers to this as 'tension points' (Fig. 7.28). Accompanying the increase in

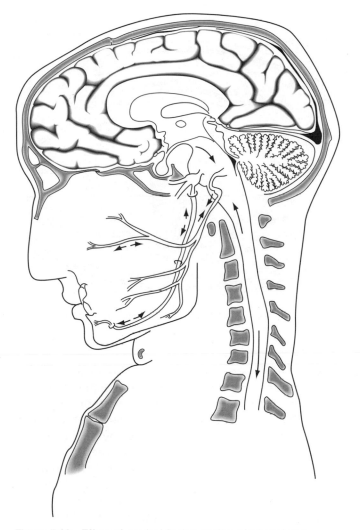

Figure 7.22 Effect of cervical flexion on the spinal cord and branches of the mandibular nerve (from von Piekartz & Bryden 2001, with permission).

length will be an increase in tissue tension (Butler 1991). It should be noted that the neuroaxis moves relative to its meningeal covering: they do not move as one (Louis 1981).

With the reverse movement, from full flexion to full extension, the spinal canal reduces its length and the contents shorten and lie more posteriorly in the spinal canal (Breig 1978). Lateral flexion movements will lengthen the spinal canal on the contralateral side and shorten it on the ipsilateral side; the neuraxis and meningeal coverings will mirror these movements.

Movements of the spine also affect the size of the intervertebral foramen, where the nerve root lies. In the lumbar spine, from a neutral start position, lumbar spine flexion has been found to increase the size of the intervertebral foramen by 12%, and extension decreases it by 15% (Inufusa et al 1996). Flexion would therefore reduce compression on the exiting nervous tissue, but would increase its tension, while extension would increase compression, but reduce tension (Adams et al 2002).

The spinal arachnoid and pia mater are continuous with the perineurium of a peripheral

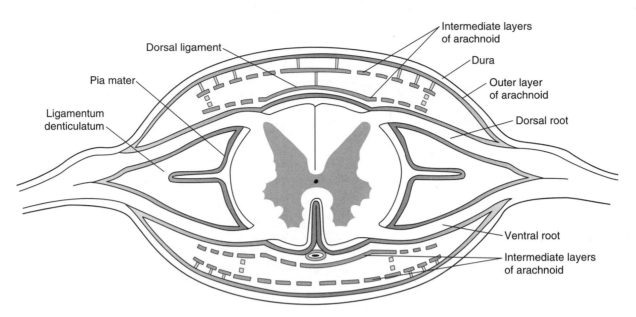

Figure 7.23 Horizontal cross section of the spinal cord with the connective tissue layers, dura mater, arachnoid and pia mater (from Williams et al 1995).

nerve, and the spinal dura mater is continuous with the epineurium of a peripheral nerve (Williams et al 1995). Thus, the cerebral meninges, spinal meninges, and perineurium and epineurium of peripheral nerves are one continuous structure.

Movement of peripheral nerves

Peripheral nerves are covered with a conjunctiva-like adventitia that allows extraneural gliding with adjacent tissues; there is also gliding between the fascicles (intraneural gliding) (Rempel et al 1999). There are many data available on peripheral nerve movement. What is provided here are a few examples of the median and ulnar nerve movement. The effects of neurodynamic test movements, as a whole, on peripheral nerve movement are addressed in Chapter 8 under neurodynamic treatment.

Nerve movement can be measured using magnetic resonance imaging (MRI) (Greening et al 1999) and by ultrasound imaging (Dilley et al 2001, Greening et al 2001, Hough et al 2000a, 2000b). Both longitudinal and transverse movements have been measured.

Movement of the fingers causes movement of the median nerve in the forearm and wrist. From full flexion of the index finger to 30 degrees extension at the interphalangeal joints, the median nerve in the forearm moves longitudinally between 1.6 and 4.5 mm (Dilley et al 2001). Under the flexor retinaculum at the wrist joint, index finger extension causes the median nerve to glide up to 2 mm in an ulnar direction (Nakamichi & Tachibana 1995).

Movement of the wrist also causes movement of the median nerve at the wrist and at the elbow. Wrist movement from 30 degrees flexion to 30 degrees extension causes the median nerve at the wrist to move approximately 3–5 mm in an ulnar direction (Greening et al 1999, 2001), and 2 mm in an anterior direction (Greening et al 2001). With rather more wrist movement, from 55 degrees flexion to 55 degrees extension, the median nerve at the elbow has been found to move distally between 10 and 21 mm (Hough et al 2000a).

Median nerve movement and tension have been measured in the upper limb in five cadavers (Wright et al 1996). As might be expected, finger hyperextension and wrist extension caused distal movement and increased tension at the wrist

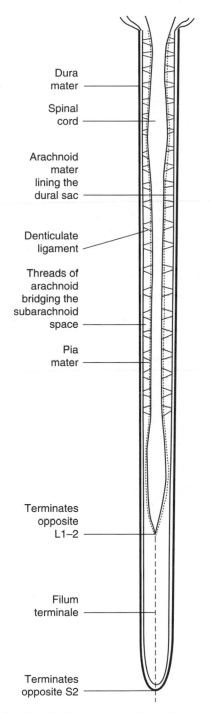

Dura mater

Spinal cord

Arachnoid mater lining the dural sac

Denticulate ligament

Threads of arachnoid bridging the subarachnoid space

Pia mater

Terminates opposite L1–2

Filum terminale

Terminates opposite S2

Figure 7.24 Longitudinal section of the spinal cord (from Palastanga et al 2002, with permission).

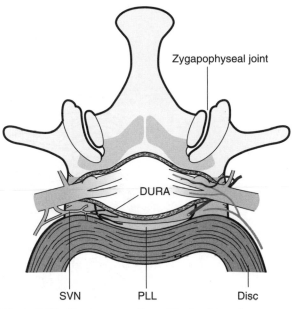

Zygapophyseal joint

DURA

SVN   PLL   Disc

Figure 7.25 Transverse section of the lumbar spine demonstrating the relationship of the dura mater, posterior longitudinal ligament (PLL) and the intervertebral disc, with sinuvertebral nerve (SVN) (after Bogduk 1997, with permission).

and, to a lesser degree, movement at the elbow (tension at the elbow was not measured). Elbow flexion caused distal movement of the median nerve at the wrist with a reduction in tension and proximal movement of the nerve at the elbow. Shoulder abduction to 110 degrees caused proximal movement and increased tension of the median nerve at both the wrist and elbow. Supination caused proximal movement at both the wrist and elbow, with increased tension at the wrist and reduced tension at the elbow; all changes in movement and tension were small. Pronation caused the median nerve to move distally, with reduced tension at the wrist, and to move proximally with increased tension at the elbow; again, all the changes in movement and tension were small. It should be remembered that these values are based on five cadavers, and greater variation may have been found if a larger number had been used. In addition, cadaveric measurements may be rather different to in vivo measurements. Nevertheless, the study provides

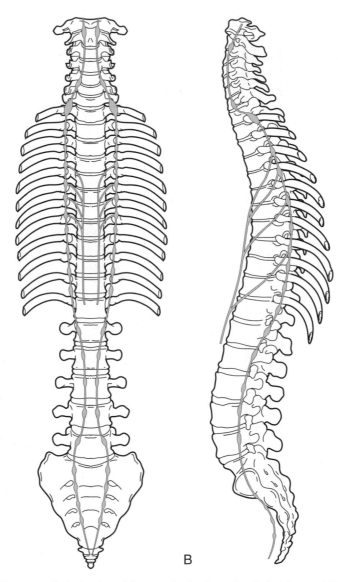

A B

Figure 7.26 Relationship of the sympathetic trunk and the vertebral column **A** anterior view and **B** lateral view (from Butler 1991, with permission).

useful information about nerve movement and provides support for some of the movements used in the upper limb tension tests (ULTT1 and 2a) to increase tension in the median nerve (Butler 2000). Shoulder abduction, wrist extension and finger hyperextension all caused an increased tension in the median nerve, at both the elbow and wrist, and supination caused an increased tension at the wrist.

In order to gain further knowledge for the management of patients with carpal tunnel syndrome, research has investigated the effect of movement and functional activities of the hand, on carpal tunnel pressure. Generally, wrist extension causes a fourfold increase, and flexion a threefold increase in carpal tunnel pressure (Hamanaka et al 1995, Rojviroj et al 1990, Seradge et al 1995). Making a fist with the hand increased

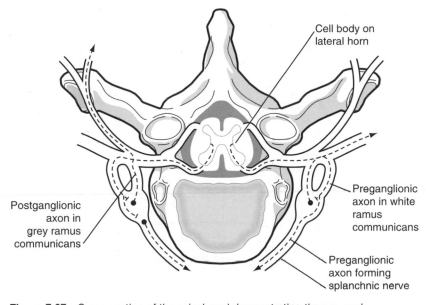

Cell body on
lateral horn

Preganglionic
axon in white
ramus
communicans

Postganglionic
axon in
grey ramus
communicans

Preganglionic
axon forming
splanchnic nerve

Figure 7.27 Cross section of the spinal cord demonstrating the pre- and postganglionic axons of the white and grey rami communicans (from Palastanga et al 2002, with permission).

carpal tunnel pressure from 24 to 234 mmHg (Seradge et al 1995); this is almost a tenfold increase. In a similar study a power grip increased carpal pressure from 43 mmHg to 167 mmHg, almost a fourfold increase (Hamanaka et al 1995), and finger and thumb pinch grip increased carpal tunnel pressure from 5 mmHg to about 50 mmHg (Keir et al 1998).

The movement of the ulnar nerve during elbow flexion and extension has also been investigated (Gelberman et al 1998). The cross-sectional area of the ulnar nerve and the cubital tunnel in which the nerve runs are reduced during elbow flexion, the ulnar nerve by up to 50%. The pressure within the nerve increased incrementally from 90 degrees to 130 degrees flexion, suggesting an increase in nerve tensioning (Gelberman et al 1998).

Summary of nerve function

The central and peripheral nervous systems are anatomically, biomechanically and physiologically linked as part of one whole system. This highly complex system not only produces move-ment of the body, through the coordinated activation of numerous muscles, but is adapted to cope with the physical stresses applied to it during these very movements.

NERVE DYSFUNCTION

Just as the functions of nerves depend on the function of joints and muscles, so dysfunction of nerves can lead to dysfunction of joints and muscles. They are dependent on each other in both normal and abnormal conditions and this is depicted in Figure 7.29. Some specific examples which follow may help to highlight how nerve dysfunction will often be accompanied by joint and/or muscle dysfunction.

Nerve dysfunction appears to accelerate joint degeneration. An experimental study on dogs found that cutting the joint nerve supply around the knee, combined with rupturing the anterior cruciate ligament, caused severe knee joint degeneration within 3 weeks, while the dogs with only the anterior cruciate ligament cut had no such degeneration (O'Connor et al 1985, Vilensky et al 1997).

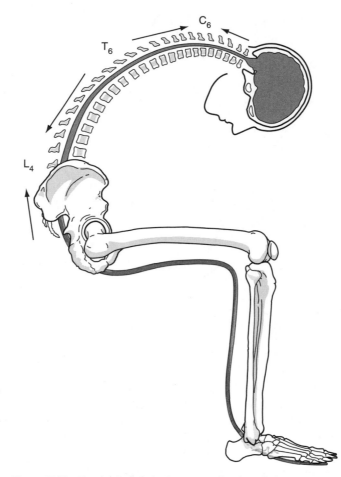

Figure 7.28 Tension points in the neuroaxis where little movement occurs (from Butler 1991, with permission).

Compression of nerves, for example, the median nerve in the carpal tunnel, can lead to a condition known as carpal tunnel syndrome. Signs and symptoms include altered sensation with numbness and paraesthesia, impaired dexterity and muscle weakness (Fuchs et al 1991), which later leads to muscle atrophy (Rempel et al 1999). End-of-range wrist movements will be avoided by the patient as these positions increase the carpal tunnel pressure, thus provoking symptoms. It can be seen then that chronic nerve compression in the long term will cause joint and muscle dysfunction.

Nerve dysfunction can be broadly classified as:

- altered nerve conduction
- reduced nerve movement
- production of symptoms.

Altered nerve conduction

As peripheral nerves are made up of sensory, motor and autonomic fibres, any disruption of nerve conduction will produce alterations in sensation, muscle activation and autonomic control. The sensory and motor alterations are tested clinically by the neurological integrity tests of sensation, isometric muscle strength and reflex testing, described in detail in the companion text (Petty & Moore 2001). Where there are changes in all three aspects of nerve function, a nerve lesion is suspected (Magee 2002). Where the findings relate to dermatome and myotome patterns, with or without reflex changes, a nerve root would be suspected. Where the findings implicate a peripheral nerve, this is termed a mononeuropa-

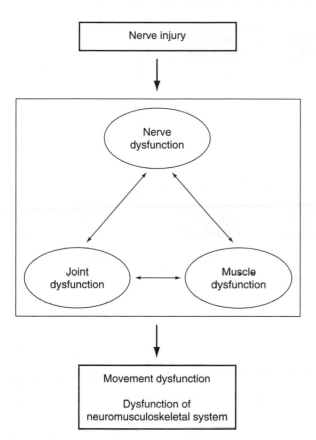

Figure 7.29 Dysfunction of nerve can produce joint and/or muscle dysfunction.

thy, where more than one peripheral nerve is involved, a polyneuropathy.

Altered nerve conduction may be due to structural damage of the nerve, and can be classified into:

- neuropraxia, where there is a temporary interruption of conduction, with or without segmental demyelination, and no structural damage to the axon
- axonotmesis, where there is structural damage to the axon and myelin sheath, but intact connective tissue
- neurotmesis, where there is structural damage to the axon, the myelin sheath and the surrounding connective tissue.

Clinical findings of a neuropraxia, at the level of the nerve root, are most commonly seen in patients with neuromusculoskeletal dysfunction.

The signs and symptoms include: altered sensation in the part of the relevant dermatome, muscle weakness in the relevant myotomes and diminished reflexes (where relevant).

Clinical findings for an axonotmesis and neurotmesis (Magee 2002) are:

- sensory changes which include: loss or abnormal sensation, the skin may be warm, flushed, scaly (early nerve lesions) or cold, white, thin and shiny (later signs of nerve lesion), loss of skin creases and alterations to nails (Magee 2002)
- motor changes, which include: muscle weakness, muscle atrophy, reduced muscle length, reduced joint range of movement and increased stiffness to movement (Magee 2002)
- autonomic function is suggested by abnormalities of temperature, colour and sweating (Scadding 2003).

Commonly, nerve damage seen by clinicians in patients with neuromusculoskeletal dysfunction involves compression and stretch injuries. These are discussed below.

Effects of nerve compression

Compression of a normal nerve root or peripheral nerve will initially not cause pain, but may cause numbness, due to nerve ischaemia (Lundborg et al 1982). Nerves are susceptible to compression, the effects of which depend on the magnitude and duration of the compression (Dahlin & McLean 1986, Rydevik & Lundborg 1977). Nerve compression usually occurs where the nerve lies in a tunnel, such as the median nerve in the carpal tunnel, the ulnar nerve at the wrist, or a spinal nerve root in the intervertebral foramina (Rempel et al 1999).

Nerve can be broadly compressed in one of two ways, either a circumferential pressure or a lateral pressure. A circumferential pressure, as the name suggests, is where the compression is applied circumferentially around the nerve, for example, with carpal tunnel syndrome and spinal stenosis. The forces applied to the nerve and the alteration in shape of the nerve are demonstrated in Figure 7.30. The main effect is at

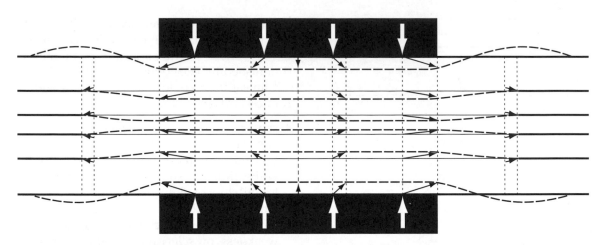

Figure 7.30 The 'edge effect' whereby a circumferential pressure is applied to a nerve with maximal effect at the edge of the compression (from Rydevik 1984, Brown and Lundborg/Pathoanatomy and pathophysiology of nerve root compression. Spine 9(1):7–15 with permission).

the edge of the compressed segment and is referred to as 'the edge effect' (Ochoa et al 1972).

A lateral pressure is where something presses on the side of a nerve causing deformation of the nerve – such as a posterolateral disc protrusion compressing an exiting nerve root (Fig. 7.31). It

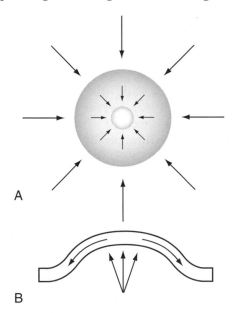

Figure 7.31 **A** Circumference pressure, such as spinal stenosis. **B** Lateral pressure on a nerve – from a prolapsed intervertebral disc for example – causing nerve deformation. (From Rydevik 1984, Brown and Lundborg/Pathoanatomy and pathophysiology of nerve root compression. Spine 9(1): 7–15 with permission.)

can be seen that the site of compression causes the nerve to be lengthened, and will increase nerve tension, if its ends are fixed (Rydevik et al 1984). It has been speculated that this lengthening of the nerve fibre membrane may alter its permeability and conductivity, which could trigger nociception (Rydevik et al 1989).

Experimental studies have investigated the effects of compression on animal peripheral nerves. The effects include mechanical injury to the blood vessels (Lundborg et al 1983) and nerve fibres (Dyck et al 1990).

The blood vessels within the epineurium of the nerve are the parts most sensitive to compression injuries (Lundborg et al 1983, Rydevik & Lundborg 1977). Compression injury of the blood vessels results in increased permeability of the vessel walls, with oedema formation (Rydevik & Lundborg 1977), ischaemic changes in the nerve (Rydevik & Lundborg 1977, Rydevik et al 1981) and a reduced blood flow (Ogata & Naito 1986). Pressures as low as 20–30 mmHg (millimetres of mercury) can reduce the blood flow to the epineurium (Rydevik et al 1981); pressures of 80 mmHg for over 4 hours are needed to cause endoneurial oedema (Lundborg et al 1983).

Mechanical injury of nerve fibres reduces the axonal transport (Dahlin & McLean 1986) and causes nerve degeneration and demyelination (Lundborg et al 1983, Powell & Myers 1986).

Pressure of about 30 mmHg held for 8 hours can cause a reduction in the slow and fast axonal transport systems (Dahlin & McLean 1986). An injury to a nerve axon will affect the whole nerve, including the cell body in the intervertebral foramen or spinal cord (Dahlin & Lundborg 1990). So, for example, compression of the common peroneal nerve at the superior tibiofibular joint will affect the nerve fibres to their distal endings and proximally in the dorsal horn of the spinal cord. Pressures of 50 mmHg held for 2 minutes (Dyck et al 1990), 30 mmHg for 2 hours (Powell & Myers 1986) and 80 mmHg for 4 hours (Lundborg et al 1983) have been shown to cause demyelination of nerve fibres and axonal damage. Fibrosis between the epineurium and adjacent muscles has been observed following a compression injury (Powell & Myers 1986); this would presumably alter the quality of nerve movement.

Nerve compression thus causes widespread mechanical and ischaemic changes in nerves, which will alter nerve conduction and nerve movement.

Chronic nerve compression, with the above changes, is thought to increase the susceptibility of nerve to additional trauma, such as the double-crush injury (Dahlin & Kanje 1992, Dahlin & McLean 1986, Dahlin & Thambert 1993, Mackinnon 1992, Nemoto et al 1987, Upton & McComas 1973) and multiple crush injuries (Mackinnon 1992), outlined in Figure 7.32.

Having discussed, in a general manner, the effects of nerve compression, a specific example now follows to help clarify the clinical presentation of a patient. The example used is carpal tunnel syndrome causing compression of the median nerve.

Carpal tunnel syndrome. The development of signs and symptoms of carpal tunnel syndrome has been linked to the effects of circumferential nerve compression, described above (Rempel et al 1999). Early signs are intermittent paraesthesia and alteration in sensation, particularly at night; this may be due to the changes in the intraneural circulation with some oedema accumulating at night and disappearing during the day (Lundborg et al 1983). Later in the progression of nerve compression there is increased numbness and paraesthesia, impaired dexterity and muscle weakness, these symptoms being present during the day as well as at night; this may be related to altered circulation and the presence of oedema (Fuchs et al 1991) along with demyelination. Minor mechanical irritation can cause radiating pain (Howe et al 1977, MacNab 1972, Rydevik et al 1984, Smyth & Wright 1958). Finally, there is constant pain, atrophy of the thenar muscles and permanent sensory changes; this may be due to a neuropraxia caused by lesions of the myelin sheath of the nerve fibres (Lundborg & Dahlin 1996). Clinical measurement of nerve conduction velocity and latency can be measured objectively; however, there is a 20% false-negative response in patients with carpal tunnel syndrome (Spindler & Dellon 1982).

The pressure within the carpal tunnel is generally increased in patients with carpal tunnel syndrome (Fuchs et al 1991, Hamanaka et al 1995, Seradge et al 1995), although there is a wide variation among individuals such that some have a reduced pressure (Hamanaka et al 1995, Seradge et al 1995). While normal subjects have a resting carpal tunnel pressure of about 24 mmHg, patients with carpal tunnel syndrome generally have pressures of 43 mmHg, with ranges between 5 and 164 mmHg (Seradge et al 1995). In a similar study, carpal tunnel pressure was found to be a little higher in asymptomatic subjects, at about 43 mmHg, but again, patients had higher pressures of up to about 60 mmHg (Hamanaka et al 1995). Patients with carpal tunnel syndrome who are regularly exposed to hand-held vibration tools have been found to have demyelination and incomplete regeneration of the dorsal interosseous nerve at the wrist (Stromberg et al 1997). This suggests that, in some patients, carpal tunnel syndrome may be caused by two mechanisms: nerve compression and nerve vibration (Stromberg et al 1997).

Experimental compression of nerves in normal subjects provides valuable information on the effect of nerve compression on clinical neurological testing. A catheter inserted into the carpal tunnel allows for controlled and accurate increases in carpal pressure to 30, 40, 50, 60, 70

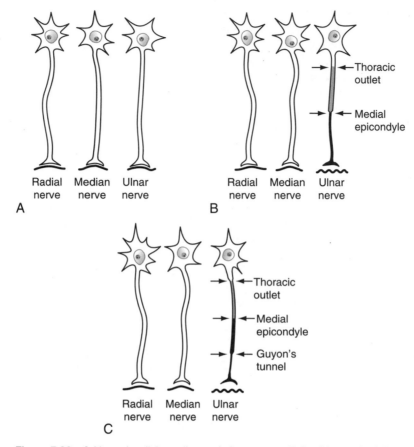

Figure 7.32 **A** Normal radial, median and ulnar nerves. **B** Double-crush of the ulnar nerve whereby compression of the ulnar nerve exiting the thoracic outlet leads to injury of the nerve at the medial epicondyle of the elbow. **C** This develops into multiple crush with injury of the deep palmer division of the ulnar nerve in the Guyon's tunnel (Sunderland 1978). The floor of Guyon's tunnel is formed by the flexor retinaculum and pisohamate ligament, the hook of the hamate forms the lateral wall, the pisiform and tendon of flexor carpi ulnaris form the medial wall, and the rather thin roof is formed by the carpal ligament and palmaris brevis (Sunderland 1978). (After Mackinnon 1992, with permission.)

and 90 mmHg (Gelberman et al 1983, Lundborg et al 1982, Szabo et al 1983). The earliest signs of nerve impairment are the subjective reporting of numbness, tingling or paraesthesia in the distribution of the median nerve (Gelberman et al 1983, Szabo et al 1983). At 40–50 mmHg sensation is completely blocked (Gelberman et al 1983), and in hypertensive subjects with a higher neural arteriole pressure, sensory block occurs at 60–70 mmHg (Szabo et al 1983). This suggests that patients with raised or lowered blood pressure may respond differently to a given amount

of nerve compression (Szabo et al 1983). At 90 mmHg paraesthesia in the hand was felt after 20 minutes, after 30–50 minutes there was a complete sensory block, and after a further 10–30 minutes there was a complete motor block (Lundborg et al 1982).

The effect of graded compression and ischaemia on the common peroneal nerve in the rabbit has been investigated (Dahlin et al 1989). The C fibres (transmitting pain) were found to be the most sensitive to ischaemia, while the large myelinated fibres, A beta, were found to be the most sensitive to compression (Dahlin et al 1989).

The most sensitive physical tests of nerve impairment are vibration sensibility (Gelberman et al 1983, Szabo et al 1983) using a 256 cycles-per-second tuning fork (Dellon 1980, 1981) or vibrameter (Goldberg & Lindblom 1979, Martina et al 1998) and pressure testing (Gelberman et al 1983, Szabo et al 1983) using von Fry monofilaments (Levin et al 1978). These sensory changes occurred before any motor changes (Gelberman et al 1983, Szabo et al 1983). Another sensory test, two-point discrimination, has been found to be an extremely insensitive measure of nerve compression (Gelberman et al 1983, Lundborg et al 1982, Szabo et al 1983). The sensitivity of vibration sensibility is supported by earlier research which found 72% of patients with symptoms of carpal tunnel syndrome had abnormal vibration sensibility (Dellon 1978). Vibration sense is more pronounced in the upper limbs compared to the lower limbs and there is a decrease in vibration threshold with increasing age (Martina et al 1998). Because of these variations the comparison of the left to right sides of a patient would seem the most reliable method of determining a difference.

The sensitivity of vibration is highlighted in keyboard workers with related upper-limb disorders who were found to have an elevated vibration threshold in the median nerve distribution (Greening & Lynn 1998). Patients with repetitive strain injury (RSI) were concluded to have signs of minor polyneuropathy of the median nerve and, to a lesser extent, the ulnar and radial nerves (Greening & Lynn 1998).

Effects of stretching nerves

Lengthening a nerve by 5–10% can reduce the blood flow in a nerve and alter nerve function (Clark et al 1992, Lundborg & Rydevik 1973). In rats, it has been found that an 8% strain of the sciatic nerve results in a 50% reduction in blood flow to the nerve, which recovers on release of the strain; a 15% strain results in an 80% reduction in blood flow which does not recover on release of the strain (Clark et al 1992). A similar

study found that a stretch of about 16% resulted in complete occlusion of the blood flow in the sciatic nerve (Ogata & Naito 1986).

The nerve injury at the limit of elasticity (Fig. 7.14) would correspond to a neuropraxia (temporary interruption of conduction, with or without segmental demyelination, but no structural damage to the axon) or an axonotmesis (structural damage to axon and myelin sheath but intact connective tissue) (Haftek 1970). Beyond the limit of elasticity the injury would correspond to a neurotmesis (structural damage to axon, myelin sheath and surrounding connective tissue) (Haftek 1970). The effects of excessive nerve stretch on one fasciculus is depicted in Figure 7.33.

Nerve regeneration

Following nerve injury the distal portion of the nerve undergoes Wallerian degeneration. Distal

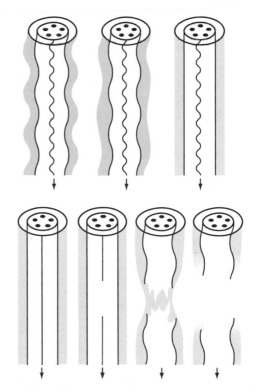

Figure 7.33 Changes to one fasciculus in a nerve as it is stretched to structural failure (from Sunderland 1990, with permission).

to the site of injury, the Schwann cells proliferate and the myelin and axoplasm disintegrate and are reabsorbed by macrophagic activity. Proximal to the site of injury axons grow a large number of sprouts, which grow at approximately 1 mm per day towards the distal segment. If the Schwann cell columns remain intact the sprouting axons will be guided to reinnervate the target organ. If the Schwann cell columns have been destroyed by the injury then sprouting axons may grow and innervate inappropriate areas, giving a poorer clinical result.

The reinnervation and sensory restoration following a myocutaneous skin flap has been investigated and highlights the clinical outcome of nerve regeneration. Some axons were found to sprout into Schwann cell columns, while a number of axons were found to be unmyelinated and associated with blood vessels (Terenghi 1995, Turkof et al 1993). The degree of sensory restoration varied widely between individuals; some flaps were totally numb while others had moderate sensation (Turkof et al 1993). From this research it seems that there is a wide variation in the functional regeneration of sensory nerves, from very poor to moderately good.

An additional effect in regeneration of nerve axons occurs at the dorsal horn within 2 weeks of a nerve injury (Doubell & Woolf 1997). C fibres, which synapse in lamina II of the dorsal horn, atrophy, and leave vacant synaptic spaces (Fig. 7.34). Large myelinated A fibres sprout into these spaces, altering the processing of mechanoreceptor input from A fibres (Woolf et al 1992, Doubell & Woolf 1997).

The repair process of the connective tissue around nerve is similar to that of ligament. Following a nerve injury, there is an increase in the collagen tissue within the perineurium and endoneurium, indicative of scar formation (Salonen et al 1985, Starkweather et al 1978). Additionally, it has been demonstrated in rat sciatic nerves that 3 weeks after a nerve injury, there is a 28% reduction in nerve length (Clark et al 1992).

Reduced nerve movement

This includes a reduced ability of a nerve to lengthen and a reduced ability of a nerve to move relative to adjacent tissues (referred to as the interface). It seems reasonable to suggest that if there is a restriction in the longitudinal movement there will be a restriction in interface movements, and vice versa. Some examples below provide illustrations of reduced nerve movement.

Patients with non-specific arm pain have been found to have reduced median nerve movement

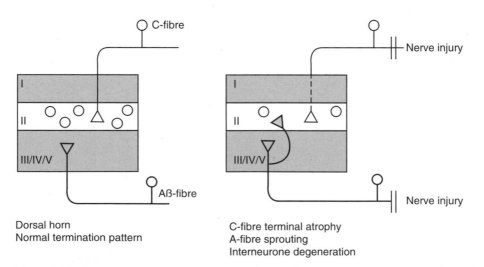

Dorsal horn
Normal termination pattern

C-fibre terminal atrophy
A-fibre sprouting
Interneurone degeneration

Figure 7.34 Sprouting of A fibres into lamina II of the dorsal horn to replace atrophied C fibres (from Doubell et al 1999, with permission).

during wrist movements (Greening et al 1999). In asymptomatic subjects, moving the wrist from 30 degrees extension to 30 degrees wrist flexion caused the median nerve to move approximately 3–5 mm in a radial direction (Greening et al l999, 2001) and 2 mm in a posterior direction (Greening et al 2001). In the patient group, the radial movement and the posterior movement were each approximately 1 mm (Greening et al l999, 2001). Interestingly, and importantly, the loss in median nerve movement correlated with the upper limb tension test (ULTT1 for the median nerve). Patients with the least radial or posterior movement of the median nerve had the most limiting ULTT range of movement – symptoms were reproduced at less than 90 degrees elbow extension; patients with rather more movement had symptoms reproduced at 90–150 degrees elbow extension (Greening et al 2001). It has been suggested that the reduced nerve mobility may be due to an increased stress on the nerve by adjacent tissues or an altered distribution of tension throughout the nerve (Greening et al 2001).

In addition, patients with carpal tunnel syndrome have reduced median nerve movement under the flexor retinaculum at the wrist, during index finger flexion and extension. In normal subjects flexion is accompanied by radial glide of the median nerve and extension by ulnar glide, the excursion being just under 2 mm; in patients with carpal tunnel syndrome this movement was reduced to less than 0.4 mm (Nakamichi & Tachibana 1995). This study suggests that reduced nerve movement may be contributing to the signs and symptoms of carpal tunnel syndrome (Nakamichi & Tachibana 1995).

In rats, experimental transection of the sciatic nerve resulted in a 4% shortening of the nerve and, at 3 weeks, a 28% shortening; this is thought to be due to an alteration in the collagen in the nerve, similar to that seen in ligament injury (Clark et al 1992). At 3 weeks, the nerve had a greater stiffness than immediately following the transection (Clark et al 1992).

An example of restricted interface movement is the adhesion formation between lumbar nerve roots and the intervertebral foramina that can reduce the ability of the nerve to move (Goddard & Reid 1965). This can be caused by local pathological changes or may occur as a result of normal age-related changes (Goddard & Reid 1965).

The above examples, of course, demonstrate minor differences in the range of nerve movement, and the clinician will almost certainly not have the instrumentation necessary to identify these small reductions in movement. The usual clinical method is to use neurodynamic tests: the slump, straight leg raise, passive knee bend, passive neck flexion and upper limb tension tests. These have been described in the companion text (Petty & Moore 2001).

Production of symptoms

Pain from a peripheral nerve can arise from its innervated connective tissue covering or from the axon itself. Where pain arises from the connective tissue it can be considered similar to pain arising from ligament or muscle – in the sense that nociceptors lying in the tissue can provoke symptoms. The pain coming from the connective tissue is therefore classified in the same way as joint and muscle pain, as mechanical or chemical pain, with chemical pain being further subdivided into inflammatory and ischaemic (Gifford 1998). Pain arising from the axon itself is termed neurogenic pain, which can be subdivided into peripheral or central neurogenic pain. Where pathology causes pain from the nerve, it can be referred to as neuropathic pain. The effects of nerve compression and carpal tunnel syndrome, discussed earlier, are examples of peripheral neurogenic or neuropathic pain.

Before discussing pain, a distinction needs to be made between nociception and pain. Nociception is the transmission of impulses from nociceptors that occurs with tissue damage. This activation, however, does not necessarily lead to pain being felt. The perception of pain occurs within the central nervous system (Grieve 1994) and is more than simply the sensation and physiological effects of tissue damage (Fig. 7.35). It includes affective factors such as mood and emotion, cognitive factors such as beliefs and knowledge, behavioural factors such as posture and

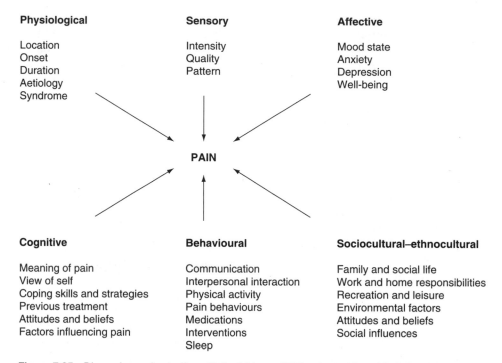

Figure 7.35 Dimensions of pain (from Petty & Moore 2001, adapted from McGuire 1995).

analgesic intake, and socio-cultural factors such as age, gender and ethnicity (Ahles & Martin 1992, McGuire 1985).

Pain has therefore been defined as 'an unpleasant sensory and emotional experience associated with actual or potential tissue damage, or described in terms of such damage' (Merskey et al 1979). This is not an entirely new idea: Descartes (1985) in the 17th century recognized that pain was accompanied by sadness. He wrote that the body is 'ill-disposed when I feel pain', while unclear of the relationship between 'the thing which causes pain and the sense of sadness to which this feeling gives rise'. In 1940 the classical Christian scholar C. S. Lewis attempted to unravel the meaning of pain (Lewis 1998), describing it as 'any experience, whether physical or mental, that the patient dislikes and is synonymous with suffering, anguish, tribulation, adversity and trouble'; he clearly associated pain with effects on emotion and thought. Indeed, what person has ever felt indifferent when experiencing pain? Most, if not all, readers will be able to testify to the sense of suffering and to an emotional response that goes hand in hand with the experience of pain. Pain is an extensive subject and cannot be covered comprehensively in this text. The reader is referred to a number of excellent books on pain, most notably a text by Wall and Melzack (1999). What follows here is an overview of how tissue damage can cause nociception and potentially cause a person to perceive pain.

The perception of pain affects the sympathetic nervous system, which has widespread effects on the respiratory, cardiovascular, gastrointestinal and genitourinary systems, and on endocrine and metabolic function (Cousins & Power 1999). These effects are listed in Table 7.3.

Pain from the connective tissue surrounding nerves

The connective tissue surrounding peripheral nerves and dorsal and ventral nerve roots contain nociceptors and can be stimulated by a nox-

Table 7.3 The effects of acute pain on respiratory, cardiovascular, gastrointestinal and genitourinary systems and on endocrine and metabolic function (Cousins & Power 1999)

Respiratory	Splinting of abdominal and thoracic muscles
	Grunting on expiration
	Small tidal volume
	Rapid respiratory rate
Cardiovascular	Increased heart rate
	Increased blood pressure
	Increased cardiac output
	Decreased blood flow in the limbs
Gastrointestinal and geniturinary	Increased intestinal secretions
	Increased smooth muscle tone
	Reduced intestinal motility
	Urinary retention
Endocrine and metabolic function	Nausea, vomiting
	Altered metabolic rate

ious mechanical force or chemical stimulus (Bahns et al 1986, Bove & Light 1995, Hromada 1963).

The effect of nociceptor activity by a mechanical or chemical stimulus alters the physiology of the nociceptor itself; in this way the nociceptor is plastic, that is, it changes. This increased sensitivity of nociceptors leads to a decreased pain threshold, an increased pain to supra-threshold stimuli – changes collectively referred to as primary hyperalgesia. If a stimulus is applied which would normally not provoke pain, such as joint movement or light touch, and pain is provoked, this is termed allodynia (Raja et al 1999). Allodynia is due to altered transmission of A beta fibres and/or

reduced threshold of nociceptor activity at the periphery (Woolf & Mannion 1999). In addition, mechanoreceptors in adjacent uninjured tissues develop the ability to evoke pain, a phenomenon known as secondary hyperalgesia (Raja et al 1999). This is thought to be due to an increase in the responsiveness of second-order nociceptor neurones in the spinal cord that become activated by mechanoreceptor activity, a response known as central sensitization (Raja et al 1999).

The pain from nerve connective tissue can be classified as mechanical or chemical nociceptive pain (Gifford 1998). Mechanical pain occurs where certain movements stress injured tissue, increasing the mechanical deformation and activation of nociceptors; other movements reduce the stress on injured tissue, reducing the mechanical deformation and activation of nociceptors. Thus, with mechanical pain, there are particular movements that aggravate and ease the pain, sometimes referred to as 'on/off pain' (Table 7.4). The magnitude of the mechanical deformation may be directly related to the magnitude of nociceptor activity; this has been found in the skin of the cat where greater forces cause greater nociceptor activity (Garell et al 1996).

Chemical nociceptive pain can be produced by the chemicals released as a result of inflammation, ischaemia or sympathetic nervous system activity (Gifford 1998). Inflammation releases noxious chemicals into the tissues, which induces or sensitizes activity of the nociceptors

Table 7.4 Clinical features of mechanical, inflammatory and ischaemic nociceptive pain (Butler 2000) and neuropathic pain

Mechanical pain	Particular movements that aggravate and ease the pain, sometimes referred to as 'on/off pain'
Inflammatory pain	Redness, oedema and heat
	Acute pain and tissue damage
	Close relationship of stimulus response and pain
	Diurnal pattern with pain and stiffness worst at night and in the morning
	Signs of neurogenic inflammation (redness, swelling or symptoms in neural zone)
	Beneficial effect of anti-inflammatory medication
Ischaemic pain	Symptoms produced after prolonged or unusual activities
	Rapid ease of symptoms after a change in posture
	Symptoms towards the end of the day or after the accumulation of activity
	Poor response to anti-inflammatory medication
	Absence of trauma
Neuropathic pain	Persistent and intractable
	Stimulus-independent pain: shooting, lancinating or burning pain
	Paraesthesia
	Dysaesthesia

(Dray 1995, Levine & Reichling 1999), that is, hyperalgesia. Clinical features of inflammatory pain are: redness, oedema and heat, acute pain and tissue damage, a close relationship of stimulus response and pain, a diurnal pattern with pain and stiffness worst at night and in the morning, signs of neurogenic inflammation (redness, swelling or symptoms in neural zone) and a beneficial effect of anti-inflammatory medication (Butler 2000).

Ischaemic nociceptive pain is caused by a lowered pH (acidosis) in tissues, which stimulates nociceptor activity (Steen et al 1995). Lowered pH level is frequently related to both painful ischaemic conditions and painful inflammatory conditions (Steen et al 1995). Ischaemia is the underlying cause of sensory and motor changes with nerve compression injuries (Lundborg et al 1982). Clinical features of ischaemic pain are thought to be: symptoms produced after prolonged or unusual activities, rapid ease of symptoms after a change in posture, symptoms towards the end of the day or after the accumulation of activity, a poor response to anti-inflammatory medication and sometimes absence of trauma (Butler 2000).

Pain from the axon: neurogenic or neuropathic pain

This is pain that arises from the axon itself and can manifest as stimulus-independent pain, or stimulus-dependent pain (Woolf & Mannion 1999).

Stimulus-independent pain is mostly characterized as a persistent and intractable pain, where there is no clear relationship between stimulus and response. Pain is felt when no physical stimulus has been applied (Woolf & Mannion 1999). The symptoms may be described as shooting, lancinating or burning pain (Woolf & Mannion 1999). The underlying mechanism for this may be generation of ectopic action potentials on the axon (Woolf & Mannion 1999) (Fig. 7.36). The constant barrage of nociceptor activity at the dorsal horn causes central sensitization (Doubell et al 1999). An alternative cause of chronic pain may be from gene transcription changes which cause an alteration in the expression of neurotransmitters and receptors (Doubell et al 1999) and an increase in synaptic strength in A delta and C fibres at the dorsal horn (Sandkuhler 2000). The growth of large myelinated fibres into lamina II of the dorsal horn, which normally contains only C fibres afferents, alters the mechanoreceptor input from A beta fibres, and may also be responsible for intractable neuropathic pain (Woolf et al 1992, Doubell & Woolf 1997). Continuous activity of C fibres is thought to provoke burning pain and continuous activity of A beta fibres as continuous paraesthesia which, later, with central sensitization, become dysaesthesias and pain. Dysaesthesias (dys meaning bad) indicates an unpleasant sensation (Butler 2000).

Neuropathic pain may also be characterized by hypersensitivity to a stimulus, so that there is a stimulus-dependent pain (Woolf & Mannion 1999). The underlying mechanism is due to hyperalgesia and allodynia. Hyperalgesia is the increase pain response to a suprathreshold noxious stimulus due to abnormal processing of nociceptive information (Woolf & Mannion 1999). Allodynia is the sensation of pain elicited from non-noxious stimuli and is due to altered transmission of A beta fibres and/or reduced threshold of nociceptor activity at the periphery (Woolf & Mannion 1999). A neuroma (swelling at the proximal end of an injured nerve) contains sensitized A and C fibres (Woolf & Mannion 1999).

Transmission of nociceptor information

There are two types of afferents transmitting pain from nociceptors (Jessell & Kelly 1991). Small-diameter, thinly myelinated, fast-conducting A delta fibres are thermal or mechanical nociceptors and give rise to sharp pricking pain. Small-diameter, unmyelinated, slow-conducting C fibres are high-threshold, mechanical, chemical and thermal nociceptors. Tissue injury causes changes in both the peripheral nervous system and the central nervous system and will be discussed under the headings of peripheral sensitization and central sensitization.

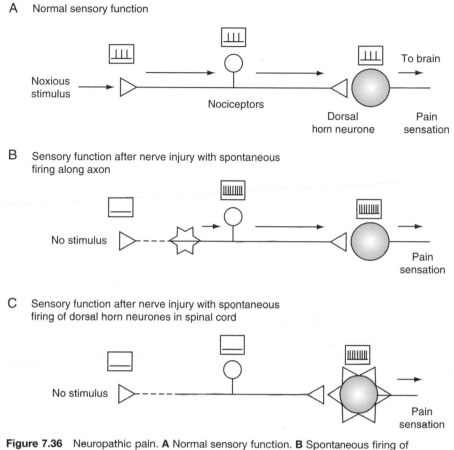

A Normal sensory function

B Sensory function after nerve injury with spontaneous firing along axon

C Sensory function after nerve injury with spontaneous firing of dorsal horn neurones in spinal cord

Figure 7.36 Neuropathic pain. **A** Normal sensory function. **B** Spontaneous firing of nociceptors along its length. **C** Spontaneous firing of dorsal horn cells. (After Woolf & Mannion 1999, with permission.)

Peripheral sensitization following tissue injury

In the normal asymptomatic and uninjured state, the nociceptive system is in a state of tonic inhibition (Stamford 1995). When tissue is damaged, there is activation of the nociceptor such that the threshold for response is lowered and there is an increased response to suprathreshold stimuli (Raja et al 1999). The clinical manifestation of this is known as primary hyperalgesia; this is a lowered pain threshold and an increased pain to suprathreshold mechanical stimuli (Raja et al 1999).

Evidence suggests that primary hyperalgesia following a mechanical injury is the result of spatial summation, reduced nociceptor inhibition by mechanoreceptor activity and chemical sensitiza-

tion of mechanical nociceptors (Box 7.1). A noxious mechanical stimulus has been found to cause A delta nociceptors (in the skin) to become spontaneously active, have a lower mechanical threshold and an expanded receptor field (Reeh et al 1987). In addition, subsequent stimuli cause a large number of nociceptors to be stimulated, producing spatial summation, and thus producing more pain (Raja et al 1999). An additional cause of

Box 7.1 Mechanisms of primary mechanical hyperalgesia

- Spatial summation
- Reduced inhibition of nociceptor activity
- Chemical sensitization of mechanical nociceptors

mechanical primary hyperalgesia may be due to a reduction in the activation of low-threshold mechanoreceptors in the area of injury (Raja et al 1999), which, in normal circumstances, inhibits pain (Bini et al 1984, Van Hees & Gybels 1981).

Injury to tissue initiates an inflammatory response, and the chemicals released into the tissues (bradykinin, histamine, serotonin, potassium, adenosine, protons, prostaglandins, leukotriences and cytokines) have been found to sensitize nociceptors (Davis et al 1993, Dray 1995, Martin et al 1987). Prostaglandins and bradykinins may also directly cause the nociceptor to fire repeatedly (Dray 1995). Peripheral sensitization may also be enhanced by tissue injury causing activation of normally silent nociceptors (Wright 1999). Silent or 'sleeping' nociceptors have been found in the skin (Handwerker 1996), joints (Schmidt 1996) and viscera (Gebhart 1996); it is not known whether they occur in the connective tissue surrounding nerve. Nociceptors are particularly sensitive to a lowered pH level, which commonly occurs with inflammation due to a raised proton level (Dray 1995). The combination of lowered pH level with inflammatory chemicals, producing an 'inflammatory soup', appears to have the most powerful effect on nociceptor sensitivity (Handwerker & Reeh 1991). Additionally, nociceptors release vasoactive neuropeptides, such as substance P, which causes vasodilation of the blood vessels and enhances the release of histamine from mast cells (Jessell & Kelly 1991), thus enhancing the inflammatory response. Therefore, primary hyperalgesia of mechanical nociceptors is thought to be due to spatial summation, reduced mechanoreceptor activity inhibiting nociceptor activity and chemical sensitization of mechanical nociceptors.

In addition, tissue damage also causes secondary hyperalgesia, where nearby uninjured tissue develops a lowered pain threshold, an increased pain to suprathreshold stimuli, and gives rise to spontaneous pain (Raja et al 1999). The stimulus in secondary hyperalgesia is mechanical, and two types have been identified: stroking hyperalgesia (pain is felt on light stroking) and punctate hyperalgesia (pain is felt with blunt pressure) (Raja et al 1999). The underlying mechanism of both stroking and punctate hyperalgesia is thought to be central sensitization, where the CNS pain pathways develop an enhanced responsiveness to stimuli (Raja et al 1999, Simone et al 1991). Stroking hyperalgesia is an enhanced responsiveness of central pain pathways to innocuous mechanoreceptor activity from large myelinated (A) afferent fibres (Torebjork et al 1992), and punctate hyperalgesia is an enhanced responsiveness to nociceptor input (Ali et al 1999) (Box 7.2).

Central sensitization following tissue injury

The sensory nerves running to the dorsal horn can be classified as A beta, A delta and C fibres. A beta fibres are large, myelinated fast-conducting axons transmitting non-noxious stimuli. Small, thinly myelinated A delta fibres and thin unmyelinated C fibres each transmit noxious mechanical and thermal stimuli (Doubell et al 1999). The afferents terminate in an organized way within the dorsal horn (Fig. 7.37), which is dependent on the threshold sensitivity and location of the afferent in the body. The A beta fibres terminate in laminar III, IV and V while high-threshold C and A delta nociceptors terminate in lamina I and II with some to lamina V (Doubell et al 1999).

The dorsal horn neurones can be classified as projecting neurones, propriospinal neurones or local interneurones. The projecting neurones transmit sensory information to the brain and are involved in the descending control systems from the brain to the spinal cord, which affect the sensitivity of the dorsal horn cells (Schaible et al 1991). Propriospinal neurones run a few segments up and down the spinal cord; their role in nociception is unclear (Doubell et al 1999). The majority are local interneurones, some of which are excitatory while others are inhibitory. They

---

Box 7.2 Mechanisms of secondary mechanical hyperalgesia

Central sensitization
(enhanced responsiveness of central pain pathways) to:
innocuous mechanoreceptor activity
nociceptor activity

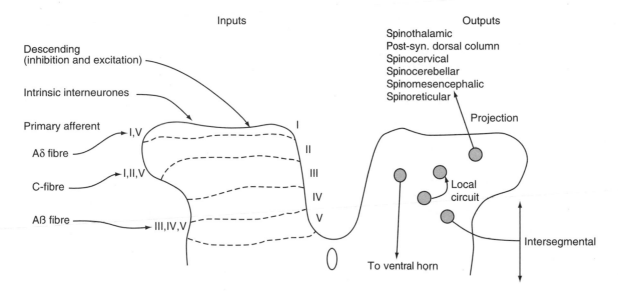

Figure 7.37 Schematic diagram of connections to and from the dorsal horn (after Doubell et al 1999, with permission).

maintain and define the receptive fields of dorsal horn neurones. The threshold of excitation of the dorsal horn cells depends on the collective input from sensory afferents and the descending control systems from the brain. If there is sufficient inhibition of the projecting neurones, when nociceptor activity is received at the spinal cord, then the threshold of the projecting neurone may be insufficient to relay nociception to the brain.

With tissue injury and peripheral sensitization, as described above, there is coactivation of spinal alpha-amino-3-hydroxyl-5-methyl-isoxazoleproprionic acid (AMPA) and metabotrophic glutamate receptors in the dorsal horn, which causes acute mechanical sensitization (Meller et al 1996). Central sensitization causes an increased excitability of wide-dynamic range cells in the dorsal horn (Woolf 1989), an increase in the size of the receptor field (Cook et al 1987) and changes in the somatic withdrawal reflexes (Woolf 1984). There is, overall, an increase in the excitability and synaptic efficacy of the dorsal horn cells, which may then affect other neurones with which they synapse (Wright 1999).

Usually the sympathetic nervous system does not communicate with afferent neurones (Janig et al 1996). However, following nerve injury, sym-

pathetic neurones can activate and sensitize primary afferents (Devor 1995, Janig et al 1996, Sato & Perl 1991). In the presence of tissue injury or inflammation, sympathetic nervous system activity can maintain the perception of pain or enhance nociception in inflamed tissue (Raja et al 1999). The nociceptors are activated by noradrenaline (norepinephrine) released by the sympathetic nervous system, which causes central sensitization. As a result of this the CNS pain pathways develop an enhanced responsiveness to innocuous mechanoreceptor activity (Raja et al 1999). Sympathetically maintained pain can occur with complex regional pain syndromes and may play a part in chronic arthritis and soft-tissue trauma (Raja et al 1999). Certainly, alterations in SNS function have been observed in patients with frozen shoulder or suspected epicondylitis (Mani et al 1989, Smith et al 1994, Thomas et al 1992).

Modulation of pain

Peripherally at the site of the tissue injury there is a natural analgesia that occurs with tissue injury and inflammation (Raja et al 1999). Inflammatory cells (lymphocytes, monocytes and macrophages, mast cells, plasma cells) have been found to contain opioid peptides (Przewlocki et al 1992, Stein et al 1990), and opioid receptors are present at afferent nerve endings (Coggeshall et al 1997, Stein et al 1990). The opioids released from the inflammatory cells activate the opioid receptors at afferent nerve endings (Stein et al 1990) and thus provide a natural analgesic effect in the tissues.

Within the central nervous system there is a descending control system that modulates nociceptive information to the brain; a useful review is provided by Stamford (1995). This system can inhibit or facilitate nociceptive transmission (Almeida et al 1996, Woolf & Slater 2000). This system may be activated by peripheral sensory input, producing counter-irritation, or by cortical input such as stress, suggestion, emotion and learned behaviour (Doubell et al 1999); thoughts, attention and motivation may also affect this system (Miron et al 1989, Zusman 2002).

The periaqueductal grey (PAG) region lies in the posterior thalamus in the mid-brain and is an important part of this descending control system (Fig 7.38). PAG receives input from various parts of the brain, including the frontal lobe, the amygdala and the hypothalamus, suggesting that it may have an ascending control of nociception (Fields & Basbaum 1999) and the dorsal horn of the spinal cord. Afferents project from PAG to the rostral ventromedial medulla (RVM which includes the nucleus raphe magnus and the reticular formation), the dorsolateral pontomesencephalic tegmentum (DLPT) and to the dorsal horn of the spinal cord, in particular from laminar I (Hylden et al 1986) where it thought to control the upward transmission of nociception (Fields 1988). The importance of PAG in pain modulation is highlighted by a study that found electrical stimulation of PAG to alleviate completely the severe pain in patients with cancer (Boivie & Meyerson 1982).

PAG has two distinct regions, the dorsolateral PAG (dPAG) and the ventrolateral PAG (vPAG).

dPAG

The dorsolateral PAG (dPAG) runs to the dorsolateral pons and ventrolateral medulla, which is

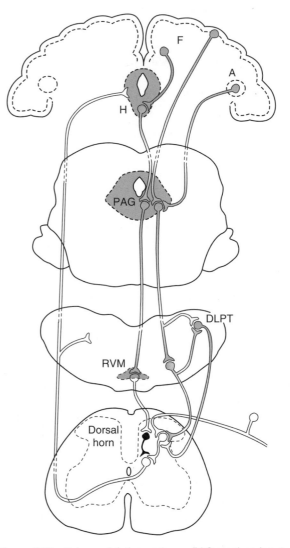

Figure 7.38 Pain-modulating pathway. PAG receives input from the frontal lobe (F), the amygdala (A) and the hypothalamus (H). Afferents from PAG travel to the rostral ventromedial medulla (RVM) and the dorsolateral pontomesencephalic tegmentum (DLPT) and on to the dorsal horn. The RVM has bidirectional control of nociceptive transmission. There are inhibitory (filled) and excitatory (unfilled) interneurones. (From Fields & Basbaum 1999, with permission.)

involved in autonomic control (Fields & Basbaum 1999). In the rat, stimulation of the dPAG causes analgesia, increased blood pressure, increased heart rate, vasodilation of the hind limb muscles and increased rate and depth of respiration, and coordinated hind limb, jaw and tail movements, suggesting increased activity of the sympathetic nervous system (SNS) and alpha motor neurones (Lovick 1991). The neurotransmitter from dPAG is noradrenaline (norepinephrine) and the analgesic effect appears to mediate morphine analgesia of mechanical nociceptor stimuli (Kuraishi et al 1983). In the dorsal horn of the spinal cord, dPAG causes inhibition of substance P from peripheral noxious mechanical stimulation (Kuraishi 1990).

vPAG

The ventrolateral PAG (vPAG) runs mainly to the nucleus raphe magnus. In the rat, stimulation of vPAG causes analgesia with decreased blood pressure, decreased heart rate, vasodilation of the hind limb muscles and reduced hind limb, jaw and tail movements, suggesting inhibition of the SNS and inhibition of alpha motor neurones (Lovick 1991). The neurotransmitter used in vPAG is serotonin and the analgesic effect appears to mediate morphine analgesia of thermal nociceptive stimuli (Kuraishi et al 1983). At the dorsal horn, vPAG inhibits the release of somatostatin, produced by peripheral noxious thermal stimulation (Kuraishi 1990). These mechanisms have been linked to the behaviour of an animal under threat, which initially acts with a sympathetic flight-or-fight response followed by recuperation (Fanselow 1991, Lovick 1991); this is summarized in Figure 7.39.

The rostral ventromedial medulla (RVM) receives a major input from PAG; electrical stimulation or injection of opioids into the RVM produces analgesia and inhibits nociceptors in the spinal cord (Fields et al 1991). This is the major pathway modulating pain (Fields & Basbaum 1999). The neurones from the RVM mostly terminate in laminae I, II and V and excite inhibitory interneurones and inhibit excitatory interneurones (Fields & Basbaum 1999). The DLPT receives input from lamina I and is connected to the RVM. Electrical stimulation of DLPT is also able to relieve pain in chronic pain patients (Young et al 1992).

Opiates are the most potent and reliable analgesic drug, the strongest being morphine (Fields 1988). The body produces its own (endogenous)

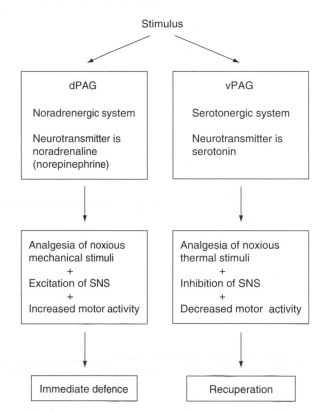

Figure 7.39 Descending inhibition of mechanical nociception from dPAG (noradrenergic system) and thermal nociception from vPAG (serotonergic system).

opioid peptides, (or 'endorphins'), which also have an analgesic effect, and these are found throughout the pain-modulating pathway, in the amygdala, hypothalamus, PAG, DLPT and RVM and superficial dorsal horn (Fields & Basbaum 1999). The chemical naloxene blocks the effect of endogenous opioids and has been used in research to investigate pain. Evidence to support the analgesic effect of endogenous opioids has come from the observation that administrating naloxene causes an increase in pain in postoperative pain patients (Levine et al 1987). Interestingly, endogenous opioids are thought to play a role in placebo analgesia (Fields & Basbaum 1999). Another transmitter considered important in pain modulation is serotonin (5HT) found in RVM neurones (Fields et al 1991, Mason & Gao 1998).

Inhibition of nociceptive transmission at the dorsal horn (Fields & Basbaum 1999) is thought to occur by:

- direct inhibition of the projection neurones
- inhibition of neurotransmitters from primary afferents produced by opioid release
- excitation of inhibitory interneurones. Stimulation of RVM stimulates some inhibitory interneurones in the dorsal horn that release inhibitory neurotransmitters, including GABA, glycine and enkephalin
- inhibition of excitatory interneurones. Opioids inhibit lamina II interneurones, which connect C fibres to lamina I projecting cells.

Activation of the descending control system

Noxious stimuli can cause activation of the descending control system (Fields & Basbaum 1999, Yaksh & Elde 1981), which can reduce or enhance nociceptive transmission. Noxious stimulation has been found to cause release of enkephalins at the supraspinal and spinal levels (Yaksh & Elde 1981). It has also been found that stimulation of the spinothalamic tract, transmitting nociceptive information from one foot, can be inhibited by noxious input from the contralateral foot, hand, face or trunk (Gerhart et al 1981). This may explain the relief of pain with acupuncture (where pain is induced) and pain behaviours such as 'biting your lip and banging your head against a wall'!(Melzack 1975).

The nucleus reticular dorsalis (NRD) has a direct link with the lamina I dorsal horn neurones; it can inhibit nociceptive transmission at the spinal cord, along with the PAG-RVM-dorsal horn pathway (Almeida et al 1996). The level of this inhibition will depend on a number of factors, including the location of the stimulus, the duration of the stimulus, the environment in which the stimulus is applied and the behavioural state (Watkins et al 1982). The nervous system is plastic, that is, it adapts, which underpins, for example, motor learning. Similarly, the nervous system will adapt to noxious input, or even a perceived threat, with learned responses (Sandkuhler 2000). In animals, it is possible to increase the activation of dorsal horn cells, which are known to transmit nociception, prior to the animal receiving a nociceptive stimulus (Duncan et al 1987). The animal learns to expect the nociceptive stimulus and this causes the neural change. This is not dissimilar to anticipatory muscle activity discussed in Chapter 5.

Functional imaging studies of the central nervous system are identifying the close relationship between areas controlling pain with areas controlling motor function, autonomic function and emotional state (Porro & Cavazzuti 1996). For example, the basal ganglia and PAG region receive nociceptive input as well as coordinating movement and motor control (Lovick 1991). Similarly, the limbic system and PAG receive nociceptive input as well as controlling autonomic function and emotional states (Chapman 1996, Hylden et al 1986, Lovick 1991). The motor centres are activated by noxious stimuli (Casey 1999), which is considered to be useful for movement to avoid the painful stimulation (Price 2000). Part of the forebrain, the anterior cingulated cortex (ACC), is considered to provide an overall sense of threat to the body from noxious input, involving integration of movement and postural planning alongside emotions and motivation (Price 2000). The ACC has been found to be sensitive to cognitive attention, that is, when humans focus on the pain this increases the perception of the pain in terms of intensity and unpleasantness (Miron et al 1989). This neurophysiological knowledge of brain function supports the definition of pain as 'an unpleasant sensory and emotional experience associated with actual or potential tissue damage, or described in terms of such damage' (Merskey et al 1979).

Nociceptive transmission can be facilitated by the descending control system to produce a more urgent, localized and rapid pain signal by inhibiting other neuronal activity (Woolf & Slater 2000). This mechanism would enhance the transmission of biologically useful pain information by removing irrelevant 'noise' from the system (Le Bars et al 1992).

Summary of nerve dysfunction

Nerve dysfunction has been broadly classified as altered nerve conduction, reduced nerve movement and symptom production. The next chapter discusses nerve treatment.

REFERENCES

Adams M A, Bogduk N, Burton K, Dolan P 2002 The biomechanics of back pain. Churchill Livingstone, Edinburgh

Ahles T A, Martin J B 1992 Cancer pain: a multidimensional perspective. In: Turk D C, Feldman C S (eds) Noninvasive approaches to pain management in the terminally ill. Haworth, New York, p 25–48

Ali Z, Ringkamp M, Hartke T V et al 1999 Uninjured C-fiber nociceptors develop spontaneous activity and alpha adrenergic sensitivity following L6 spinal nerve ligation in monkey. Journal of Neurophysiology 81:455–466

Almeida A, Tjolsen A, Lima D et al 1996 The medullary dorsal reticular nucleus facilitates acute nociception in the rat. Brain Research Bulletin 39(1):7–15

Bahns E, Ernsberger U, Janig W, Nelke A 1986 Discharge properties of mechanosensitive afferents supplying the retroperitoneal space. Pflügers Archiv 407:519–525

Bini G, Cruccu G, Hagbarth K-E et al 1984 Analgesic effect of vibration and cooling on pain induced by intraneural electrical stimulation. Pain 18:239–248

Bisby M A 1982 Functions of retrograde axonal transport. Federation Proceedings 41(7):2307–2311

Bogduk N 1997 Clinical anatomy of the lumbar spine and sacrum, 3rd edn. Churchill Livingstone, New York

Boivie J, Meyerson B A 1982 A correlative anatomical and clinical study of pain suppression by deep brain stimulation. Pain 13:113–126

Bove G M, Light A R 1995 Unmyelinated nociceptors of rat paraspinal tissues. Journal of Neurophysiology 73(5):1752–1762

Breig A 1978 Adverse mechanical tension in the central nervous system. Almqvist & Wiksell, Stockholm

Breig A, Marions O 1963 Biomechanics of the lumbosacral nerve roots. Acta Radiologica 1:1141–1160

Butler D S 1991 Mobilisation of the nervous system. Churchill Livingstone, Melbourne

Butler D S 2000 The sensitive nervous system. Noigroup, Adelaide

Casey K L 1999 Forebrain mechanisms of nociception and pain: analysis through imaging. Proceedings of the National Academy of Sciences of the USA 96:7668–7674

Chapman C R 1996 Limbic processes and the affective dimension of pain. In: Carli G, Zimmermann M (eds) Progress in Brain Research vol 110, Elsevier Science, Amsterdam, ch 5, p 63–81

Clark W L, Trumble T E, Swiontkowski M F, Tencer A F 1992 Nerve tension and blood flow in a rat model of immediate and delayed repairs. Journal of Hand Surgery 17A:677–687

Coggeshall R E, Zhou S, Carlton S M 1997 Opioid receptors on peripheral sensory axons. Brain Research 764:126–132

Cook A J, Woolf C J, Wall P D, McMahon S B 1987 Dynamic receptive field plasticity in rat spinal cord dorsal horn following C-primary afferent input. Nature 325(8):151–153

Cousins M, Power I 1999 Acute and postoperative pain. In: Wall P D, Melzack R (eds) Textbook of pain, 4th edn. Churchill Livingstone, Edinburgh, ch 19, p 447–491

Crow J L, Haas B M 2001 The neural control of human movement. In: Trew M, Everett T (eds) Human Movement, an introductory text, 4th edn. Churchill Livingstone, Edinburgh, ch 4, p 69

Dahlin L B, Kanje M 1992 Conditioning effect induced by chronic nerve compression. An experimental study of the sciatic and tibial nerves of rats. Scandinavian Journal of Plastic and Reconstructive Surgery and Hand Surgery 26:37–41

Dahlin L B, Lundborg G 1990 The neurone and its response to peripheral nerve compression. Journal of Hand Surgery 15B(1):5–10

Dahlin L B, McLean W G 1986 Effects of graded experimental compression on slow and fast axonal transport in rabbit vagus nerve. Journal of the Neurological Sciences 72:19–30

Dahlin L B, Thambert C 1993 Acute nerve compression at low pressures has a conditioning lesion effect on rat sciatic nerves. Acta Orthopaedica Scandinavica 64(4):479–481

Dahlin L B, Shyu B C, Danielsen N, Andersson S A 1989 Effects of nerve compression or ischaemia on conduction properties of myelinated and non-myelinated nerve fibres. An experimental study in the rabbit common peroneal nerve. Acta Physiologica Scandinavica 136: 97–105

Davis K D, Meyer R A, Campbell J N 1993 Chemosensitivity and sensitization of nociceptive afferents that innervate the hairy skin of monkey. Journal of Neurophysiology 69(4):1071–1081

Dellon A L 1978 The moving two-point discrimination test: clinical evaluation of the quickly-adapting fiber/receptor system. Journal of Hand Surgery 3:474–481

Dellon A L 1980 Clinical use of vibratory stimuli to evaluate peripheral nerve injury and compression neuropathy. Plastic and Reconstructive Surgery 65(4):466–476

Dellon A L 1981 Evaluation of sensibility and re-education of sensation in the hand. Williams and Wilkins, Baltimore

Descartes R 1985 Discourse on method and the meditations. Penguin, Middlesex, 6th meditation p 150–169

Devor M 1995 Peripheral and central mechanisms of sympathetic related pain. The Pain Clinic 8(1):5–14

Dilley A, Greening J, Lynn B, Leary R, Morris V 2001 The use of cross-correlation analysis between high-frequency ultrasound images to measure longitudinal median nerve movement. Ultrasound in Medicine and Biology 27(9):1211–1218

Doubell T P, Woolf C J 1997 Growth-associated protein 43 immunoreactivity in the superficial dorsal horn of the rat spinal cord is localized in atrophic C-fiber, and not in sprouted A-fiber, central terminals after peripheral nerve injury. Journal of Comparative Neurology 386:111–118

Doubell T P, Mannion R J, Woolf C J 1999 The dorsal horn: state-dependent sensory processing, plasticity and the generation of pain. In: Wall P D, Melzack R (eds) Textbook of pain, 4th edn. Churchill Livingstone, Edinburgh, ch 6, p 165–181

Dray A 1995 Inflammatory mediators of pain. British Journal of Anaesthetics 75:125–131

Duncan G H, Bushnell M C, Bates R, Dubner R 1987 Task-related responses of monkey medullary dorsal horn neurons. Journal of Neurophysiology 57(1):289–310

Dyck P J, Lais A C, Giannini C, Engelstad J K 1990 Structural alterations of nerve during cuff compression. Proceedings of the National Academy of Sciences of the USA 87:9828–9832

Epstein B S 1966 An anatomic, myelographic and cinemyelographic study of the dentate ligaments. American Journal of Roentgenography 98(3):704–712

Fanselow M S 1991 The midbrain periaqueductal gray as a coordinator of action in response to fear and anxiety. In: Depaulis A, Bandler R (eds) The midbrain periaqueductal gray matter. Plenum Press, New York, p 151–173

Fields H L 1988 Sources of variability in the sensation of pain. Pain 33:195–200

Fields H L, Basbaum A I 1999 Central nervous system mechanisms of pain modulation. In: Wall P D, Melzack R (eds) Textbook of pain, 4th edn. Churchill Livingstone, Edinburgh, ch 11, p 309–329

Fields H L, Heinricher M M, Mason P 1991 Neurotransmitters in nociceptive modulatory circuits. Annual Review of Neuroscience 14:219–245

Freeman M A R, Wyke B 1967 Articular reflexes at the ankle joint: an electromyographic study of normal and abnormal influences of ankle joint mechanoreceptors upon reflex activity in the leg muscles. British Journal of Surgery 54(12):990–1001

Fuchs P C, Nathan P A, Myers L D 1991 Synovial histology in carpal tunnel syndrome. Journal of Hand Surgery 16A(4):753–758

Gandevia S C, Hall L A, McCloskey D I, Potter E K 1983 Proprioceptive sensation at the terminal joint of the middle finger. Journal of Physiology (Lond) 335:507–517

Garell P C, McGillis S L B, Greenspan J D 1996 Mechanical response properties of nociceptors innervating feline hairy skin. Journal of Neurophysiology 75(3):1177–1189

Gebhart G F 1996 Visceral polymodal receptors. In: Kumazawa T, Kruger L, Mizumura K (eds) Progress in Brain Research, Elsevier, Amsterdam, 113, ch 6, p 101–112

Gelberman R H, Szabo R M, Williamson R V, Dimick M P 1983 Sensibility testing in peripheral-nerve compression syndromes, an experimental study in humans. Journal of Bone and Joint Surgery 65A(5):632–638

Gelberman R H, Yamaguchi K, Hollstien S B et al 1998 Changes in interstitial pressure and cross-sectional area of the cubital tunnel and of the ulnar nerve with flexion of the elbow, an experimental study in human cadavera. Journal of Bone and Joint Surgery 80A(4):492–501

Gerhart K D, Yezierski R P, Giesler G J, Willis W D 1981 Inhibitory receptive fields of primate spinothalamic tract cells. Journal of Neurophysiology 46(6):1309–1325

Gifford L 1998 Pain. In: Pitt-Brooke J, Reid H, Lockwood J, Kerr K (eds) Rehabilitation of movement, theoretical basis of clinical practice. W B Saunders, London, ch 5, p 196–232

Goddard M D, Reid J D 1965 Movements induced by straight leg raising in the lumbo-sacral roots, nerves and plexus, and in the intrapelvic section of the sciatic nerve. Journal of Neurology, Neurosurgery and Psychiatry 28:12–18

Goldberg J M, Lindblom U 1979 Standardised method of determining vibratory perception thresholds for diagnosis and screening in neurological investigation. Journal of Neurology, Neurosurgery and Psychiatry 42:793–803

Grafstein B, Forman D S 1980 Intracellular transport in neurons. Physiological Reviews 60(4):1167–1283

Greening J, Lynn B 1998 Vibration sense in the upper limb in patients with repetitive strain injury and a group of at-risk office workers. International Archives of Occupational and Environmental Health 71:29–34

Greening J, Smart S, Leary R et al 1999 Reduced movement of median nerve in carpal tunnel during wrist flexion in patients with non-specific arm pain. Lancet 354:217–218

Greening J, Lynn B, Leary R et al 2001 The use of ultrasound imaging to demonstrate reduced movement of the median nerve during wrist flexion in patients with non-specific arm pain. Journal of Hand Surgery 26B(5):401–406

Grieve G P 1994 Referred pain and other clinical features. In: Grieve's modern manual therapy, the vertebral column, 2nd edn. Boyling J D, Palastanga N (eds) Churchill Livingstone, Edinburgh, ch 19, p 271–292

Haftek J 1970 Stretch injury of peripheral nerve, acute effects of stretching on rabbit nerve. Journal of Bone and Joint Surgery 52B(2):354–365

Hamanaka I, Okutsu I, Shimizu K et al 1995 Evaluation of carpal canal pressure in carpal tunnel syndrome. Journal of Hand Surgery 20A(5):848–854

Handwerker H O 1996 Sixty years of C-fiber recordings from animal and human skin nerves: historical notes. In: Kumazawa T, Kruger L, Mizumura K (eds) Progress in Brain Research, Elsevier, Amsterdam, 113, ch 3, p 39–51

Handwerker H O, Reeh P W 1991 Pain and inflammation. In: Bond M R, Charlton J E, Woolf C J (eds) Pain research and clinical management. Proceedings of the VIth World Congress on Pain, Elsevier, Amsterdam, ch 7, p 59–70

Hough A, Moore A, Jones M 2000a Doppler ultrasound measurement of median nerve motion. International Federation of Orthopaedic Manipulative Therapists 7th Scientific Conference Proceedings Abstract 62, p 56

Hough A D, Moore A P, Jones M P 2000b Peripheral nerve motion measurement with spectral Doppler sonography: a reliability study. Journal of Hand Surgery 25B(6):585–589

Howe J F, Loeser J D, Calvin W H 1977 Mechanosensitivity of dorsal root ganglia and chronically injured axons: a physiological basis for the radicular pain of nerve root compression. Pain 3:25–41

Hromada J 1963 On the nerve supply of the connective tissue of some peripheral nervous system components. Acta Anatomica 55:343–351

Hylden J L K, Hayashi H, Dubner R, Bennett G J 1986 Physiology and morphology of the lamina I spinomesencephalic projection. Journal of Comparative Neurology 247:505–515

Indahl A, Kaigle A, Reikeras O, Holm S 1995 Electromyographic response of the porcine multifidus musculature after nerve stimulation. Spine 20(24):2652–2658

Indahl A, Kaigle A M, Reikeras O, Holm S 1997 Interaction between the porcine lumbar intervertebral disc, zygapophysial joints, and paraspinal muscles. Spine 22(24):2834–2840

Inman V T, Saunders J B 1942 The clinico-anatomical aspects of the lumbosacral region. Radiology 38:669–678

Inufusa A, An H S, Lim T-H et al 1996 Anatomic changes of the spinal canal and intervertebral foramen associated with flexion-extension movement. Spine 21(21):2412–2420

Janig W, Levine J D, Michaelis M 1996 Interactions of sympathetic and primary afferent neurons following nerve injury and tissue trauma. In: Kumazawa T, Kruger L, Mizumura K (eds) Progress in Brain Research, Elsevier, Amsterdam, 113, ch 10, p 161–184

Jessell T M, Kelly D D 1991 Pain and analgesia. In: Kandel E R, Schwartz J H, Jessell T M (eds) Principles of neural science, 3rd edn. Elsevier, New York, ch 27, p 385–399

Keir P J, Bach J M, Rempel D M 1998 Fingertip loading and carpal tunnel pressure: differences between a pinching and a pressing task. Journal of Orthopaedic Research 16(1):112–115

Kimura J 1983 Electrodiagnosis in diseases of nerve and muscle: principles and practice. F A Davies, Philadelphia, ch 5, p 83–104

Kuraishi Y 1990 Neuropeptide-mediated transmission of nociceptive information and its regulation. Novel mechanisms of analgesics. Yakugaku Zasshi 110(10):711–726

Kuraishi Y, Harada Y, Aratani S, Satoh M, Takagi H 1983 Separate involvement of the spinal noradrenergic and serotonergic systems in morphine analgesia: the differences in mechanical and thermal algesic tests. Brain Research 273:245–252

Le Bars D, Villanueva L, Bouhassira D, Willer J-C 1992 Diffuse noxious inhibitory controls (DNIC) in animals and in man. Pathological, Physiological and Experimental Therapy 4:55–65

Levin S, Pearsell G, Ruderman R J 1978 Von Frey's method of measuring pressure sensibility in the hand: an engineering analysis of the Weinstein-Semmes pressure aesthesiometer. Journal of Hand Surgery 3:211–216

Levine J D, Reichling D B 1999 Peripheral mechanisms of inflammatory pain. In: Wall P D, Melzack R (eds) Textbook of pain, 4th edn. Churchill Livingstone, Edinburgh

Levine J D, Gordon N C, Jones R T, Fields H L 1978 The narcotic antagonist naloxene enhances clinical pain. Nature 272:826–827

Lewis C S 1998 The problem of pain. Fount, HarperCollins

Louis R 1981 Vertebroradicular and vertebromedullar dynamics. Anatomica Clinica 3:1–11

Lovick T 1991 Interactions between descending pathways from the dorsal and ventrolateral periaqueductal gray matter in the rat. In: Depaulis A, Bandler R (eds) The midbrain periaqueductal gray matter. Plenum Press, New York, p 101–120

Lundborg G 1975 Structure and function of the intraneural microvessels as related to trauma, edema formation, and nerve function. Journal of Bone and Joint Surgery 57A:938–948

Lundborg G, Dahlin L B 1996 Anatomy, function, and pathophysiology of peripheral nerves and nerve compression. Hand Clinics 12(2):185–193

Lundborg G, Rydevik B 1973 Effects of stretching the tibial nerve of the rabbit. A preliminary study of the intraneural circulation and the barrier function of the perineurium. Journal of Bone and Joint Surgery 55B(2):390–401

Lundborg G, Gelbermann R H, Minteer-Convery M et al 1982 Median nerve compression in the carpal tunnel: functional response to experimentally induced controlled pressure. Journal of Hand Surgery 7(3):252–259

Lundborg G, Myers R, Powell H 1983 Nerve compression injury and increased endoneurial fluid pressure: a 'miniature compartment syndrome'. Journal of Neurology, Neurosurgery and Psychiatry 46:1119–1124

Lundborg G, Rydevik B, Manthorpe M et al 1987 Peripheral nerve: the physiology of injury and repair. In: Woo S L-Y, Buckwalter J A (eds) Injury and repair of the musculoskeletal soft tissues. American Academy of Orthopaedic Surgeons, Park Ridge, Illinois, ch 7, p 295–352

McCloskey D I, Macefield G, Gandevia S C, Burke D 1987 Sensing position and movements of the fingers. News in Physiological Science 2:226–230

Macefield G, Gandevia S C, Burke D 1990 Perceptual responses to microstimulation of single afferents innervating joints, muscles and skin of the human hand. Journal of Physiology (Lond) 429:113–129

McGuire D B 1995 The multiple dimensions of cancer pain: a framework for assessment and management. In: McGuire D B, Yarbro C H, Ferrell B R (eds) Cancer pain management, 2nd edn. Jones and Bartlett, Boston, ch 1, p 1–17

Mackinnon S E 1992 Double and multiple 'crush' syndromes, double and multiple entrapment neuropathies. Hand Clinics 8(2):369–390

MacNab I 1972 The mechanism of spondylogenic pain. In: Hirsch C, Zotterman Y (eds) Cervical pain. Pergamon Press, Oxford p 89–95

Magee D J 2002 Orthopaedic physical assessment, 4th edn. Saunders, Philadelphia

Mani R, Cooper C, Kidd B L et al 1989 Use of laser Doppler flowmetry and transcutaneous oxygen tension electrodes to assess local autonomic dysfunction in patients with frozen shoulder. Journal of the Royal Society of Medicine 82:536–538

Marieb E N 1995 Human anatomy and physiology, 3rd edn. Benjamin/Cummings, California

Martin H A, Basbaum A I, Kwiat G C et al 1987 Leukotriene and prostaglandin sensitization of cutaneous high-threshold C- and A-delta mechanononociceptors in the hairy skin of rate hindlimbs. Neuroscience 22(2):651–659

Martina I S J, van Koningsveld R, Schmitz P I M et al 1998 Measuring vibration threshold with a graduated tuning fork in normal aging and in patients with polyneuropathy. Journal of Neurology, Neurosurgery and Psychiatry 65:743–747

Mason P, Gao K 1998 Raphe magnus serotonergic neurons tonically modulate nociceptive transmission. Pain Forum 7(3):143–150

Meller S T, Dykstra C, Gebhart G F 1996 Acute mechanical hyperalgesia in the rat can be produced by coactivation of spinal ionotrophic AMPA and metabotrophic glutamate receptors, activation of phospholipase A_2 and generation of cyclooxygenase products. In: Carli G, Zimmermann M (eds) Progress in Brain Research vol 110. Elsevier Science, Amsterdam p 177–192

Melzack R 1975 Prolonged relief of pain by brief, intense transcutaneous somatic stimulation. Pain 1:357–373

Merskey R, Albe-Fessard D G, Bonica J J et al 1979 Pain terms: a list with definitions and notes on usage. Pain 6:249–252

Miron D, Duncan G H, Bushnell M C 1989 Effects of attention on the intensity and unpleasantness of thermal pain. Pain 39:345–352

Moberg E 1983 The role of cutaneous afferents in position sense, kinaesthesia, and motor function of the hand. Brain 106:1–19

Nakamichi K, Tachibana S 1995 Restricted motion of the median nerve in carpal tunnel syndrome. Journal of Hand Surgery 20B(4):460–464

Nemoto K, Matsumoto N, Tazaki K-i, Horiuchi Y, Uchinishi K-i, Mori Y 1987 An experimental study on the 'double crush' hypothesis. Journal of Hand Surgery 12A(4):552–559

Ochoa J, Fowler T J, Gilliatt R W 1972 Anatomical changes in peripheral nerves compressed by a pneumatic tourniquet. Journal of Anatomy 113(3):433–455

O'Connor B L, Palmoski M J, Brandt K D 1985 Neurogenic acceleration of degenerative joint lesions. Journal of Bone and Joint Surgery 67A(4):562–572

Ogata K, Naito M 1986 Blood flow of peripheral nerve effects of dissection, stretching and compression. Journal of Hand Surgery 11B(1):10–14

Oliver J, Middleditch A 1991 Functional anatomy of the spine. Butterworth-Heinemann, Oxford

Palastanga N, Field D, Soames R 2002 Anatomy and human movement – structure and function, 4th edn. Butterworth-Heinemann, Oxford

Panjabi M M 1992 The stabilizing system of the spine. Part 1. Function, dysfunction, adaptation, and enhancement. Journal of Spinal Disorders 5(4):383–389

Panjabi M M, White A A 2001 Biomechanics in the musculoskeletal system. Churchill Livingstone, New York

Petty N J, Moore A P 2001 Neuromusculoskeletal examination and assessment, a handbook for therapists, 2nd edn. Churchill Livingstone, Edinburgh

Porro C A, Cavazzuti M 1996 Functional imaging studies of the pain system in man and animals. In: Carli G, Zimmermann M (eds) Progress in Brain Research vol 110. Elsevier Science, Amsterdam, p 47–62

Powell H C, Myers R R 1986 Pathology of experimental nerve compression. Laboratory Investigation 55(1):91–100

Price D D 2000 Psychological and neural mechanisms of the affective dimension of pain. Science 288: 1769–1772

Przewlocki R, Hassan A H S, Lason W et al 1992 Gene expression and localization of opioid peptides in immune cells of inflamed tissue: functional role in antinociception. Neuroscience 48(2):491–500

Raja S N, Meyer R A, Ringkamp M, Campbell J N 1999 Peripheral neural mechanisms of nociception. In: Wall P D, Melzack R (eds) Textbook of pain, 4th edn. Churchill Livingstone, Edinburgh, ch 1, p 11–84

Reeh P W, Bayer J, Kocher L, Handwerker H O 1987 Sensitization of nociceptive cutaneous nerve fibers from the rat's tail by noxious mechanical stimulation. Experimental Brain Research 65:505–512

Rempel D, Dahlin L, Lundborg G 1999 Pathophysiology of nerve compression syndromes: response of peripheral nerves to loading. Journal of Bone and Joint Surgery 81A(11):1600–1610

Rojviroj S, Sirichativapee W, Kowsuvon W et al 1990 Pressures in the carpal tunnel, a comparison between patients with carpal tunnel syndrome and normal subjects. Journal of Bone and Joint Surgery 72B(3):516–518

Rydevik B, Lundborg G 1977 Permeability of intraneural microvessels and perineurium following acute, graded experimental nerve compression. Scandinavian Journal of Plastic and Reconstructive Surgery and Hand Surgery 11:179–187

Rydevik B, Lundborg G, Bagge U 1981 Effects of graded compression on intraneural blood flow. An in vivo study on rabbit tibial nerve. Journal of Hand Surgery 6:3–12

Rydevik B, Brown M D, Lundborg G 1984 Pathoanatomy and pathophysiology of nerve root compression. Spine 9(1):7–15

Rydevik B, Lundborg G, Skalak R 1989 Biomechanics of peripheral nerves. In: Nordin M, Frankel V H (eds) Basic biomechanics of the musculoskeletal system, 2nd edn. Lea & Febiger, Philadelphia, ch 4, p 75–87

Salonen V, Lehto M, Vaheri A, Aro H, Peltonen J 1985 Endoneurial fibrosis following nerve transection. Acta Neuropathologica 67:315–321

Sandkuhler J 2000 Learning and memory in pain pathways. Pain 88:113–118

Sato J, Perl E R 1991 Adrenergic excitation of cutaneous pain receptors induced by peripheral nerve injury. Science 251:1608–1610

Scadding J W 2003 Complex regional pain syndrome. In: Melzack R, Wall P D (eds) Handbook of pain management, a clinical companion to Wall and Melzack's textbook of pain. Churchill Livingstone, Edinburgh, ch 18, p 275–288

Schaible H-G, Neugebauer V, Cervero F, Schmidt R F 1991 Changes in tonic descending inhibition of spinal neurons with articular input during the development of acute arthritis in the cat. Journal of Neurophysiology 66(3):1021–1032

Schaumburg H H, Spencer P S, Ochoa J 1983 The aging human peripheral nervous system. In: Katzman R, Terry R (eds) The neurology of aging. F A Davies, Philadelphia, ch 5, p 111–122

Schmidt R F 1996 The articular polymodal nociceptor in health and disease. In: Kumazawa T, Kruger L, Mizumura K (eds) Progress in Brain Research. Elsevier, Amsterdam, 113, ch 4, p 53–81

Schwartz J H 1991 Synthesis and trafficking of neuronal proteins. In: Kandel E R, Schwartz J H, Jessell T M (eds) Principles of neural science, 3rd edn. Elsevier, New York, ch 4, p 49–65

Seradge H, Jia Y-C, Owens W 1995 In vivo measurement of carpal tunnel pressure in the functioning hand. Journal of Hand Surgery 20A:855–859

Simone D A, Sorkin L S, Oh U et al 1991 Neurogenic hyperalgesia: central neural correlates in responses of spinothalamic tract neurons. Journal of Neurophysiology 66(1):228–246

Smith R W, Papadopolous E, Mani R, Cawley M I D 1994 Abnormal microvascular responses in lateral epicondylitis. British Journal of Rheumatology 33:1166–1168

Smyth M J, Wright V 1958 Sciatica and the intervertebral disc, an experimental study. Journal of Bone and Joint Surgery 40A(6):1401–1418

Solomonow M, Zhou B-H, Harris M, Lu Y, Baratta R V 1998 The ligamento-muscular stabilizing system of the spine. Spine 23(23):2552–2562

Spindler H A, Dellon A L 1982 Nerve conduction studies and sensibility testing in carpal tunnel syndrome. Journal of Hand Surgery 7(3):260–263

Stamford J A 1995 Descending control of pain. British Journal of Anaesthesia 75:217–227

Starkweather R J, Neviaser R J, Adams J P, Parsons D B 1978 The effect of devascularization on the regeneration of lacerated peripheral nerves: an experimental study. Journal of Hand Surgery 3(2):163–167

Steen K H, Issberner U, Reeh P H 1995 Pain due to experimental acidosis in human skin: evidence for non-adapting nociceptor excitation. Neuroscience Letters 199:29–32

Stein C, Hassan A H S, Przewlocki R et al 1990 Opioids from immunocytes interact with receptors on sensory nerves to inhibit nociception in inflammation. Proceedings of the National Academy of Sciences of the USA 87:5935–5939

Stromberg T, Dahlin L B, Brun A, Lundborg G 1997 Structural nerve changes at wrist level in workers exposed to vibration. Occupational and Environmental Medicine 54:307–311

Sunderland S 1978 Nerves and nerve injuries, 2nd edn. Churchill Livingstone, Edinburgh, ch 2, p 39 and ch 53, p 680

Sunderland S 1990 The anatomy and physiology of nerve injury. Muscle and Nerve 13:771–784

Sunderland S, Bradley K C 1961 Stress-strain phenomena in human peripheral nerve trunks. Brain 84:102–119

Szabo R M, Gelberman R H, Williamson R V, Hargens A R 1983 Effects of increased systemic blood pressure on the tissue fluid pressure threshold of peripheral nerve. Journal of Orthopaedic Research 1(2):172–178

Tencer A F, Allen B L, Ferguson R L 1985 A biomechanical study of thoracolumbar spine fractures with bone in the canal, part III, mechanical properties of the dura and its tethering ligaments. Spine 10(8):741–747

Terenghi G 1995 Peripheral nerve injury and regeneration. Histology and Histopathology 10:709–718

Thomas D, Siahamis G, Marion M, Boyle C 1992 Computerised infrared thermography and isotopic bone scanning in tennis elbow. Annals of the Rheumatic Diseases 51:103–107

Torebjork H E, Lundberg L E R, LaMotte R H 1992 Central changes in processing of mechanoreceptive input in capsaicin-induced secondary hyperalgesia in humans. Journal of Physiology (London) 448:765–780

Turkof E, Jurecka W, Sikos G, Piza-Katzer H 1993 Sensory recovery in myocutaneous, noninnervated free flaps: a morphologic, immunohistochemical, and electron microscopic study. Plastic and Reconstructive Surgery 92:238–247

Upton A R M, McComas A J 1973 The double crush in nerve-entrapment syndromes. Lancet ii:359–362

Van Hees J, Gybels J 1981 C nociceptor activity in human nerve during painful and non painful skin stimulation. Journal of Neurology, Neurosurgery and Psychiatry 44:600–607

Vilensky J A, O'Connor B L, Brandt K D et al 1997 Serial kinematic analysis of the canine hindlimb joints after deafferentation and anterior cruciate ligament transection. Osteoarthritis and Cartilage 5:173–182

von Piekartz H & Bryden L 2001 Craniofacial dysfunction and pain: manual therapy, assessment and management. Butterworth-Heinemann, Oxford

Wall P D, Melzack R 1999 Textbook of pain, 4th edn. Churchill Livingstone, Edinburgh

Wall E J, Massie J B, Kwan M K et al 1992 Experimental stretch neuropathy. Changes in nerve conduction under tension. Journal of Bone and Joint Surgery 74B(1):126–129

Watkins L R, Cobelli D A, Mayer D J 1982 Classical conditioning of front paw and hind paw footshock induced analgesia (FSIA): naloxene reversibility and descending pathways. Brain Research 243:119–132

Williams P L, Warwick R 1980 Gray's Anatomy, 36th edn. Churchill Livingstone, Edinburgh

Williams P L, Bannister L H, Berry M M et al 1995 Gray's anatomy, 38th edn. Churchill Livingstone, New York

Woolf C J 1984 Long term alterations in the excitability of the flexion reflex produced by peripheral tissue injury in the chronic decerebrate rat. Pain 18:325–343

Woolf C J 1989 Recent advances in the pathophysiology of acute pain. British Journal of Anaesthetics 63:139–146

Woolf C J, Mannion R J 1999 Neuropathic pain: aetiology, symptoms, mechanisms, and management. Lancet 353:1959–1964

Woolf C J, Slater M W 2000 Neuronal plasticity: increasing the gain in pain. Science 288:1765–1768

Woolf C J, Shortland P, Coggeshall R E 1992 Peripheral nerve injury triggers central sprouting of myelinated afferents. Nature 355(2):75–77

Wright A 1999 Recent concepts in the neurophysiology of pain. Manual Therapy 4(4):196–202

Wright T W, Glowczewskie F, Wheeler D et al 1996 Excursion and strain of the median nerve. Journal of Bone and Joint Surgery 78A(12):1897–1903

Yaksh T L, Elde R P 1981 Factors governing release of methionine enkephalin-like immunoreactivity from mesencephalon and spinal cord of the cat in vivo. Journal of Neurophysiology 46(5):1056–1075

Young R F, Tronnier V, Rinaldi P C 1992 Chronic stimulation of the Kolliker-Fuse nucleus region for relief of intractable pain in humans. Journal of Neurosurgery 76:979–985

Zoech G, Reihsner R, Beer R, Millesi H 1991 Stress and strain in peripheral nerves. Neuro-Orthopaedics 10:73–82

Zusman M 2002 Forebrain-mediated sensitization of central pain pathways: 'non-specific' pain and a new image for MT. Manual Therapy 7(2):80–88

8

Principles of nerve treatment

There is no pure treatment for nerves, that is, treatment cannot be isolated to nerve alone, it will always, to a greater or lesser extent, affect joint and/or muscle tissues. Some sort of classification system for treatment is needed in order to have meaningful communication among and between clinicians, and this text follows the traditional classification of nerve, joint and muscle treatment. In this text a 'nerve treatment' is defined as a 'treatment to effect a change in nerve'; that is, the intention of the clinician is to produce a change in nerve and therefore it is described as a nerve treatment. Similarly, where a technique is used to effect a change in a joint, it will be referred to as a 'joint treatment' and where a technique is used to effect a change in muscle, it will be referred to as a 'muscle treatment'. Thus, techniques are classified according to which tissue the clinician is predominantly attempting to affect. This relationship of treatment of nerve, joint and muscle is depicted in Figure 8.1.

An example may help to illustrate the impurity of a nerve treatment technique. With the subject in supine, the clinician takes the hip into flexion, with the knee extended, and applies an oscillatory dorsiflexion movement to the ankle, with a view to mobilizing the posterior tibial nerve/sciatic nerve. Further analysis of this movement reveals that this technique is not purely a nerve treatment: it also involves joints and muscles. There will be a sustained lengthening of the hip extensor and knee flexors. The oscillatory movement into dorsiflexion will cause talocrural dorsiflexion, which will cause

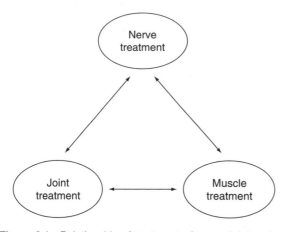

Figure 8.1 Relationship of treatment of nerve, joint and muscle.

movement at the inferior and superior tibiofibular joints. The movement will also cause oscillatory lengthening of the ankle plantarflexor muscles. It can readily be seen that this simple straight leg raise technique (SLR), which might be described as a neurodynamic (i.e. movement of nerve) treatment, also affects joint and muscle tissues. For this reason the technique could be used to effect a change in joint and/or muscle. The therapeutic affect of the SLR technique is likely to be a combined effect on nerve, joint and muscle.

There is a variety of nerve treatments. Treatments are categorized in this text from the dysfunctions identified in the previous chapter, namely, altered nerve conduction, reduced nerve

movement and production of symptoms (Table 8.1). From this, a classification of nerve treatment can be identified: to alter nerve conduction, increase nerve movement and reduce symptoms. The reader is reminded that there is a number of precautions and contraindications to nerve mobilization treatments and these are given in Chapter 2 on assessment. A variety of techniques for addressing each of these treatments is also given in Table 8.1. For further information on treatment of nervous tissue the reader is referred to Butler (2000).

The aims of nerve treatment can be broadly classified as:

- to alter nerve conduction
- to increase nerve range of movement
- to reduce symptoms.

TO ALTER NERVE CONDUCTION

Altered nerve conduction will be manifested by an alteration in sensation, isometric muscle strength and reflex changes. Treatment will depend on the degree of altered nerve conduction. Where there appears to be severe or complete disruption, for example carpal tunnel syndrome, a steroid injection into the carpal tunnel or a surgical decompression may be required.

Commonly seen are symptoms suggesting mild disruption of nerve conduction. Treatment will often be indirect, that is, treatment will be directed at the tissues causing the alteration in nerve con-

Table 8.1 Nerve dysfunction: aim of nerve treatment and treatment techniques

Nerve dysfunction	Aim of nerve treatment	Nerve treatment technique
Altered nerve conduction	Alter nerve conduction	Joint, muscle or nerve treatment techniques to affect the suspected interface tissue responsible for altered nerve conduction
		Electrotherapy
Reduced nerve movement	Increase length	Passive or active lengthening of nerve
		Soft-tissue mobilizations
		PNF
	Increase movement with interface tissue	Joint mobilizations
		Soft-tissue mobilizations
Production of symptoms	Reduce symptoms	Joint, muscle or nerve treatment techniques to affect nerve tissue
		Soft-tissue mobilizations
		Electrotherapy

duction. For example, a patient may have signs of L5 nerve root compression, comprising pain in the lumbar spine with posterolateral calf pain, reduced sensation to fine touch over the posterolateral calf, together with weakness of the big toe extensors. The SLR test position of hip flexion, knee extension and foot dorsiflexion may be limited to 45 degrees hip flexion, reproducing the patient's pain, with the pain increased on cervical flexion, giving a positive SLR. In addition, there may be positive findings on passive accessory movements of the lumbar spine; for example, the patient's back and calf pain may be reproduced with a unilateral posteroanterior pressure on L5 with a caudad inclination. A neurodynamic treatment could be used for this patient, or passive accessory movements to the lumbar spine could be used to treat this patient. It might be speculated that the pain is emanating from the nerve root as it exits the intervertebral foramen at L5/S1 level and so the accessory movement is being used as a neurodynamic interface treatment. Alternatively, a neurodynamic lengthening movement to the restricted SLR could be used, with hold–relax for example, if it is felt that muscle is limiting the movement. Finally, a simple oscillatory movement to a component of the SLR test movement could be used to affect the nerve. Whichever technique is selected, treatment may alter the neurological integrity signs of altered sensation and reduced muscle strength. The neurological integrity signs will be reassessed following treatment to determine the ability of the chosen technique to effect a change. In this way, the neurological integrity signs are not treated directly but may be affected indirectly by affecting tissues around the nerve.

Another example may be treatment of a patient whose symptoms suggest a mild carpal tunnel syndrome. Treatment may be aimed at increasing the space within the carpal tunnel to reduce the compression on the median nerve. For example, joint accessory movements may be applied to the carpal bones (Tal-Akabi & Rushton 2000). Interestingly, 1 minute of wrist and finger flexion and extension at a rate of 30 cycles per minute has been found to reduce carpal tunnel pressure for up to 15 minutes (Seradge et al

1995). If this effect occurred in a patient group it could reduce symptoms.

In the case of a Bell's palsy, with paralysis of the muscles supplied by the facial nerve, the clinician may apply massage over the muscles, use electrotherapy and encourage the patient to exercise the facial muscles in front of a mirror. In this case, with a primary nerve problem, treatment addresses the tissue to be re-innervated in an attempt to facilitate recovery. A similar management occurs for peripheral nerve injuries.

TO INCREASE NERVE RANGE OF MOVEMENT

Examination of neurodynamic tests may suggest that there is a reduced range of nerve movement. These examination procedures have been described in the companion text (Petty & Moore 2001) and can readily be converted to a treatment technique by choosing a particular dose given below.

It may be worth clarifying the variety of terminology that can be used with nerve movement. For the purposes of this text, the following terms can be considered synonymous: adverse mechanical tension tests or treatment = neurodynamic tests or treatment = pain provocation tests or treatment. For the upper limb: upper limb tension tests or treatment = brachial plexus tension tests or treatment = neural tissue provocation tests or treatment.

Nervous tissue can be lengthened passively by the clinician, or by the patient.

Passive lengthening by the clinician

A passive stretch can be performed in much the same way as a passive stretch to a joint or a muscle, that is, the clinician applies a static or oscillatory force to lengthen the nerve. The dose of passive stretch incorporates a number of factors, and is outlined in Table 8.2.

Position

This includes the general position of the patient, such as lying, sitting or standing, and the specific

Table 8.2 Treatment dose for passive lengthening by the clinician and active lengthening by the patient

Factors	Passive stretching by the clinician	Active stretching by the patient
Patient's position	e.g. supine	e.g. sitting, standing with heel of foot on a stool with knee extended
Direction of movement	e.g. hip flexion	e.g. active knee extension
Magnitude of force applied	Related to therapist's perception of resistance: grades I to V	Related to patient's perception of stretch
Amplitude of oscillation	Static or small or large	Static or small or large
Speed	Slow or fast	Slow or fast (if fast may be referred to as ballistic)
Rhythm	Smooth or staccato	Smooth or staccato
Time	Of repetitions and number of repetitions	Of repetitions and number of repetitions
Temperature	Room temperature or heat with short-wave diathermy	Room temperature
Symptom response	Short of symptom production	Short of symptom production
	Point of onset or increase in resting symptom	Point of onset or increase in resting symptom
	Partial reproduction of symptom	Partial reproduction of symptom
	Full reproduction of symptom	Full reproduction of symptom

position of the body part – for example, the hip may be placed in medial rotation and then flexed. The nervous system is one whole organ from the head to the toes and to the hands, and so the clinician needs to consider carefully the positioning of the whole body. The choice of general and specific positioning will depend on a number of factors:

- the comfort and support of the patient
- the comfort of the clinician applying the technique
- accurate application of the technique
- the desired effect of the treatment
- whether weight-bearing or non-weight-bearing is desired
- to what extent the movement is to be functional
- to what extent symptoms are to be produced.

Direction of movement

The predominant direction of movement can be broadly divided into longitudinal movement and transverse movement. An example of a predominantly longitudinal movement would be foot plantarflexion/dorsiflexion movement to effect a change in the common peroneal nerve, where the movement of plantarflexion will lengthen and dorsiflexion will shorten the nerve. An example of a transverse movement would be

a force applied across the nerve, for example, a posteroanterior glide of the superior tibiofibular joint to effect a change in the common peroneal nerve. The transverse movement, in this case, is applied to a joint and is therefore an indirect method of affecting nerve tissue. Because of this, it is commonly referred to as an interface treatment. Soft-tissue mobilizations, described below, may apply forces to adjacent muscle in order to have an effect on nervous tissue; again, this would be described as an interface treatment.

Peripheral nerves follow an elaborate and variable pathway through the tissues of the body and therefore the clinician needs to explore nerve length fully in both examination and treatment. For example, the classical SLR test of hip flexion, adduction and medial rotation may need to be altered by using lateral rotation instead of medial rotation. The textbook descriptions of neurodynamic tests, for example Petty & Moore (2001) and Butler (2000), are useful as a guideline that then needs to be adapted for each individual patient.

Magnitude of force

The force applied by the clinician may be described using grades of movement (Magarey 1985, 1986, Maitland et al 2001) in the same way as joint mobilizations. As a nerve is passively lengthened, resistance to movement will be felt by the clinician and this can be depicted on a movement diagram (Petty & Moore 2001). With physiological movements that lengthen nerve there is often minimal resistance early in the range of movement. For example, during the SLR, hip flexion will have little resistance in the early part of the range and the clinician may mark the onset of resistance (R_1) somewhere towards the end of the movement (Fig. 8.2). Grades of movement are then defined according to the resistance curve. The grades of movement as defined in this text are shown in Table 8.3; they are modified from Maitland et al (2001) and Magarey (1985, 1986). The modification allows every possible position in range to be described (cf. Magarey 1985, 1986), and each grade to be distinct from one another (cf. Maitland et al 2001). The choice of magnitude of force, like every other factor of treatment dose, depends on what the clinician is attempting to achieve.

Amplitude of oscillation

The movement can be a sustained or oscillatory force. If the force is oscillated it is described as having a small or large amplitude, which is relative to the available range of any movement. The amplitude of oscillatory movement is described

Table 8.3 Grades of movement

Grade	Definition
I	Small-amplitude movement short of resistance
II	Large-amplitude movement short of resistance
III–	Large-amplitude movement in the first third of resistance
IV–	Small-amplitude movement in the first third of resistance
III	Large-amplitude movement in the middle third of resistance
IV	Small-amplitude movement in the middle third of resistance
III+	Large-amplitude movement in the last third of resistance
IV+	Small-amplitude movement in the last third of resistance

within the definition of grades of movement: grades I and IV are small-amplitude movements and grades II and III are large-amplitude movements. It is impossible for a truly sustained force to be applied to the tissues as there will always be some variation in the force, albeit very small. For this reason it is sometimes referred to in research articles as a quasistatic force; however, for the purposes of clinical practice the term static is used. Where a clinician applies a sustained force, the written clinical notes may use grades I, IV–, IV or IV+ with the word 'sustained' written prior to the grade; for example, treatment notes would read 'sustained grade IV–'. In this case the grade of movement is used only to denote where in resistance the force is applied. Alternatively, the clinician may write in words where in range they applied a sustained force. What is important, however, is not the choice of notation but the full description of the treatment dose.

It can be seen that, with an oscillatory force, grades of movement describe the magnitude of the force and the amplitude of oscillation. The choice of grade of movement is determined by the relationship of pain (or other symptom) and resistance through the range of movement. Where resistance limits the range of movement and there is minimal pain, a grade III+ or IV+ might be appropriate (Fig. 8.3A). Where pain

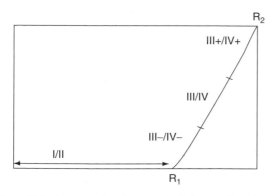

Figure 8.2 A movement diagram depicting grades of movement for straight leg raise (hip flexion, adduction and medial rotation, with knee extension). The onset of resistance (R_1) may be felt by the clinician somewhere towards the end of the movement, with R_2 depicting the end of range.

limits the range of movement and there is minimal resistance, a grade I or II may be appropriate (Fig. 8.3B), so that no pain is produced. A grade III– or IV– may be chosen if the pain is not severe and not irritable and there is no caution related to the nature of the disorder. Where resistance limits the movement, and there is a significant amount of pain, or where pain limits the movement and there is a significant amount of resistance, the choice of grade will depend on the degree to which symptoms can be provoked (Fig. 8.3C and D). For example, in Figure 8.3C, if a grade IV is chosen at about 50% of resistance, this would provoke an intensity of pain for the patient of about 3 out of 10 (where A is 0 and C is 10). If a grade IV is chosen for 8.3D, this would provoke about 4 out of 10, which may or may not be acceptable to the patient.

Speed and rhythm of movement

The speed of the movement can be described as slow or fast, and the rhythm as smooth or staccato (jerky); of course, these terms will apply only to oscillatory forces. Speed and rhythm go hand in hand: movements will tend to be slow and smooth, fast and smooth, or fast and staccato; it would be difficult to apply a slow staccato movement. The connective tissue in nerve is viscoelastic and is therefore sensitive to the speed of the applied force (Sunderland & Bradley 1961). A force applied quickly will produce less movement, provoking a greater stiffness; that is, the gradient of the resistance curve will be steep; on the other hand, a force applied more slowly will cause more movement as the stiffness is relatively less. If the intention of treatment is to maximize range of movement by lengthening

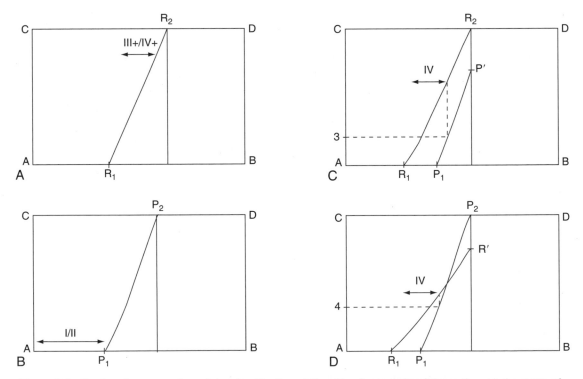

Figure 8.3 Grades of movement are determined by the relationship of pain and resistance through the range of movement; this is depicted on a movement diagram. **A** Resistance limiting movement. **B** Pain limiting movement. **C** Resistance limiting movement with a significant amount of pain. **D** Pain limiting movement with a significant amount of resistance.

connective tissue then a slow speed would seem preferable.

Time

In terms of treatment dose, time relates to the amount of time the nervous tissue is placed on a stretch, the number of times this is repeated, and the frequency of the appointments.

Temperature

Temperature influences the mechanical behaviour of connective tissue under tensile load. As temperature rises to about 40–45° C, stiffness decreases and extensibility increases (Rigby 1964). Increasing the temperature of a nerve will depend on its depth: it will obviously be easier to heat more superficial nerves.

Short-wave diathermy and ultrasound have been found to increase muscle and tendon temperature (Lehmann et al 1966, Millard 1961). The temperature of nerve has not been investigated, but it seems reasonable to assume that nerve temperature will follow a course similar to that of muscle temperature. Twenty minutes of short-wave diathermy has been shown to raise muscle temperature by as much as 4° C (Millard 1961). If normal muscle temperature is assumed to be the same as normal body temperature, 37° C, then this would raise the temperature of muscle to 41° C, sufficient to enhance the effect of stretching. Ultrasound at a frequency of 1 MHz with a 12.5 cm^2 head at an intensity of 1 w/cm^2 for 7 minutes caused the muscle temperature (3.5 cm below the surface of the skin) to rise to 40° C (Lehmann et al 1966). If the temperature of nerve connective tissue follows that of muscle then heating with short-wave diathermy or ultrasound may enhance the effect of lengthening nerve.

Symptom response

The clinician decides which, and to what extent, each symptom is to be provoked during treatment. Choices include:

- no provocation
- provocation to the point of onset, or increase in resting symptoms
- partial reproduction
- total reproduction.

The decision as to what extent symptoms are provoked during treatment depends on the severity and irritability of the symptom(s) and the nature of the condition. If the symptoms are severe, that is, the patient is unable to tolerate the symptom being produced, the clinician would choose not to provoke the symptoms. The clinician may also choose not to provoke symptoms if they are irritable, that is, once symptoms are provoked they take some time to ease. If, however, the symptoms are not severe and not irritable, then the clinician is able to reproduce the patient's symptoms during treatment, and the extent to which symptoms are reproduced will depend on the tolerance of the patient. The nature of the condition may limit the extent to which symptoms are produced, such as a recent traumatic injury.

Treatment is progressed or regressed by altering appropriate aspects of the treatment dose: the patient's position, movement, direction of force, magnitude of force, amplitude of oscillation, speed, rhythm, time, temperature or symptom response. Progression and regression of each aspect of the treatment dose can be used (Table 8.4).

It is suggested that inexperienced clinicians alter only one aspect of treatment dose at an attendance so that they fully understand the value of the alteration; in this way they will quickly develop valuable clinical experience and clinical mileage, which will contribute to growth in their clinical learning skills. The immediate and more long-term effect of the alteration can then be evaluated by reassessment of the subjective and physical asterisks. Table 8.5 provides an example of how a treatment dose may be progressed and regressed. It can be seen in the last example that both speed and rhythm have been altered; these two factors are very closely linked and can be considered separately or together. Other aspects of treatment dose that are closely

Table 8.4 Progression and regression of treatment dose

Treatment dose	Progression	Regression
Position	Joint towards end of available range	Joint towards beginning of available range
Direction of force	More provocative	Less provocative
Magnitude of force	Increase	Decrease
Amplitude of oscillation	Decreased	Increased
Rhythm	Staccato	Smoother
Time	Longer	Shorter
Speed	Slower or faster	Slower
Symptom response	Allowing more symptoms to be provoked	Allowing fewer symptoms to be provoked

Table 8.5 Examples of how a neurodynamic treatment dose can be progressed and regressed

Regression	Dose	Progression	Explanation
In cervical extension: did central PA C4 IV ×3 (1 min) slowly & smoothly to partial reproduction of patient's neck pain	In cervical neutral did: central PA C4 IV ×3 (1 min) slowly & smoothly to partial reproduction of patient's neck pain	In cervical flexion did: central PA C4 IV ×3 (1 min) slowly & smoothly to partial reproduction of patient's neck pain	The starting position has been altered. It might be assumed that extension is a position of ease and flexion a more provocative position
In 90 degrees knee flexion did: medial glide tibiofemoral joint I ×3 (1 min) slowly & smoothly short of P1	In 90 degrees knee flexion did: medial glide tibiofemoral joint II slowly & smoothly ×3 (1 min) short of P1	In 90 degrees knee flexion did: medial glide tibiofemoral joint III− ×3 (1 min) slowly & smoothly short of P1	The grade of movement has been altered
Physiological plantarflexion III ×3 (1 min) slowly & smoothly to full reproduction of ankle pain	Physiological plantarflexion III+ ×3 (1 min) slowly & smoothly to full reproduction of ankle pain	Physiological plantarflexion III+ ×3 (1 min) fast & staccato to full reproduction of ankle pain	Grade has been altered as a regression Speed and rhythm have been altered as a progression

linked are the length of time for each repetition and the number of repetitions; these, together, provide a dose of time and so can be considered separately or together.

Passive nerve lengthening by the patient

The patient can actively lengthen a nerve. The factors defining the treatment dose are exactly the same as the clinician passively lengthening a nerve (Table 8.2). The only difference is that, with passive lengthening by the patient, the patient is in total control of the movement and relies on their own perception of stretch and symptom production to determine the way the movement is carried out. The patient needs to be fully informed as to how to carry out the movement, that is, how forceful to be and to what extent they

should reproduce the symptoms. The clinician in this case takes on a more educational and advisory role.

An analysis of each neurodynamic test is provided below to offer a biomechanical basis for the use of these tests as treatment techniques.

The underlying effect of lengthening nerve

The effect of certain movements on nerve length and tension is largely a matter of logical deduction, based on the position of a nerve relative to the axis of the movement. If a nerve lies anterior to the axis of movement and the movement reduces the angle between the bones then it seems reasonable to suggest that the nerve will be slackened and tension will be reduced; if the movement increases the angle between the bones, then the nerve will be lengthened and the tension will be increased. Having said this, there are variations in the pathway of nerves between individuals (e.g. Adkison et al 1991), and the presence of pathology may further alter the response of tests and treatment (Butler 1991). For this reason, the clinician is wise to be cautious in assigning treatment to a particular nerve, or root level, and may often need to examine and treat patients in non-standard positions.

While it is known that lengthening a nerve beyond 15% (Clark et al 1992) of its resting length results in nerve pathology, it is difficult to assess what percentage change in length is occurring during neurodynamic examination and treatment. It is conceivable that a change in nerve conduction would occur if lengthening of greater than 15% occurred during the technique. This does not seem to occur in asymptomatic individuals (Ridehalgh et al 2004). Vibration threshold testing was performed on 30 asymptomatic subjects before, during, and after a three-repetition, 30-second treatment of straight leg raise with plantar flexion and inversion. Significant differences ($P<0.05$) were not found between readings, suggesting that conduction of the large-diameter afferents (the first to show signs of minor nerve injury) was not altered; therefore, it seems unlikely that such detrimental changes in length occur during neurodynamic assessment and treatment.

There is not necessarily a direct relationship between length and tension; the degree to which lengthening increases tension, or shortening reduces tension, will depend on the ability of the nerve to move. If, for example, a nerve is fixed at one end, and is then pulled, there will be an increase in length with a gradual build up in tension. If, on the other hand, a nerve is not fixed at either end, and a longitudinal pull is applied, the whole nerve may be free to move, relative to adjacent tissues, and until there is some resistance to this movement tension within the nerve may not rise appreciably. This freedom of nerve to move relative to adjacent tissues is thought to be greater where a nerve is passing through tissues, and is least where nerve branches or where it pierces muscle or runs around a bone (Sunderland 1978).

The following provides a useful anatomical and biomechanical basis of neurodynamic tests and treatment – but that is all it is: it does not necessarily explain the response of a test or treatment of a particular patient. The clinician applies this knowledge to patients and, using the concept of the permeable brick wall (Maitland et al 2001), believes the response of the patient, regardless of whether or not it fits with anatomical or biomechanical knowledge of nerve movement. In this way, the clinician is free to explore movement fully and to treat any movement dysfunction that the patient may present with.

Passive neck flexion

Cervical flexion has been found to:

- reduce the length of the cervical region of the sympathetic trunk
- lengthen the spinal canal and neuroaxis in the cervical region (Reid 1960, Tencer et al 1985)
- increase the tension in the neuroaxis in the cervical region (Reid 1960, Tencer et al 1985)
- increase tension of the dural sac (Reid 1960, Tencer et al 1985)
- move and tension the lumbosacral nerve roots (Breig 1978, Breig & Marions 1963).

Neurodynamic testing of the mandibular nerve involves upper cervical flexion and lateral flexion, with the addition of depression and contralateral deviation of the mandible for the lingual and mental nerves, and transverse movement of the mandible for the buccal and auriculotemporal nerves (von Piekartz & Bryden 2001). Neurodynamic testing of the facial nerve involves upper cervical flexion and lateral flexion, with ipsilateral rotation (von Piekartz & Bryden 2001). Further details are given elsewhere (von Piekartz & Bryden 2001).

Straight leg raise

The movement of hip flexion with knee extension, with variable amounts of hip adduction and medial rotation, will lengthen and tension the sciatic nerve, the CNS neuroaxis as far as the brain, the upper limb nervous system, and the sympathetic trunk (Breig 1978, Butler 1991). During SLR the L5–S1 nerve roots have been found to move distally between 0 and 5 mm, and the sciatic nerve at the exit from the pelvis between 3 and 10 mm (Goddard & Reid 1965, Smith et al 1993). The nerve roots are lengthened about 2–4% from neutral to 60 degrees SLR (Smith et al 1993). Movement of the sciatic nerve has been found to occur immediately the foot is lifted up from the horizontal position, with little movement after 70 degrees hip flexion (Goddard & Reid 1965). Moving the knee from flexion to extension is thought to cause the nervous system, distal to the knee, to move in a cephalad direction, and the nervous tissue proximal to the knee to move in a caudad direction (Fig. 8.4). Behind the knee there is little movement, and this is considered to be a 'tension point'. Foot dorsiflexion, eversion and a combination of dorsiflexion and

eversion have been found to increase the tension of the posterior tibial nerve (Daniels et al 1998).

The addition of medial rotation has been found to cause the sacral plexus to move 0–1 cm towards the greater sciatic foramen and to increase its tension (Breig & Troup 1979).

Passive knee bend (PKB)

Side lie slump, hip extension with the knee flexed, lengthens the femoral nerve (L2/3/4 nerve roots) and will also apply tension to the neuroaxis and meninges (Davidson 1987, Dyck 1976). The hypothesized movement of the femoral nerve and neuroaxis during the slump PKB is shown in Figure 8.5.

Slump

The full slumped position – sitting with the cervical spine and trunk in flexion, and with the hip in flexion, knee in extension and foot in dorsi-

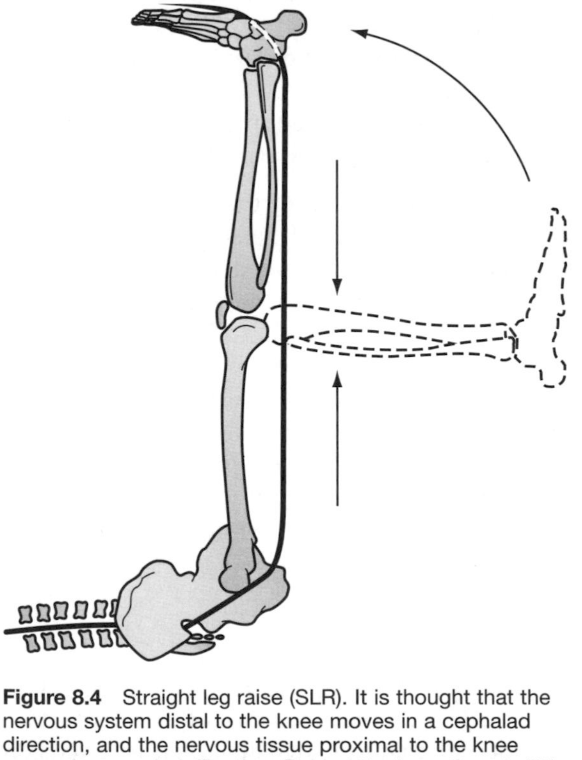

Figure 8.4 Straight leg raise (SLR). It is thought that the nervous system distal to the knee moves in a cephalad direction, and the nervous tissue proximal to the knee moves in a caudad direction. Behind the knee there is little movement, and this is considered to be a tension point. (After Butler 1991, with permission.)

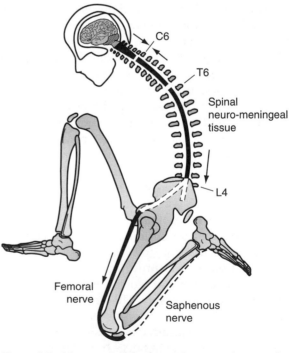

Figure 8.5 Movement of the femoral nerve and neuroaxis during the slump PKB (from Davidson 1987, with permission).

flexion – is thought to lengthen fully and tension the CNS and posterior tibial portion of the sciatic nerve. There is some evidence to suggest that the slump has a greater potential for lengthening and tensioning the nervous system compared with the PNF or SLR movements (Massey 1986).

In asymptomatic subjects, the addition of foot dorsiflexion, hip medial rotation and cervical flexion were all found to reduce the available knee extension range of movement (Johnson & Chiarello 1997). No measurement was made of nerve movement or tension, so while the study provides some support for these components in the slump it does not validate their use.

Examination of slump and its consequent use as a treatment modality is highlighted by a study of Australian Rules football players with signs of a hamstring tear (Kornberg & Lew 1989). A large majority of players (76%) were found to have a positive slump test. All the players were treated with traditional muscle treatment techniques, with one group also receiving slump treatment. The players who were treated with slump had a greater functional improvement than those treated only with traditional methods. In a later study, the slump test was found to cause an increase in sympathetic outflow to the lower limbs, causing vasodilation, and it was speculated that this may have been the underlying effect of the slump treatment of the Australian Rules footballer players (Kornberg & McCarthy 1992).

Patients with symptoms suggestive of frozen shoulder, who were treated with a unilateral posteroanterior pressure to T6 for 1 minute in the sympathetic slump position, were found to have an increase in sympathetic nervous system activity in the affected hand (Slater 1995). Interestingly, the treatment did not affect pain scores, pressure pain thresholds or neurodynamic testing.

Similarly, a positive slump test was found in patients with an ankle inversion sprain (Pahor & Toppenberg 1996), and while the effect of treatment with slump was not carried out in the study it seems reasonable to suggest that this would need to be addressed in the management of such patients.

The sympathetic slump test is carried out in long sitting with the trunk in left lateral flexion and rotation, and the cervical spine in left lateral flexion to affect the right side of the sympathetic trunk (Fig. 8.6; Butler & Slater 1994). It has been shown in asymptomatic subjects that this position for 1 minute causes a large increase in skin conductance and a small decrease in temperature (compared to a placebo and control group), indicative of an increase in vasomotor activity and an increase in sympathetic activity (Slater et al 1994).

Upper-limb tension tests (ULTT)

The following analysis of the effects of the upper-limb tension tests on nerve tension and nerve length uses a mixture of anatomical knowledge and research findings.

1. Cervical contralateral lateral flexion has been shown to increase the strain at the C5–T1 nerve roots (Reid 1987, Selvaratnam et al 1988) and to alter the onset of pain in asymptomatic subjects (van der Heide et al 2001). It has also been found to reduce the movement of the median nerve at the elbow by 5% (Hough et al 2000).

2. Shoulder girdle depression has not been found to increase the tension in the brachial plexus (Ginn 1988, Reid 1987), although when this is eliminated from the upper-limb tension test there is a large reduction in the developing tension in all the cords of the brachial plexus. Shoulder girdle depression with glenohumeral abduction increases the tension in the brachial plexus (Butler 1991, Lord & Rosati 1971).

3. Glenohumeral joint abduction causes an increase in the tension of the brachial plexus (Ginn 1988, Reid 1987) and causes about 15 mm of movement of the brachial plexus (Wilgis & Murphy 1986).

4. Horizontal extension at 90 degrees glenohumeral abduction causes a slight reduction in tension in the brachial plexus (Ginn 1988).

5. Lateral rotation at 90 degrees glenohumeral abduction causes a large reduction in the tension in all the cords of the brachial plexus (Ginn 1988, Reid 1987). The reduction in tension with lateral

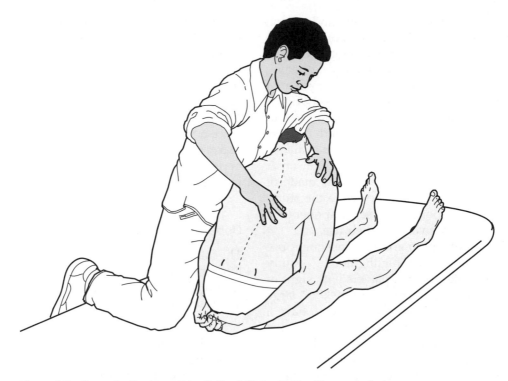

Figure 8.6 Sympathetic slump (from Butler & Slater 1994, with permission).

rotation is accompanied by an increase in tension in the biceps brachii muscle and, for this reason, is recommended as part of the test (Ginn 1988). Medial rotation has been found to reduce the tension in the ulnar nerve (Reid 1987).

6. Elbow extension increases the tension in the radial and median nerves, which lie anterior to the axis of rotation, while it decreases tension in the ulnar nerve (Reid 1987), as it lies posterior to the axis of rotation. The converse will occur: elbow flexion will increase tension in the ulnar nerve and decrease tension in the radial and median nerves (Butler 1991, Reid 1987).

7. Forearm supination and wrist extension each increase the tension on the median nerve at both the elbow and the wrist (Kleinrensink et al 1995). From a neutral wrist position to 55 degrees extension, the median nerve at the elbow has been found to move distally between 6 and 13 mm (Hough et al 2000).

8. Wrist and finger extension will increase the length and tension of the median and ulnar

nerves, and decrease tension in the radial nerve, and vice versa. Wrist extension has been found to increase the tension in the median nerve at both the elbow and wrist (Kleinrensink et al 1995). The median nerve in the upper arm has been found to move distally about 7 mm on wrist and finger extension (McLellan & Swash 1976).

These studies support the component movements used in the upper-limb tension test for the median nerve. The use of horizontal extension does not appear to be useful to increase tension in the brachial plexus (Ginn 1988).

Using buckle force transducers around the median nerve, just distal to the axilla of five cadavers, the typical order of movements of the ULTT1 was carried out while measuring the tension within the median nerve (Lewis et al 1998). The position of neutral cervical spine position, shoulder girdle depression, glenohumeral joint abduction and external rotation and forearm supination failed to cause an increase in median nerve tension (Lewis et al 1998). When the addition of elbow extension was added there was an increase in median nerve tension, and this was further increased with wrist extension and cervical contralateral lateral flexion.

Further support for the components of ULTT1 comes from an in vivo study of asymptomatic subjects (Coppieters et al 2001). A starting position of 30 N longitudinal force to shoulder girdle depression, 90 degrees glenohumeral abduction and external rotation was used. Additions of wrist extension, contralateral cervical lateral flexion, and wrist extension with contralateral cervical lateral flexion each progressively reduced the available elbow extension and provoked more stretch or paraesthesia, mostly localized to the hand (Coppieters et al 2001). No measurement was made of nerve movement or tension, so while the study provides some support for these components in the ULTT1 it does not validate their use.

In asymptomatic subjects, the range of each component of arm movement during the ULTT1 (median nerve bias) of the left and right sides has been found to be the same (van der Heide et al 2001). Treatment may be indicated therefore in patients with asymmetry (van der Heide et al 2001). In addition, it is worth noting that, in this asymptomatic subject group, the onset of pain was correlated with an increased EMG activity of the upper fibres of trapezius. Treatment of nervous tissue, in this case, may need to address this muscle component.

The viscoelastic nature of nerve was observed in one small study using two cadavers (Reid 1987). Repeated movements resulted in a reduction in nerve tension and the tension did not return to its original level, indicating the phenomenon of stress relaxation and hysteresis. It is not known whether this occurs with neurodynamic treatments.

Proprioceptive neuromuscular facilitation (PNF)

The aim of this type of treatment is to cause a relaxation of the contractile unit of muscle in order to increase muscle length, which may indirectly increase nerve length. Proprioceptive neuromuscular facilitation (PNF) is advocated to achieve this muscle relaxation (Knott & Voss 1968, Waddington 1999). These are hold–relax, contract–relax and agonist–contract.

Hold–relax

The muscle is positioned in its stretched position, either actively or passively. A strong isometric contraction of the muscle is achieved by the clinician providing manual resistance. The muscle contraction needs to be carefully controlled by the clinician. This is achieved by saying to the patient 'don't let me move you' or 'hold' and by slowly and smoothly increasing the manual resistance up to a maximum contraction. Following contraction, the patient is asked to relax, the clinician gradually reduces the resistance, and time is allowed for muscle relaxation to occur. The clinician then moves further into range, to increase the length of the muscle. The procedure of contraction followed by relaxation is then repeated until no further increase in muscle length can be achieved.

Contract–relax

This is the same as hold–relax except that, following the isometric contraction, the patient actively contracts to further lengthen the antagonistic muscle, rather than the clinician passively lengthening the muscle. For example, to lengthen quadriceps the patient isometrically contracts the quadriceps at, for example, 60 degrees flexion for 3–6 seconds. The patient is then asked to relax and to contract their hamstrings actively in an attempt to increase knee flexion and to stretch the quadriceps muscle group. As in hold–relax, the procedure is repeated in the new range of movement and repeated until no further increase in muscle length is achieved.

Agonist–contract

The muscle is put in a position of stretch and a contraction of the agonist attempts to increase movement and thus increase stretch of the muscle.

The clinician facilitates this movement by carefully applying a passive force. For example, to lengthen quadriceps the knee is positioned 60 degrees flexion. The patient actively contracts the hamstrings in an attempt to increase knee flexion and stretch the quadriceps muscle group. The clinician applies a force to the lower leg to enhance this movement.

Soft-tissue mobilization of nerve

Hunter (1998) has coined the phrase 'specific soft tissue mobilization' (SSTM). It is essentially the application of manual force to soft tissue, which can be considered to include nerve as well as skin, fascia, ligament, muscle and tendon.

There are three types of treatment technique: physiological SSTM, accessory SSTM and combined SSTM (physiological and accessory).

1. Physiological SSTM involves full exploration of all anatomical regions of nervous tissue by a combination of physiological movements. For example, to explore the common peroneal nerve fully, the SLR with hip adduction and medial rotation and ankle plantarflexion may need to be combined with foot inversion.

2. Accessory SSTM involves applying manual force to the nervous tissue. It is recommended that the force be applied in the plane of the nerve (Fig. 8.7) and at right angles to the site of dysfunction (Hunter 1998). For example, accessory SSTM may be applied over the piriformis muscle to effect a change in the sciatic nerve, or may be applied directly onto a superficial nerve such as the ulnar nerve in the upper arm. Manual force can be applied with the nerve relaxed or

with isometric, concentric or eccentric muscle contraction.

3. Combined accessory and physiological SSTM involves the nerve in a lengthened position while an accessory force is applied. For example, in a position that tensions the nerve, such as SLR with plantarflexion, an accessory movement is carefully applied to the common peroneal nerve, medial to the biceps femoris muscle, behind the knee. With ankle plantarflexion and inversion, the superficial peroneal nerve can also be mobilized on the dorsum of the foot.

Treatment dose

The decisions to be made by the clinician, in terms of treatment dose include: the patient's position, movement, direction, magnitude of force applied, amplitude of oscillation, speed and rhythm of movement, time and symptom response. Table 8.6 provides a summary of the treatment options, and is identical to the treatment dose for joint and muscle.

The underlying effect of soft-tissue mobilization is not yet known. Soft-tissue mobilization is considered to be appropriate following soft-tissue injury, especially during the regeneration and remodelling phase of healing (Hunter 1998), details of which are given below with nerve injury. During the regeneration and remodelling phases, soft-tissue mobilization is thought to enhance collagen synthesis and cross-linkage development, promote the orientation of collagen fibres along functional lines of stress, and promote 'normal' viscoelastic behaviour (Hunter 1998). It is also proposed that SSTM is beneficial for degenerative lesions by stimulating an inflammatory response that initiates healing (Hunter 1998).

TO REDUCE SYMPTOMS

A useful premise for the clinician to consider is that the symptoms are whatever the patient says they are, existing whenever the patient says they are (McCaffery 1979). This was originally used for pain, but can be widened to any symptom the patient feels.

Accessory SSTM

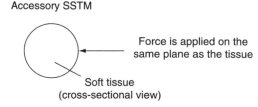

Force is applied on the same plane as the tissue

Soft tissue (cross-sectional view)

Figure 8.7 Direction of force and position of force for accessory specific soft-tissue mobilization to a nerve (from Hunter 1998, with permission).

Table 8.6 Treatment dose for specific soft-tissue mobilization

Factors	Variables
Patient's position	e.g. prone, side lie, sitting
Movement	Physiological movement
	Accessory movement or a mixture of accessory and physiological
Direction of force applied	e.g. medial transverse, lateral transverse, AP, PA, caudad, cephalad
Magnitude of force applied	Related to therapist's perception of resistance: grades I to V
Amplitude of oscillation	None: sustained (quasistatic)
	Small: grades I and IV
	Large: grades II and III
Speed	Slow or fast
Rhythm	Smooth or staccato
Time	Of repetition and number of repetitions
Symptom response	Short of symptom production
	Point of onset or increase in resting symptom
	Partial reproduction of symptom
	Full reproduction of symptom

The assumption in this text is that the cause of the nerve pain is from some sort of injury to the nerve. In this situation, the pain may be a result of mechanical and/or chemical irritation of the nociceptors within the connective tissue surrounding peripheral nerves, or peripheral neurogenic/neuropathic pain where the pain is generated from the nerve axon itself. There are two general approaches that can be used to reduce the experience of pain, either interrupt the nociceptive pathway and/or mimic the natural endogenous inhibitory system (Doubell et al 1999). Placebo analgesia is thought to occur via stimulation of endogenous opioids, which are found throughout the descending pain-modulation pathways (Fields & Basbaum 1999).

The subjective information from the patient, particularly the behaviour of symptoms and mechanism of injury, may enable the clinician to identify whether the pain is mechanical or chemical nociceptive pain from the connective tissue of nerve, or whether it is neurogenic/neuropathic pain from the axon itself. For example, an overstretch injury, with no neurological integrity signs and an intermittent ache, may be considered mechanical nociceptive pain, whereas constant, lancinating pain, with neurological integrity signs (reduced sensation, reduced isometric muscle strength and reduced tendon

reflexes) may indicate pain from an injury to the nerve axon (Woolf & Mannion 1999).

Reducing mechanical or chemical nociceptive pain

Various palpatory techniques can be used to reduce symptoms emanating from mechanical or chemical nociceptive pain and include: massage, specific soft-tissue mobilizations, connective tissue massage, and electrotherapy. Specific soft-tissue mobilization has been described above. Electrotherapy is beyond the scope of this text; the reader is referred to other texts such as Low & Reed (1990) as well as an excellent review by Watson (2000).

Massage can be applied to reduce pain, using: stroking, effleurage, kneading, picking up, wringing and skin rolling. Additional effects are thought to include: an increase in the flow of the circulation, muscle relaxation, lengthening of tissues and an increased tissue drainage and pain relief (Thomson et al 1991). For further details see Thomson et al (1991).

Connective tissue massage (CTM) involves applying specific strokes to the skin and subcutaneous tissues from the lumbar spine to the upper limbs or from the lumbar spine to the lower limbs. It has been suggested that it affects the autonomic nervous system and, via this system, increases circulation, which aids healing and eases pain (Thomson et al 1991). For further details see Thomson et al (1991).

The mechanism by which pain is relieved with each of these manual techniques is still unclear. Large-diameter afferents are distributed throughout skin, joint, muscle and tendon and are stimulated by pressure. It is possible that the manual techniques described above may stimulate these afferents and cause a reflex inhibition of the type IV nociceptors according to the pain gate theory (Melzack & Wall 1965). The pain may also be reduced via a descending inhibitory system; further information can be found later in this chapter.

The sympathetic slump position in asymptomatic subjects has been shown to cause a large increase in skin conductance and a small decrease in temperature (compared to a placebo and control group), indicative of an increase in sympathetic activity (Slater et al 1994). Similarly, the slump position sustained for just 7 seconds was also considered to affect sympathetic outflow to the lower limb (Kornberg & McCarthy 1992). An increase in sympathetic activity, together with hypoalgesia, is considered to be part of a powerful descending pain control system (Lovick 1991). The reduction in pain following neural, as well as joint, treatment techniques is thought to be due, at least in part, to activation of this system (Wright 1995). An outline of this descending system is given below to explain this proposed mechanism of pain relief.

Descending inhibition of pain

The periaqueductal grey (PAG) area has been found to be important in the control of nociception. PAG projects to dorsal horn, having a descending control of nociception (Fig. 8.8). It also projects upwards to the medial thalamus and orbital frontal cortex, suggesting that it may have an ascending control of nociception (Fields & Basbaum 1999). The PAG has two distinct regions: the dorsolateral PAG (dPAG) and the ventrolateral PAG (vPAG).

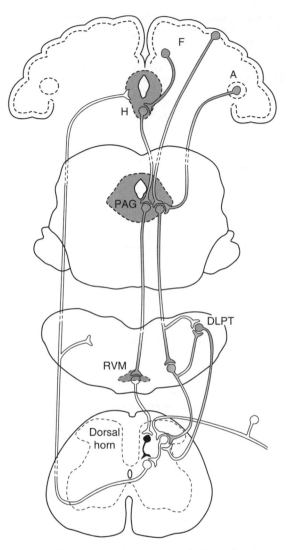

Figure 8.8 Pain-modulating pathway. PAG receives input from the frontal lobe (F), the amygdala (A) and the hypothalamus (H). Afferents from PAG travel to the rostral ventromedial medulla (RVM) and the dorsolateral pontomesencephalic tegmentum (DLPT) and on to the dorsal horn. The RVM has bidirectional control of nociceptive transmission. There are inhibitory (filled) and excitatory (unfilled) interneurones. (From Fields & Basbaum 1999, with permission.)

dPAG

The dorsolateral PAG (dPAG) runs to the dorsolateral pons and ventrolateral medulla, which is involved in autonomic control (Fields & Basbaum 1999). In the rat, stimulation of the dPAG causes analgesia, increased blood pressure, increased heart rate, vasodilation of the hind limb muscles and increased rate and depth of respiration, and coordinated hind limb, jaw and tail movements, suggesting increased activity of the sympathetic nervous system (SNS) and alpha motor neurones (Lovick 1991). The neurotransmitter from dPAG is noradrenaline (norepinephrine) and the analgesic effect appears to mediate morphine analgesia of mechanical nociceptor stimuli (Kuraishi et al 1983). At the spinal cord dPAG causes inhibition of substance P from peripheral noxious mechanical stimulation (Kuraishi 1990).

vPAG

The ventrolateral PAG (vPAG) mainly runs to the nucleus raphe magnus. In the rat, stimulation of vPAG causes analgesia with decreased blood pressure, decreased heart rate, vasodilation of the hind limb muscles and reduced hind limb, jaw and tail movements suggesting inhibition of the SNS and inhibition of alpha motor neurones (Lovick 1991). The neurotransmitter used in vPAG is serotonin and the analgesic effect appears to mediate morphine analgesia of thermal nociceptive stimuli (Kuraishi et al 1983). At the dorsal horn vPAG inhibits the release of somatostatin produced by peripheral noxious thermal stimulation (Kuraishi 1990). These mechanisms have been linked to the behaviour of an animal under threat, which initially acts with a defensive flight-or-fight response followed by recuperation (Fanselow 1991, Lovick 1991); this is summarized in Figure 8.9.

Noxious stimuli can cause activation of the descending control system (Fields & Basbaum 1999, Yaksh & Elde 1981), which may reduce nociceptive transmission. Noxious stimulation has been found to cause release of enkephalins at the supraspinal and spinal levels (Yaksh & Elde 1981). It has also been found that stimulation of the spinothalamic tract, transmitting nociceptive information from one foot, can be inhibited by noxious input from the contralateral foot, hand, face or trunk (Gerhart et al 1981). It has been suggested that this may explain the relief of pain with acupuncture and pain behaviours such as

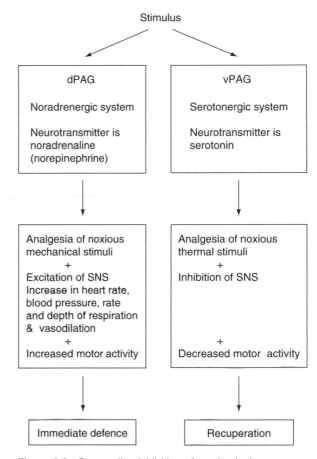

Figure 8.9 Descending inhibition of mechanical nociception from dPAG (noradrenergic system) and thermal nociception from vPAG (serotonergic system).

biting your lip and banging your head against a wall (Melzack 1975). Production of pain during neurodynamic treatment may also activate the descending control system.

The proposed mechanism by which nerve mobilizations relieve pain is outlined in Figure 8.10 (Wright 1995). It is suggested that nerve mobilizations almost immediately stimulate the dPAG to cause hypoalgesia, and a few minutes later vPAG is stimulated (Takeshige et al 1992). There are a number of research studies that support the proposal by Wright (1995); these studies have investigated the immediate effects of joint mobilization on noxious mechanical and thermal thresholds and sympathetic nervous system activity. In a number of the studies noxious

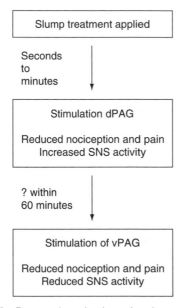

Figure 8.10 Proposed mechanism whereby a neurodynamic treatment, such as a slump, reduces pain (Wright 1995).

mechanical thresholds have been measured using a digital pressure algometer, and noxious thermal thresholds have used a contact thermode system (Wright 1995). Increased sympathetic nervous system (SNS) activity has been measured indirectly by measuring a decrease in skin temperature and an increase in skin conductance (due to a decrease in skin resistance). Skin temperature has been measured using an AT42 skin temperature monitor (Autogenic Advanced Technology, Chicago) and skin conductance has been measured using an AT64 skin conductance monitor (Autogenic Advanced Technology, Chicago).

A number of studies have found that joint mobilizations have an immediate hypoalgesic effect on mechanical nociceptor activity and/or increased sympathetic nervous system (SNS) activity. It may be that the nerve treatment techniques have a similar effect.

Addressing the biopsychosocial aspects of symptoms

Injury, or the perception of injury, produces anxiety and fear (Craig 1999). Who has ever injured themselves, however minimally, and not experienced an emotional reaction? The psychological aspects of pain sometimes focus on 'emotional individuals' or on chronic pain patients. However, all of us will have a cognitive and emotional response to injury, because injury interrupts our lives. There is never a right time for an injury: it will always be, to a greater or lesser degree, a nuisance to us. That 'nuisance' will drive our emotional reactions. It seems reasonable to suggest, therefore, that all patients with neuromusculoskeletal dysfunction will have thoughts and feelings about their problem, and it would be an oversight on the part of the clinician not to enquire about this. This enquiry involves the clinician understanding the patient's thoughts and feelings. This is no easy task, and to do it well requires a high level of skill in active listening. Active listening involves putting our own thoughts, beliefs and feelings to one side and choosing instead to hear what the patient has to say. It involves trying to understand the patient and their world, through their eyes, and trying to avoid the all-too-easy error of re-interpreting through our eyes. It requires the clinician to listen with compassion, patience, and without judgement. It involves the clinician using words carefully and meaningfully, and using open-ended questions, to search for information, until understanding is reached. It involves sensitive verbal and non-verbal communication, thus encouraging safe and open communication. This is a tall order, but the benefits of truly being able to come alongside the patient will far outweigh the effort of developing these skills.

The use of 'yellow flags' was devised specifically for acute low-back pain to identify beliefs, emotions and behaviours that may contribute to long-term disability (Watson & Kendall 2000). Screening questionnaires (e.g. Main & Waddell 1999) have been devised; these, like all questionnaires, have major limitations. Questions provide a superficial, and sometimes false, understanding of the problem – as anyone who has filled in any questionnaire knows only too well. For example, while a question may ask 'how much have you been bothered by feeling depressed in the last week' and the recipient answers on a

0 to 10 scale from 'not at all' to 'extremely', little information is gleaned from this; there may be a wide variety of factors underlying the given score. For this reason, if a questionnaire is used, a discussion with the patient will also be necessary to understand the problems faced by the patient (Watson & Kendall 2000). The questionnaire can be useful to provide the clinician with aspects to discuss with the patient; however, there is a danger that it becomes a mechanistic form-filling exercise. It is worth remembering that the clinical management of patients is fundamentally based on human relationships, which are not normally enriched by form filling!

Following the enquiry of the patient as to their thoughts and feelings two further steps are recommended: education and exposure (Vlaeyen & Crombez 1999). Education involves the clinician carefully facilitating the patient's understanding of the problem. The way this is carried out with patients will vary according to a number of factors – such as the patient's prior knowledge, thoughts and beliefs and how they feel about the problem. All the listening skills discussed above will be imperative in this process. The ability of the clinician to be honest is important. The clinician needs to explain the problem to the patient in a careful way. There is a world of difference between 'the pain in your back is from the disc' and 'I think the pain in your back could be coming from the disc'. The former explanation suggests that you know that the pain is coming from the disc, and yet there is overwhelming evidence that you cannot make such claims; it has been estimated that a definite diagnosis of the pathology can be made in only about 15% of cases (Waddell 1999). Furthermore, there is a long-term problem with being so confident as the patient may, in the future, have a recurrence of the same pain and may see another clinician who may say 'the pain in your back is from your sacroiliac joint'. The patient is aware that this is a repeat episode and now, quite rightly, begins to have doubts about the ability of these two clinicians. This will be a familiar story to experienced clinicians who will have come across patients who have received perhaps three, four or even more confident 'diagnoses' of the same problem and

who come to you depressed, cynical and disillusioned with the medical profession.

The final aspect is exposure, which involves careful and graded exposure to the movements or postures that provoke pain (Vlaeyen & Crombez 1999). While this is designed for chronic-pain patients who learn to avoid movements and posture through fear (Moseley 2003, Waddell & Main 1999), it may also be an important part of the treatment of acute tissue damage. Using movements and postures in a careful, controlled and graded way may help to avoid long-term movement dysfunctions.

To reduce neuropathic pain

At present there are no ideal therapeutic approaches to relieve neuropathic pain. The pain may be caused by ectopic action potentials in nociceptors, it may be due to central sensitization, or it may be due to altered connections in lamina II of the dorsal horn (Doubell et al 1999). Use is made of sodium channel blockers for preventing nociceptor activity entering the spinal cord, opiates for suppressing C-fibre activity, and N-methyl-D-asparate (NMDA) receptor antagonists for inhibiting central sensitization – but these agents have major limitations (Doubell et al 1999).

MODIFICATION, PROGRESSION AND REGRESSION OF TREATMENT

The continuous monitoring of the patient's subjective and physical asterisks guides the entire treatment and management programme of the patient. The clinician judges the degree of change with treatment and relates this to the expected rate of change from the prognosis – then decides whether or not a treatment needs to be altered in some way. The nature of this alteration can be to modify the technique in some way, to progress the treatment or regress the treatment. Regardless of which alteration is made, the clinician makes every effort to determine what effect this alteration has on the patient's subjective and physical asterisks. In order to do this, the clinician alters one aspect of treatment at a time and reassesses immediately to determine the value of the alteration.

Modification of treatment

The clinician may modify the treatment given to a patient by altering an existing treatment, adding a new treatment or stopping a treatment. At all times the treatment should have the functional goals of the patient in mind. Altering an existing treatment involves altering some aspect of the treatment dose, discussed earlier. The immediate and more long-term effect of the alteration is then evaluated by reassessment of the subjective and physical asterisks; this process is outlined in Figure 8.11. The clinician then decides whether, overall, the patient is better, the same or worse, relating this to the prognosis. For instance, if a quick improvement was expected, but only some improvement occurred, the clinician may progress treatment. If the patient is worse after treatment, the dose may be regressed in some way, and if the treatment made no difference at all, then a more substantial modification may be made. Before discarding a treatment it is worth making sure that it has been fully utilized, as it may be that a much stronger or much weaker treatment dose may be effective.

Summary

This chapter has outlined the principles of nerve treatment. Treatment is only a part of the overall management of a patient; the reader is therefore encouraged to go now to Chapter 9 where the principles of management are discussed.

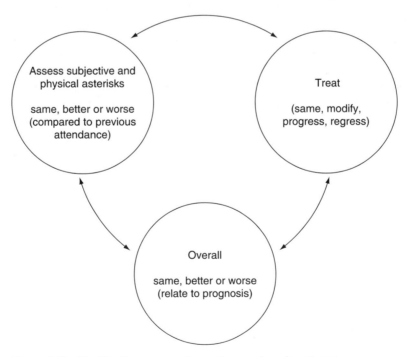

Figure 8.11 Modification, progression and regression of treatment.

REFERENCES

Adkison D P, Bosse M J, Gaccione D R, Gabriel K R 1991 Anatomical variations in the course of the superficial peroneal nerve. Journal of Bone and Joint Surgery 73A(1):112–114

Breig A 1978 Adverse mechanical tension in the central nervous system. Almqvist & Wiksell, Stockholm

Breig A, Marions O 1963 Biomechanics of the lumbosacral nerve roots. Acta Radiologica 1:1141–1160

Breig A, Troup J D G 1979 Biomechanical considerations in the straight-leg-raising test, cadaveric and clinical studies of the effects of medial hip rotation. Spine 4(3):242–250

Butler D S 1991 Mobilisation of the nervous system. Churchill Livingstone, Melbourne

Butler D 2000 The sensitive nervous system. Noigroup, Adelaide

Butler D S, Slater H 1994 Neural injury in the thoracic spine: a conceptual basis for manual therapy. In: Grant R (ed) Physical therapy of the cervical and thoracic spine, 2nd edn. Churchill Livingstone, New York, ch 15, p 313–338

Clark W L, Trumble T E, Swiontkowski M F, Tencer A F 1992 Nerve tension and blood flow in a rat model of immediate and delayed repairs. Journal of Hand Surgery 17A:677–687

Coppieters M W, Stappaerts K H, Everaert D G, Staes F F 2001 Addition of test components during neurodynamic testing: effect on range of motion and sensory responses. Journal of Orthopaedic and Sports Physical Therapy 31(5):226–237

Craig K D 1999 Emotions and psychobiology. In: Wall P D, Melzack R (eds) Textbook of pain, 4th edn. Churchill Livingstone, Edinburgh, ch 12, p 331–343

Daniels T R, Lau J T-C, Hearn T C 1998 The effects of foot position and load on tibial nerve tension. Foot and Ankle International 19(2):73–78

Davidson S 1987 Prone knee bend: an investigation into the effect of cervical flexion and extension. In: Dalziell B A, Snowsill J C (eds) Proceedings of the Manipulative Therapists' Association of Australia, 5th Biennial Conference, p 236–246

Doubell T P, Mannion R J, Woolf C J 1999 The dorsal horn: state-dependent sensory processing, plasticity and the generation of pain. In: Wall P D, Melzack R (eds) Textbook of pain, 4th edn. Churchill Livingstone, Edinburgh, ch 6, p 165–181

Dyck P 1976 The femoral nerve traction test with lumbar disc protrusions. Surgical Neurology 6:163–166

Fanselow M S 1991 The midbrain periaqueductal gray as a coordinator of action in response to fear and anxiety. In: Depaulis A, Bandler R (eds) The midbrain periaqueductal gray matter. Plenum Press, New York, p 151–173

Fields H L, Basbaum A I 1999 Central nervous system mechanisms of pain modulation. In: Wall P D, Melzack R (eds) Textbook of pain, 4th edn. Churchill Livingstone, Edinburgh, ch 11, p 309–329

Gerhart K D, Yezierski R P, Giesler G J, Willis W D 1981 Inhibitory receptive fields of primate spinothalamic tract cells. Journal of Neurophysiology 46(6):1309–1325

Ginn K 1988 An investigation of tension development in upper limb soft tissues during the upper limb tension test. In: Proceedings of the International Federation of Orthopaedic Manipulative Therapists' Conference, Cambridge, England, p 25–26

Goddard M D, Reid J D 1965 Movements induced by straight leg raising in the lumbo-sacral roots, nerves and plexus, and in the intrapelvic section of the sciatic nerve. Journal of Neurology, Neurosurgery and Psychiatry 28:12–18

Hough A, Moore A, Jones M 2000 Doppler ultrasound measurement of median nerve motion. International Federation of Orthopaedic Manipulative Therapists 7th Scientific Conference Proceedings, Abstract 62, p 56

Hunter G 1998 Specific soft tissue mobilization in the management of soft tissue dysfunction. Manual Therapy 3(1):2–11

Johnson E K, Chiarello C M 1997 The slump test: the effects of head and lower extremity position on knee extension. Journal of Orthopaedic and Sports Physical Therapy 26(6):310–317

Kleinrensink G J, Stoeckart R, Vleeming A et al 1995 Mechanical tension in the median nerve. The effects of joint positions. Clinical Biomechanics 10(5):240–244

Knott M, Voss D E 1968 Proprioceptive neuromuscular facilitation. Harper Row, New York

Kornberg C, Lew P 1989 The effect of stretching neural structures on grade one hamstring injuries. Journal of Orthopaedic and Sports Physical Therapy 6:481–487

Kornberg C, McCarthy T 1992 The effect of neural stretching technique on sympathetic outflow to the lower limbs. Journal of Orthopaedic and Sports Physical Therapists 16(6):269–274

Kuraishi Y 1990 Neuropeptide-mediated transmission of nociceptive information and its regulation. Novel mechanisms of analgesics. Yakugaku Zasshi 110(10):711–726

Kuraishi Y, Harada Y, Aratani S et al 1983 Separate involvement of the spinal noradrenergic and serotonergic systems in morphine analgesia: the differences in mechanical and thermal algesic tests. Brain Research 273:245–252

Lehmann J F, DeLateur B J, Silverman D R 1966 Selective heating effects of ultrasound in human beings. Archives of Physical Medicine and Rehabilitation 47:331–339

Lewis J, Ramot R, Green A 1998 Changes in mechanical tension in the median nerve: possible implications for the upper limb tension test. Physiotherapy 84(6):254–261

Lord J W, Rosati L M 1971 Thoracic outlet syndromes. In: CIBA Clinical Symposia, Ciba Pharmaceutical, New Jersey, 23(2):20–23

Lovick T 1991 Interactions between descending pathways from the dorsal and ventrolateral periaqueductal gray matter in the rat. In: Depaulis A, Bandler R (eds) The midbrain periaqueductal gray matter. Plenum Press, New York, p 101–120

Low J, Reed A 1990 Electrotherapy explained, principles and practice. Butterworth-Heinemann, London

McCaffery M 1979 Nursing the patient in pain. Harper & Row, London

McLellan D L, Swash M 1976 Longitudinal sliding of the median nerve during movements of the upper limb. Journal of Neurology, Neurosurgery and Psychiatry 39:566–570

Magarey M E 1985 Selection of passive treatment techniques. In: Proceedings of 4th Biennial Conference of the Manipulative Therapists' Association of Australia, Brisbane, p 298–320

Magarey M E 1986 Examination and assessment in spinal joint dysfunction. In: Grieve G P (ed) Modern manual therapy of the vertebral column. Churchill Livingstone, Edinburgh, ch 44, p 481–497

Main C J, Waddell G 1999 Psychological distress. In: Waddell G (ed) The back pain revolution. Churchill Livingstone, Edinburgh, ch 11 p 173–186

Maitland G D, Banks K, English K, Hengeveld E, 2001 Maitland's vertebral manipulation, 6th edn. Butterworth-Heinemann, Oxford

Massey A E 1986 Movement of pain-sensitive structures in the neural canal. In: Grieve G P (ed) Modern manual therapy of the vertebral column. Churchill Livingstone, Edinburgh, ch 18 p 182–193

Melzack R 1975 Prolonged relief of pain by brief, intense transcutaneous somatic stimulation. Pain 1:357–373

Melzack R, Wall P D 1965 Pain mechanisms: a new theory. Science 150:971–979

Millard J B 1961 Effect of high-frequency currents and infra-red rays on the circulation of the lower limb in man. Annals of Physical Medicine 6(2):45–66

Moseley L 2003 A pain neuromatrix approach to patients with chronic pain. Manual Therapy (in press)

Pahor S, Toppenberg R 1996 An investigation of neural tissue involvement in ankle inversion sprains. Manual Therapy 1(4):192–197

Petty N J, Moore A P 2001 Neuromusculoskeletal examination and assessment, a handbook for therapists, 2nd edn. Churchill Livingstone, Edinburgh

Reid J D 1960 Effects of flexion-extension movements of the head and spine upon the spinal cord and nerve roots. Journal of Neurology, Neurosurgery and Psychiatry 23:214–221

Reid S A 1987 The measurement of tension changes in the brachial plexus: In: Proceedings of the fifth Biennial Conference of the Manipulative Therapists' Association of Australia, Melbourne, p 79–90

Ridehalgh C, Greening J B, Petty N J 2004 The effect of straight leg raise examination and treatment on vibration threshold in the lower limb. Manual Therapy (in press)

Rigby B J 1964 The effect of mechanical extension upon the thermal stability of collagen. Biochimica et Biophysica Acta 79 (SC 43008):634–636

Selvaratnam P J, Glasgow E F, Matyas T 1988 The strain at the nerve roots of the brachial plexus. Journal of Anatomy 161:260

Seradge H, Jia Y-C, Owens W 1995 In vivo measurement of carpal tunnel pressure in the functioning hand. Journal of Hand Surgery 20A:855–859

Slater H 1995 An investigation of the physiological effects of the sympathetic slump on peripheral sympathetic nervous system function in patients with frozen shoulder. In: Shacklock M O (ed) Moving in on pain. Butterworth-Heinemann, Australia

Slater H, Vicenzino B, Wright A 1994 'Sympathetic slump': the effects of a novel manual therapy technique on peripheral sympathetic nervous system function. Journal of Manual and Manipulative Therapy 2(4):156–162

Smith S A, Massie J B, Chesnut R, Garfin S R 1993 Straight leg raising, anatomical effects on the spinal nerve root without and with fusion. Spine 18(8):992–999

Sunderland S 1978 Nerves and nerve injuries, 2nd edn. Churchill Livingstone, Edinburgh

Sunderland S, Bradley K C 1961 Stress–strain phenomena in human peripheral nerve trunks. Brain 84:102–119

Takeshige C, Sato T, Mera T, Hisamitsu T, Fang J 1992 Descending pain inhibitory system involved in acupuncture analgesia. Brain Research Bulletin 29:617–634

Tal-Akabi A, Rushton A 2000 An investigation to compare the effectiveness of carpal bone mobilisation and neurodynamic mobilisation as methods of treatment for carpal tunnel syndrome. Manual Therapy 5(4):214–222

Tencer A F, Allen B L, Ferguson R L 1985 A biomechanical study of thoracolumbar spine fractures with bone in the canal, part III, mechanical properties of the dura and its tethering ligaments. Spine 10(8):741–747

Thomson A, Skinner A, Piercy J 1991 Tidy's Physiotherapy, 12th edn. Butterworth-Heinemann, Oxford

van der Heide B, Allison G T, Zusman M 2001 Pain and muscular responses to a neural tissue provocation test in the upper limb. Manual Therapy 6(3):154–162

Vlaeyen J W S, Crombez G 1999 Fear of movement/(re)injury, avoidance and pain disability in chronic low back pain patients. Manual Therapy 4(4):187–195

von Piekartz H & Bryden L 2001 Craniofacial dysfunction and pain: manual therapy, assessment and management. Butterworth-Heinemann Oxford

Waddell G 1999 Diagnostic triage. In: Waddell G (ed) The back pain revolution. Churchill Livingstone, Edinburgh, ch 2 p 9

Waddell G, Main C J 1999 Beliefs about back pain. In: Waddell G (ed) The back pain revolution. Churchill Livingstone, Edinburgh, ch 12 p 187–202

Waddington P J 1999 In: Hollis M & Fletcher-Cook P (ed) Practical exercise therapy, Blackwell Scientific, Oxford

Watson T 2000 The role of electrotherapy in contemporary physiotherapy practice. Manual Therapy 5(3):132–141

Watson P, Kendall N 2000 Assessing psychological yellow flags. In: Gifford L (ed) Topical issues in pain 2, biopsychosocial assessment and management relationships and pain. CNS, Kestral, ch 3, p 111–129

Wilgis E F S, Murphy R 1986 The significance of longitudinal excursion in peripheral nerves. Hand Clinics 2(4):761–766

Woolf C J, Mannion R J 1999 Neuropathic pain: aetiology, symptoms, mechanisms, and management. Lancet 353:1959–1964

Wright A 1995 Hypoalgesia post-manipulative therapy: a review of a potential neurophysiological mechanism. Manual Therapy 1(1):11–16

Yaksh T L, Elde R P 1981 Factors governing release of methionine enkephalin-like immunoreactivity from mesencephalon and spinal cord of the cat in vivo. Journal of Neurophysiology 46(5):1056–1075

9

Principles of patient management

Ann P. Moore

INTRODUCTION

There can be no greater privilege bestowed on a clinician than the unqualified trust of individual patients who are seeking to maintain or improve their health status. As clinicians, we are potentially in this position throughout our working lives. It is the responsibility of every clinician to ensure that this trust is well founded by maintaining excellence in all aspects of the clinician's role.

This book has set out to help clinicians along the sometimes complex road of clinical decision making by offering the reader a comprehensive background to joint, muscle and nerve function and dysfunction. It also reviews and contextualizes the principles of the treatment strategies that may be employed by a clinician when aiding patients recovering from either single or multiple tissue dysfunction.

This chapter is devoted to exploring the principles of patient management in its broadest sense. It commences with an overview of terminology used in the 'treatment context', explores the patient–clinician relationship, the responsibilities within the relationship and the issues surrounding this relationship. The chapter then expands to include a discussion of the treatment event itself, and it concludes with an overview and analysis of the factors necessary for promoting ongoing good practice and professional development for clinicians.

It is not possible within a single chapter to deal comprehensively with all the issues raised. Rather, this chapter is concerned with raising the profile of concepts, idealisms and philosophies not usually harmonized in pure neuromusculoskeletal therapy courses or textbooks. It is hoped that this chapter will help to enrich the clinician's practice by presenting an eclectic approach to overall patient management.

By the end of this chapter readers may be struck by the complexity of the role encompassed by the clinician, and some may view the process of maturation into an expert clinician as a difficult journey. An old Taoist saying may be helpful here!

'A thousand mile journey starts with one small step' (cited by Hoff 1982)

The stimulus constantly provided by patients, their carers and relatives, and the integration of the varied concepts addressed in this chapter, may help to sustain the reader in their journey and ease the apprehension in these first early steps. It is important that each clinician enjoys the privilege of working with patients and also reaps every benefit that these working relationships have to offer both the patient and clinician.

PATIENT MANAGEMENT DEFINED

In this text the term 'patient management' has been used throughout. It is important here to clarify what is meant by this term. Synonyms for management include: administration, care, command, conduct, control, direction, guidance, handling, manipulation and supervision (Collins Thesaurus 1995). It is acknowledged that the term 'patient management', and the majority of synonyms associated with it, implies a very passive role for the patient and a paternalistic approach to the patient by the clinician. This is not the philosophy held by the author, and the term 'patient management' is used only in recognition of the common usage of these terms in general clinical practice. The context of debate surrounding 'patient management' is explored further in this chapter. The author's preferred approach is for patient-focused care with a strong emphasis on the therapeutic relationship.

Synonyms for 'therapeutic' are ameliorative, beneficial, corrective, good, healing, remedial and restorative, and synonyms for relationship include association, bond, communication, conjunction, exchange, kinship, liaison, link and rapport (Collins Thesaurus 1995). These words would seem to imply more active participation from both parties engaged in the therapeutic relationship and celebrate the positive benefits which may occur from that working relationship.

The central importance of patients to the health service and healthcare providers has gained political momentum in the United Kingdom since the publication in 1997 of the government's white paper 'The NHS Modern and Dependable' (Secretary of State for Health 1997) and, later, the NHS Plan (Department of Health 2000) which affirmed that patients are the most important people in the health service. This document also acknowledged that, for patients, their importance in the health arena may not always be apparent and that patients often feel 'talked at rather than listened to' (Department of Health 2000, p. 88). The recommendations set out in the NHS plan, and of relevance to this chapter, were for:

- more information for patients
- greater patient choice
- health services to become more patient-centred.

Later in the same year the National Health Service document (NHSE2000) 'Meeting the Challenge – a Strategy for the Allied Health Professions' further emphasized the need for patient-focused care. From April 1st, 1999, in the United Kingdom all NHS bodies had a new statutory duty of clinical governance placed upon them. Clinical governance places a duty on all health professionals to ensure that the level of service they 'deliver' to patients is satisfactory, consistent and responsive. Essentially, clinical governance is about health service providers ensuring and guaranteeing quality of health care through a system of processes which include (Secretary of State for Health 1998):

- clear lines of responsibility and accountability being in place for the overall quality of clinical care

- a comprehensive programme of quality improvement activities being in place, including support for the use of evidence and the application of evidence-based practice in everyday healthcare activities
- continuing professional development being available for all health workers
- programmes being in place which are aimed at meeting the development needs of individual health professionals and the service needs of the organization, which are regularly monitored
- effective monitoring of clinical care with high-quality systems for clinical record keeping and the collection of relevant information
- processes being in place for assuring the quality of clinical care
- clear policies aimed at managing risk in health care
- procedures for all professional groups for identifying and remedying poor performance.

In essence, all health professionals have an individual and statutory responsibility to engage with clinical governance. For individuals this means taking a lead in the delivery of quality care, demonstrating that quality of care is being provided and sharing initiatives and ideas for best practice with others. It also means that individual practitioners have a duty to undertake continuing professional development (NHS Executive 1999) and that patients and health care organizations will increasingly expect practitioners to base their practice on the best quality evidence available.

Clinical governance sits alongside a number of other NHS policies, for example:

- National Service frameworks
- NHS performance and assessment frameworks
- Health improvement programmes.

Clinical governance policy also sits alongside two statutory bodies that are outside the NHS but closely associated with it. They are: The National Institute for Clinical Excellence (NICE), which provides national evidence-based clinical guidelines and information on good practice,

and the Commission for Health Improvements (CHI). CHI has been set up to provide national leadership in the principles of clinical governance and to undertake a programme of reviews within each NHS Trust to ensure that clinical governance arrangements are in place and are working (Swage 2000).

All health professionals now have a statutory duty to acquaint themselves with the quality systems/clinical governance arrangements existing within their own area of practice. For up-to-date information on clinical governance procedures readers are advised to visit the NHS Executive or the Department of Health websites or, alternatively, to use their local hospital trust's website or clinical governance office.

STANDARDS OF PROFICIENCY – THE HEALTH PROFESSIONS COUNCIL

In most countries there are minimum standards of proficiency that must be met in order for an individual practitioner to enter and/or be maintained on the health professions/physiotherapy register. In the United Kingdom the standards of proficiency have been developed in order to protect members of the public and to ensure high standards of care. These standards place the patient at the centre of practice and include statements relating to:

- professional autonomy and accountability
- professional relationships, including working and communicating with patients and their carers
- identification and assessment of health and social care needs
- formulation and delivery of plans and strategies for meeting health and social care needs
- critical evaluation of the impact of, or response to, the registrant's actions.

The standards also indicate that registrants must have knowledge, understanding and skills of profession-specific practice and be able to modify these for specific individuals and understand the need to establish and maintain a safe practice environment (Health Professions Council 2003a).

The Chartered Society of Physiotherapy and other national professional bodies relating to physiotherapy who publish their own rules of professional conduct (Chartered Society of Physiotherapy 2002) also include a strong emphasis on patient-focused care.

The need for the patient to be the central focus of any clinical interaction is therefore underpinned by a body of government legislation, regulatory body standards and professional standards and guidelines. All clinicians need to be acquainted with, and to engage fully with, these frameworks, which are laid down in order to ensure safe and competent clinical practice.

MODELS OF CARE

Historically, physiotherapy practice was well rooted in the medical/biological model of care, and paternalism was a strong characteristic of clinical behaviour within the therapeutic relationship. Paternalism has been defined as 'a refusal to accept or acquiesce in another person's wishes, choices or actions for that person's benefit' (Singleton & McLaren 1995). Historically, paternalism has been associated with individual patients being the passive recipients of health care. Clearly, with the growth of consumerism, the dramatic rise in the availability of health-related information, and the political frameworks in which health services function, the paternalistic/biomedical model of care has given way to an autonomy model which emphasizes the rights of individuals in decision making (Singleton & McLaren 1995). This situation, in which trust and respect for an individual's autonomy exist, would appear to be a vital foundation of the therapeutic relationship; hence, joint decision making (between the patient and clinician) with regard to treatment strategies, and short- and long-term goal setting, are becoming the norm in physiotherapy and in other health care practices. The benefits of the shift to more joint decision making are increasingly being demonstrated. For example, Neistadt (1995) showed that collaboration on treatment goal set-

ting can reduce the length of hospital stays and achieve better outcomes in attaining goals.

In practice there is probably a spectrum of paternalistic and autonomous activities which take place in each clinical intervention involving both clinicians and patients. Occasionally it may be necessary for the clinician to assume a paternalistic role, focusing on the patient's condition with the patient's interests at heart and with very little importance placed on the patient's concerns, issues and or beliefs. In modern health care practices this may be seen most frequently when clinicians are dealing with emergency situations in which time is of the essence in order to save life.

Barr & Threlkeld (2000) believe that the more contemporary view of health care is to see patients and clinicians as partners in designing interventions to achieve the best outcome while contextualizing the problem within the patient's life situation. Clinicians dealing with patients with neuromusculoskeletal dysfunction are in an excellent position to develop such partnerships with patients because of the nature of the work that they do, i.e. having a strong focus on helping patients return to their pre-injury, or pre-pathological states and because largely their patients do not need emergency interventions.

Patient-centred care and clinician-centred care lie at two ends of a continuum. There may be times – for example, if a patient is very ill or in considerable pain – when clinician-centred care is the only option in the initial stages, leading to more patient-centred care later in the treatment programme when the patient takes full responsibility for managing their own condition. The balance between patient and clinician centredness between these two ends of the continuum is complex and varies from patient to patient and clinician to clinician and is perhaps best demonstrated diagrammatically in Figure 9.1, which illustrates the patient care continuum.

Stewart & Roter (1989) described several different types of doctor–patient relationship (Fig. 9.2). These authors observed that paternalism has been, in the past, the most common model adopted by doctors but that, in the late 1980s, greater patient control was taking place and thus

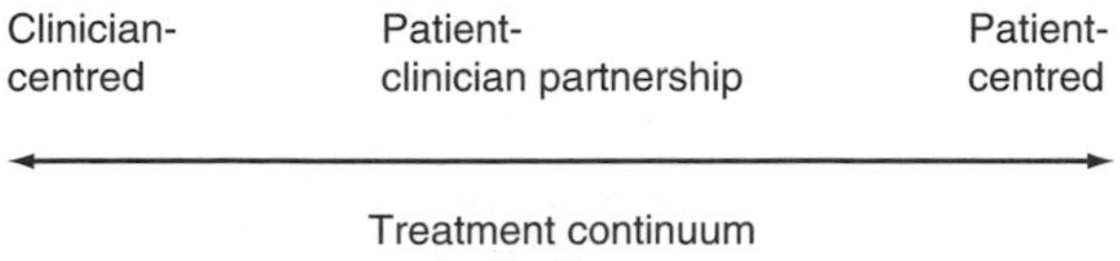

Clinician-centred	Patient-clinician partnership	Patient-centred

<——>

Treatment continuum

Figure 9.1 The patient care continuum.

more mutuality occurred when both doctors and patients brought knowledge, experience and expectations to the relationship. Similar developments have occurred in other health care practices – not least in neuromusculoskeletal therapy. The clinician, in Stewart & Roter's model, also brings clinical skills and clinical knowledge, and the clinical interaction can be seen as a joint venture with both parties exchanging information and ideas. In some circumstances the relationship may be reversed – producing, what Stewart & Roter (1989) described as a consumerist relationship in which the patient takes a more active role and the doctor a fairly passive role, for example, when patients request a second opinion. A fourth type of relationship occurs when the patient continues to be in a passive role while the doctor also attempts to reduce some of their control of the consultation. Stewart & Roter (1989) indicate that different types of relationship may be appropriate at different stages of illness/treatment, as previously described. In the context of patient-focused care, in the early stages, the interaction may be more clinician-centred, moving later into a patient–clinician partnership mode. The interaction then becomes more exclusively patient-centred as the patient learns to take control of their condition. At this point both the clinician and the patient prepare for the patient's discharge and future self-management (if necessary), either to

maintain symptoms and signs at an acceptable level or to keep the condition from re-occurring. The patient-centred model emphasizes the physical, personal and social aspects of the patient's condition (Jette 1994).

Ewles & Simnett (2003) proposed a number of ways in which clinicians can help their patients to take more control over their health and develop more autonomy. First, they can encourage individuals to make decisions and resist the urge to 'take over'. Second, they can encourage individuals to think things out for themselves (this may take much longer than simply telling them!). Third, they can respect any unusual ideas that individuals may have about their health. In addition, Ewles & Simnett (2003) advocated 'acceptance' of individuals rather than 'judging' them.

According to Ewles & Simnett (2003), when we accept an individual it means the following:

- recognizing that the individual's knowledge and beliefs have emerged from their own life experiences, whereas the clinician's have been modified and extended by their professional education and experience
- understanding one's own knowledge, beliefs, values and standards
- understanding the patient's knowledge, beliefs, values and standards from their own (the patient's) point of view
- recognizing that you (the clinician), the patients, and others you work with, may differ in knowledge, beliefs, values and standards
- recognizing that these differences do not imply that you, as the clinician, are a person of greater worth than your patients/clients.

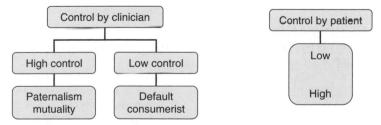

Figure 9.2 Clinician–patient therapeutic relationships (adapted from Stewart & Roter 1989).

A partnership between a clinician and a patient can exist only if there is an atmosphere of mutual trust and openness, and this can be brought about by encouraging patients to ask questions and discuss issues openly. It is also important to ask patients for their views and opinions about treatment and related matters which the clinician then accepts and respects. Often it is helpful to let patients know that you, as a clinician, have learnt something from them, however small that may be. Finally, Ewles & Simnett (2003) believe that encouraging and fostering patients to share knowledge and experience with each other, if possible, is very helpful and appropriate in helping them to become more informed participants in the therapeutic partnership.

The importance of understanding and interacting with patients and their belief systems in order to highlight the relationship between psychosocial aspects of care and the biomedical aspects of care was emphasized by Jones et al (2002) who discussed two contemporary models of health and disability: a model for organizing clinical knowledge and a model for aiding reasoning strategies within the clinician. Additionally, the reader is referred to Waddell's biopsychosocial model of back pain (Fig. 9.3), which can be applied to many neuromusculoskeletal dysfunctional states.

This model shows clearly the relationship between pain, the patient's attitudes and beliefs, psychological distress, and the illness behaviours, which may emanate from chronic pain states and the interaction and possible influences of the social environment. The importance of this model is that it highlights the need for clinicians to explore as many of the identified dimensions as possible with their patients during the course of their interactions with them.

THE PATIENT'S NEEDS AND EXPECTATIONS OF TREATMENT AND MANAGEMENT

Patients consulting clinicians will do so bringing with them expectations of the clinician, the therapy they will receive, the outcome of treatment, the position of the clinician within the multidis-

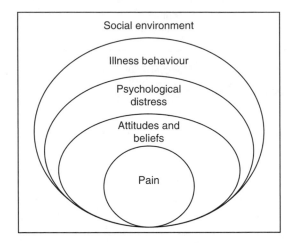

Figure 9.3 A biopsychosocial model of the clinical presentation and assessment of low back pain and disability at one point in time. (Reproduced from Waddell et al 1984, British Medical Journal 289:739–741, with permission from the BMJ Publishing Group.)

ciplinary team, the hospital, their own role within their treatment and rehabilitation and expectations about other issues.

For clinicians, it is important to understand that patients will have varied expectations which may differ from the clinician's own expectations in relation to the proposed treatment and its outcome.

When establishing a therapeutic relationship between the clinician and the patient, the patient must feel comfortable in sharing their expectations and beliefs about their condition and the therapy they may receive. Clinicians should use both non-verbal and verbal communication when trying to identify what their patients' expectations are and the needs that they hope will be fulfilled during treatment – at an early stage in the patient–clinician consultation (Jensen & Lorish 1994).

The patient's needs

Patients may have specific needs which they hope will be fulfilled by their treatment and by the clinician. The concept of need is brought to the fore mainly in the health-promotion literature. Ewles & Simnett (2003), citing Bradshaw

(1972), presented three types of need which are appropriate to discuss here:

- normative need
- felt need
- expressed need.

Normative need

Normative need is usually defined for patients by experts (in this case, the clinician), based on their own value judgements. Opinions regarding normative need, however, will vary from expert to expert. For example, safe lifting and handling information – which is thought by experts to be a need for one occupational group – may not be transferable from one working environment to another and the opinions of the experts may differ from those of the patients who may use this information.

Felt need

Felt needs are the needs in which people identify what they want. For example, a patient with low back pain may feel the need for some information on lifting and handling procedures. Felt needs, however, are limited to people's knowledge about what could be available to them. For example, patients may not know about all the types of therapy that are available to them as they have not been exposed to information about the full range of treatments that currently exist (Ewles & Simnett 2003).

Expressed need

Expressed need is what people say they need, i.e. a felt need which has been turned into an expressed request or demand. For example, a patient may demand exercises to help with low back pain (Ewles & Simnett 2003).

It is important to note here that not all of the patient's felt needs will be turned into expressed needs as the patient may lack motivation or assertiveness to do this. In some situations, in which the clinician adopts a paternalistic approach to care, the patient may not be given the opportunity to express their needs fully.

It is also important to note that patients may have based their expressed needs on a limited amount of information, or on misinformation, and the expressed needs may conflict with the clinician's perceived normative needs! For example, a patient may have decided that they need a certain form of therapy suggested by a friend who appears to have a similar problem, but the clinician may feel that the kind of therapy demanded is inappropriate. It is therefore essential that, in the spirit of partnership, these expressed needs are discussed in full to enable each party to understand fully the view of the other and come to a consensus decision about the most appropriate way forward.

Evidence is growing that patients who are well informed about their treatment, and the reasons for it, and who are involved in decisions about their care, do better than those who do not share in the decision making process (Brody et al 1989). However, there is also evidence that clinicians may not be taking full advantage of the potential for patient participation in their own care – for example, in goal setting (Baker et al 2001).

The patient's expectations

There has been a small amount of work published relating to patients' expectations of treatment but more work is needed in this area as well as in the area of felt and expressed patient needs, in physiotherapy practice generally.

It appears from a clinical trial investigating acupuncture and massage (Kalauokalani et al 2001) that patients' expectations may influence clinical outcome independently of the treatment itself. For example, in the study of Kalauokalani et al (2001) patients who expected to receive greater benefit from massage, compared with acupuncture, were more likely to experience better outcomes with massage than with acupuncture, and vice versa. This study has implications for future clinical trials and the need to control within research studies for patients' expectations.

Grimmer et al (1999) investigated expectations of patients with acute low back pain and found differences between naïve (new) patients and experienced patients. All patients expected to be relieved of symptoms after their first treatment but naïve patients decided to return for more treatments based on the relationship that they had established with the clinician. More experienced patients expected advice to be given during their first consultation (Grimmer et al 1999). The authors concluded that there is a need for a quality partnership to be established with patients on their first visit, a relationship that patients can trust and value, and a need to determine and interpret patients' expectations, to ensure that patients have enough information to become active participants in their own care and to understand the need for further treatment, if required. Also, it appeared that patients needed enough information to manage their own condition effectively in a time-efficient and sensitive manner (Grimmer et al 1999).

One study has focused on patients' expectations of chiropractic treatment. Sigrell (2001) found that patients expected the chiropractor to 'find' the problem and explain the problem to them. They also expected to be symptom-free, to feel better after the first consultation and to have been given advice and exercises. In a follow-up study, Sigrell (2002) concluded that patients expected to consult a knowledgeable professional with good communication skills who could provide effective treatment that resulted in a positive outcome.

In a study of satisfaction with physiotherapy among patients with low back pain, May (2001) identified five dimensions of care that patients found important:

• the personal and professional manner of the clinician – for example, whether they were skilled, thorough, inspired confidence, friendly and sympathetic and whether they listened and were respectful
• the explanation and teaching which occurred during care, i.e. about the problem itself, the patient's role in care, the treatment process and possible prognosis
• how much of the treatment was based on a consultative process. Patients valued being consulted on effectiveness of treatment and the

treatment being related to the individual's own self-help needs. Patients were concerned about the quality of listening (on the clinician's part) that took place within the treatment sessions, how the clinician responded and what kind of responses they made to patients' questions
• the structure that shaped access to and the time with the clinician. For example, patients appreciated fast local access to therapy, wanted scope to return to the clinician at a later date following discharge should a flare-up in their condition occur (an SOS appointment) and wanted enough quality time with the clinician in order to engage with them fully
• the outcome which ensued, i.e. whether treatment was effective and whether the patient gained self-help strategies.

In patients who had undergone hip replacement surgery it was found by Heaton et al (2000) that patients wished rehabilitation therapy and advice to be tailored to their own specific needs, particularly those with multiple impairments. Patients also felt that they should have the opportunity to carry out their rehabilitation exercises in a supportive environment where clinicians could assess their progress, address their concerns and provide ongoing advice and reassurance.

In a more recent study involving the expectations of patients with acute and chronic low back pain, Hitchcock & Moore (unpublished research) carried out a qualitative study the findings of which demonstrated six key emerging themes. The expectations of both the acute and chronic low back pain sufferers were very similar. The patients expected:

• that a diagnosis would be given and the condition would be explained to them fully
• that advice should be offered, i.e. about how to deal with the problem, how to manage pain states, how to avoid aggravating pain and how to relieve it
• that a cure would be provided (usually patients had expectations that a cure would be provided early in treatment)
• that a greater understanding of the clinician's role would be gained

- that they would be given reassurance about their condition
- that they would be enabled to set meaningful personal goals for the future.

Several patients, who had all been referred by local general practitioners, did not understand how the role of the physiotherapist integrated with that of the general practitioner or, for that matter, with other health professionals. They did not understand the full clinical remit of the physiotherapist to examine and assess them independently and to offer treatment as they saw fit in liaison with the patient. Some patients felt uneasy as they had been told by their general practitioner that they would be given a certain form of therapy which had then not been offered by the physiotherapist. Patients felt that their confidence was shaken in 'the system', particularly as some believed that only their general practitioner could prescribe or change physiotherapy-related treatments.

Patients in this study were keen to know what they could do to help themselves – for example, what exercises they could do and what activities would be best for them. It was important for patients to be able to set goals and look to the future. Anecdotally, some clinicians feel that their time should be spent on 'hands-on treatment' rather than spending time communicating fully with patients. All the previous studies, however, have offered information which supports the importance of the establishment of a patient–clinician relationship as vital to the maintenance of a stable and effective clinical partnership. In such a partnership, patients' expectations, needs and perspectives on care can be heard, explored, acted upon, and treatment and goals can be planned and developed by mutual agreement. Therefore, it is important that clinicians plan and allocate time for this to occur.

COMMUNICATION

Rose et al (1992) highlighted the relief that patients feel when they can talk about the condition with someone who understands their problem. In busy outpatient settings clinicians sometimes fail to allow time for effective communication and it is clear that this can lead to frustration, demoralization and loss of confidence in the clinician by the patient. It may also lead to poor outcome. Richardson & Moran (1995) asserted that 'appropriate, timely and effective communication with patients can in turn improve the effectiveness of care' and indicated that communication is at the heart of health care delivery because it can enhance dialogue and ensure active participation in decision making. It can also promote informed choice, and can promote evidence-based health care by ensuring that patients' preferences are noted.

Further, Richardson & Moran (1995) indicated that effective communication with patients can lead to:

- patient empowerment
- enhancement of the quality of care
- improved patient satisfaction
- improved health outcomes
- modification in professional practice in response to patients' needs.

Empowerment

The concept of empowerment is not new in the health-promotion literature but has entered the health-professional literature only in the last decade. Defined by Rodwell (1996), empowerment is the process of enabling or imparting power transfer from one individual to another; it includes the elements of power, authority, choices and permission.

The concept has useful attributes for clinicians, which include:

- being a helping process, which enables individuals to change a situation, giving them the skill, resources and opportunities to do so
- it embodies partnership which values self and others
- it aims to develop a positive belief in self and the future
- it encompasses mutual decision making using resources, opportunity and authority

- it gives individuals freedom to make choices and accept responsibilities for those choices
- it recognizes that power originates from self esteem.

These attributes are essentially the basis of patient-focused care; however, it is not possible for health professionals to empower patients but patients can empower themselves. Patients can be helped towards empowerment by an empowerment process facilitated by health professionals who can provide (i) resources, such as information, knowledge, reassurance, therapeutic skills' and (ii) opportunities, for example a safe physical environment and an open environment in which patients' questions, issues and experiences, needs and expectations can be shared and which can be used by patients to develop a sense of control.

However, for empowerment to be accomplished, patients must possess motivation, participate fully and have a mutual commitment to the process (Labonte 1989).

There may be a range of other factors which influence individuals' abilities to motivate themselves, participate fully and exhibit mutual commitment. These factors may relate to age, gender, ethnicity, previous experiences of healthcare, the nature and or success of the therapeutic relationship and health beliefs. All of these factors should be considered by the clinician in relation to patient empowerment.

Self efficacy

A further concept which has gained popularity in the healthcare systems in the USA, Australia and South Africa, and which is beginning to rise in popularity in the United Kingdom, is the concept of self efficacy. Self efficacy enables a bridge to be built between the person (the patient) and their social world in which the individual must make changes to their behaviour in order to maintain or improve their health or disability status (Rollnick et al 1999).

Self efficacy is different from self esteem (which is important for empowerment) as self efficacy relates to an individual's confidence in their ability to make a specific behavioural change. Self esteem relates more to the individual's general sense of well being.

Self-efficacy systems are based on the work of Bandura & Walter (1963) who developed, a social learning theory based on research. Rollnick et al (1999) have suggested some practical guidelines for developing self efficacy based on the work of Bandura (1977) and others.

1. Self efficacy in individuals varies across situations. Patients can have high self efficacy in some areas of behaviour, which should be praised and encouraged, but may have low self efficacy in others where they may need help in finding different approaches in order to gain confidence to change situations. For example, this can apply to a patient with a neuromusculoskeletal lower limb dysfunction who has mastered crutch walking in the house and in the gymnasium but now needs to gain confidence in walking on the street.

2. 'Doing' is the best way to enhance self efficacy, and as many bridges as possible must be built between the clinical treatment setting and the patient's everyday life; sometimes it helps for a patient to keep a diary or a record of events so that they can reflect on this and see what their successes have been and what has worked well for them. It can also help for patients to bring a friend or relative to treatment sessions, to take part in discussions, and who can then be part of the bridge between the clinical setting and the patient's social setting.

3. People need to have skills to succeed. These skills may be present but may lie dormant; sometimes these skills need to be built up and confidence gained. Such skills could be learning skills, psychomotor skills or interpersonal skills.

4. Feedback needs to be given about deficiencies in the patient's performance so that they can improve.

5. People learn best by modelling themselves on others; therefore there is value in patients' talking to, and about, friends or other patients who have succeeded in similar tasks. For example, attending self-help groups – such as arthritis support groups – can be helpful (Rollnick et al 1999).

In some situations self-help groups are run entirely by patients who talk about their experiences and successes in changing their life situations and teach others in similar situations about exercises or activities or adaptions in the home which they have found helpful.

Summary

From the patient-focused perspective, Box 9.1 summarizes what needs to be considered in relation to overall patient management.

Readers who wish to know more about changing health behaviours are referred to an excellent text: 'Health Behaviour Change' (Rollnick et al (1999).

THE MULTIFACETED ROLE OF THE CLINICIAN

This chapter has thus far been concerned with the political and professional context of practice and an overview of patient-focused care and its implications for the clinician. It is important that patient-focused care has been addressed early in this chapter as, increasingly, patients are, and should be, the central focus of care and decision making within our health services and our health practices. The patients' perspective has been presented foremost in this chapter to highlight their importance in the therapeutic relationship. What now follows is an overview of the multifaceted role of the clinician within the neuromusculoskeletal field.

The clinician functions within political, managerial service and professional frameworks and every clinician needs to be politically aware of new initiatives in these arenas. They must also know how these initiatives will affect, or have the potential to affect, their practice. Clinicians would be wise to read their professional journals and newsletters and visit National Health Service, professional body and special-interest group websites on a regular basis in order to keep up to date with initiatives which may affect practice.

The current major influences and considerations for practice which are emphasized in clinical governance procedures are:

- the rise in emphasis on patient-focused care (already addressed in the early part of this chapter)
- the requirement for practice to be based on the best available evidence, i.e evidence based practice (EBP)
- the increasing number of treatment modalities becoming available both with and without evidence to support them
- the professional and statutory requirements for all health professionals to engage in continuing professional development
- the emphasis within the health service on efficiency and effectiveness of care as well as cost effectiveness.

The multifaceted nature of the clinician's role and its complexities were acknowledged by Moore & Jull (2002). The skills of the competent clinician should include those shown in Box 9.2.

Box 9.1 A summary of patient-focused care

Patient-focused care means:
- Building a balanced therapeutic partnership/relationship which consists of trust, respect and understanding for patients ideas, beliefs, knowledge and values
- Increasing patient autonomy
- Involving patients in decision making
- Working within the biopsychosocial model of care
- Sharing and dealing with patients' expectations
- Sharing and dealing with patients' needs and encouraging their felt needs to be expressed
- Clinicians should demonstrate good knowledge, therapeutic skills and communication skills, including listening skills
- Clinicians should offer high-quality explanations, education and advice to patients
- Clinicians must offer clear guidance on the physiotherapist's role
- A consultative process within the treatment sessions should be adopted
- A flexible appointment system with SOS appointment availability is important
- Patients should be facilitated to empower themselves
- Self efficacy should be facilitated
- Clinicians should give time to patient-focused care
- Good outcomes must be achieved
- Professional practice needs to be modified as needed and required in response to the developing therapeutic relationship

---

Box 9.2 Skills of the clinician

- The ability to apply fundamental science, art and professional practical applications of physiotherapy/physical therapy (a prerequisite for practice and registration
- Good listening skills
- High-level interpersonal skills, including emotional intelligence and good communication skills
- Education skills, including skills in assessment of learning and evaluation of learning
- High-level clinical reasoning skills
- Skill in the appropriate use of evidence to support practice
- Skill in the use of clinical guidelines for neuromusculoskeletal therapy
- Expertise in examination and assessment of patients with joint, nerve and muscle dysfunction
- Competence and/or expertise in the treatment and management of patients with neuromusculoskeletal dysfunction
- Skills in reflective practice
- Motivation and skills in personal professional development
- Time management skills
- Skills in the use of information technology
- Team playing/leadership skills

Competent application of the fundamental science, art and professional practice in physiotherapy

These skills (Box 9.2) are a fundamental prerequisite to qualification and registration as a physiotherapist in the United Kingdom (Health Professions Council 2003b) and therefore are not dealt with here but suffice to say that every clinician has a duty to ensure that skills in these areas are continually refreshed, updated and reinforced (Moore & Jull 2002).

LISTENING SKILLS AND THE CLINICIAN

The importance of listening to patients' needs, expectations and beliefs has already been addressed in this chapter in relation to the therapeutic relationship. However, it is important here to stress the need for careful listening skills to be applied throughout examination and treatment processes so that appropriate treatment/management strategies can be defined in association with the patient so as to achieve a successful outcome to treatment.

Being a good listener enables the clinician to pick up new avenues of potential fruitful enquiry in the examination process from the odd gesture or a single word spoken or uttered by the patient. In this sense it may be possible to identify that patients have worries and/or fears and felt needs that they have not yet verbalized, and it gives the clinician the opportunity to help the patient express these issues fully. It may simply be that patients fail to mention facts or symptoms associated with their condition because they feel that such facts or symptoms are either unimportant or unrelated. The good listener will capitalize on these nuances and use them to best effect in their clinical reasoning processes (Moore & Jull 2001).

It is imperative that clinicians interpret what patients say in a valid way, hence the importance of discussion between the clinician and their patient in order to ensure that the interpretation of what has been said is sound and that facts have been clearly understood (Maitland et al 2001).

Listening skills are an essential part of communication in general (Maitland et al 2001). Communication consists of two components, verbal, including the tone of voice, and non-verbal (Maitland et al 2001). It is important for the clinician to recognize their own non-verbal communication as well as being observant of patient's non-verbal behaviours, which, because they are a reflex action can be more genuine and can reflect more subtly their true feelings.

Clinicians should observe patients carefully, making eye contact and exhibiting an open posture, which makes them more approachable to patients. Clinicians should watch the patient's facial expressions carefully as well as their body movements as they may give much needed messages about how the patient is really feeling. The clinician also needs to be aware of their own state of mind as this may influence how he or she interprets patient's non-verbal communication (Maitland et al 2001).

Communication

Clear verbal communication is also of vital importance to a successful therapeutic relationship. The clinician must ask questions in a clear and uncomplicated way in order to understand fully the patient's symptoms, how they are reacting to the physical examination and what effect treatment is having. The clinician should give clear scope for the patient to enter into discussions and voice their opinions, fears, anxieties, needs and expectations. Important pointers in communication are highlighted by Maitland et al (2001, p. 26):

- 'Speak slowly'
- 'Speak deliberately'
- 'Keep questions short'
- 'Ask one question at a time'.

The ideal results of the clinician's effective communication with the patient are as shown in Box 9.3.

Finally in this section on communication, an example of how important it is to ascertain fully that the patient understands any terminology that is used. There are many terms in the neuromusculoskeletal field which, to the lay person, are very similar – for example, spondylitis, spondylosis, spondylolisthesis, spondylolysis. Patients now have full access via the Internet to

---

Box 9.3 The ideal results of effective patient–clinician communication (from Moore et al 1995, with permission)

- A full understanding of the patient's condition and how it is affecting the patient is gained
- A full and accurate clinical picture is obtained through the examination process
- Patient's feelings, needs, expectations, fears and anxieties have been discussed and explored
- An understanding of the patient's confidence in taking responsibility for their condition is obtained
- The patient knows what role the clinician has in their treatment and management
- The patient understands what neuromusculoskeletal therapy is and what it aims to achieve
- The patient understands what effects may be expected from treatment
- The patient understands what their treatment will consist of
- The patient understands what treatment options there are
- The patient understands how long treatment will last and how many treatments will be necessary
- The patient understands what part they have to play in their treatment and home management, both during treatment and after discharge

---

health information and so ensuring that they have the right terminology and they have understood fully the meaning is essential. An example from practice highlights the issues. A patient having assumed as a result of a rushed conversation with their general practitioner that they had ankylosing spondylitis came to treatment in a worried and tormented fashion having consulted the medical literature. They had heard the term 'spondy.....' and no more and had assumed on coming across 'ankylosing spondylitis' that they were suffering from a progressive disease. The patient was much relieved on hearing that actually their condition had been diagnosed by their general practitioner as being spondylosis (Moore & Jull 1997).

Interpersonal skills

Interpersonal skills include listening and communication components but how we relate to individuals depends on our own attitudes, values, beliefs, knowledge and experience which become fused together in our own personal philosophy and view of life. Life changes at any time; for example, personal bereavements, divorce, illness and other life events can change our philosophy of life and therefore how we react and relate to other people (Moore et al 1997). It is important for therapists to recognize how their own interpersonal skills may be affected at any one time and make adaptions by developing necessary coping strategies, if possible, to change their interpersonal skills if they appear to be influencing a therapeutic relationship negatively. Often, voicing issues with a colleague or a mentor can help; this is important as Trede (2000) has indicated how much patients value a good interpersonal relationship with their clinician.

Golemann's (1996) work on emotional intelligence identifies five domains which may be helpful to the practitioner in terms of dealing with other people. First, knowing one's own emotions is important; managing one's own emotions is also important, and motivating oneself to recognize emotions in others are essential attributes – as is being able to handle relationships.

Golemann defines emotional intelligence as 'a capacity for recognizing our own feelings and those of others, for motivating ourselves and for managing emotions well in ourselves and in our relationships' (Golemann 1998, p. 317).

Application of neuromusculoskeletal examination and clinical skills

The reader is referred to Petty & Moore (2001) for details of the application of relevant examination procedures and to the chapters in this text dealing with the treatment and management of joint, muscle and nerve dysfunctions. This section deals with fundamental principles of patient management only.

The overall examination and treatment processes are depicted in the flow chart in Figure 9.4, created to show the treatment process together with the development of the therapeutic relationship.

Figure 9.4 shows the examination, treatment and discharge continuum. Good communication and interpersonal skills are vital at each stage of this continuum. On the right hand side of the figure the effective patient–clinician relationship develops into a continuum, with the patient empowering themselves and later developing high self efficacy. On the left hand side of the diagram, examination and assessment findings are discussed with the patient and a contract is drawn up with the patient (some NHS Hospital Trusts have standard formats for these). As part of the contract the clinician fully explains the examination and assessment findings to the patient, discusses and agrees treatment and management strategies and prognosis, including an explanation of treatment options, and finally agrees treatment and management goals with the patient together with suitable circumstances for discharge and how the overall outcome of treatment will be measured. At the end of treatment, when discharge is agreed, a follow-up (SOS) appointment may also be agreed (if offered within the clinician's home department's framework). The contract should be fully documented and signed by both the patient and the clinician.

TREATMENT

Treatment approaches can be summarized as in Figure 9.5, which depicts a multimodal physiotherapy approach to treatment. Treatment is carried out in the context of the patient's

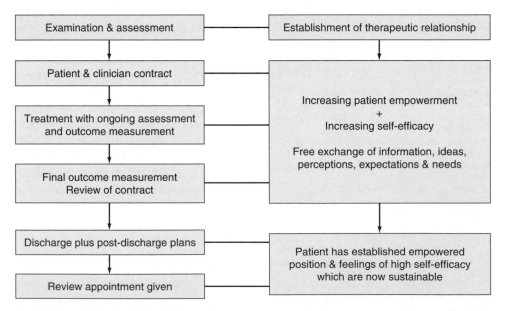

Figure 9.4 Patient-focused examination and treatment continuum.

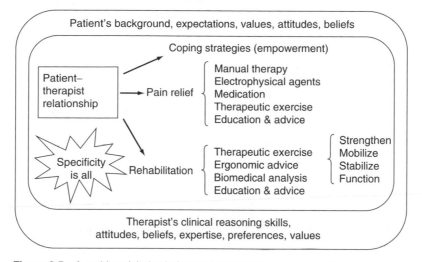

Figure 9.5   A multimodal physiotherapy/physical therapy approach.

background, their social circumstances, expectations, values, attitudes, beliefs and expressed needs and preferences and also within the clinician's code of practice, expertise and preferences for treatment modalities (which may relate to their own physique, size, shape and personal physical ability or dysfunction).

The patient–clinician relationship is integral to the multimodal approach, and management aims at developing coping and management strategies with the patient to facilitate the development of self efficacy and 'to bridge the gap' between the clinical and social environments. It also includes emphasis on pain relief and rehabilitation of dysfunctional states. Pain-relieving strategies have already been dealt with earlier in this text but include: manual therapy, electrophysical procedures, therapeutic exercise and education and advice with respect to pain-relieving postures and activities. Information on what pain-provoking activities to avoid, and enhancing the understanding of the problem and how modalities/the medication being used by the patient may help in pain relief, are also important. Also included in this aspect of treatment is the development of coping strategies with the patient for the management of pain at home by the use of exercises, positioning and/or the use of ice therapy and/or other modalities as appropriate.

Rehabilitation may include therapeutic exercise to affect muscle, joint and or nerve and may be aimed at strengthening muscle tissue, mobilizing joints and soft tissues to restore range of movement, re-education of muscle function in order to stabilize joints or regions of the body and re-education of muscle activity in active joint movement in functional activities.

Rehabilitation may also include ergonomic advice, for example, with regard to seating postures, sleeping surfaces and working postures. Biomedical intervention includes the detailed analysis of movement and dysfunction and re-education to normality. This is often undertaken in a laboratory-based setting where movement-analysis equipment is freely available.

Education within the context of rehabilitation should include home management programmes – for example, exercises and or activity programmes which will enable the patient to continue their rehabilitation at home during the treatment phase and after discharge if necessary.

The important feature here is that treatment must be made specific to the patient's condition as identified in the examination and assessment components of the management programme; in other words, the specificity of approach is all-important.

Initially, it's necessary to decide what symptoms/signs are predominating and, if pain predominates, then pain is usually treated first and a pain-relieving modality may be used. The pain-relieving modality, however, must be applied accurately to an appropriate joint or soft tissue and applied so as to produce relief of pain, taking into account the severity, irritability and nature of the condition (Petty & Moore 2001). The reader is also referred to Chapters 4, 6 and 8 of this text for more details on pain-relieving strategies.

As the condition improves, the technique that has been used for pain relief may be applied more forcefully or the technique may be changed for another following re-assessment of signs and symptoms as perhaps pain no longer predominates and the need now to increase joint range predominates. The need for specificity in the application of treatment cannot be overstated.

It is important also to note the positive effect that the patient's psychological processes may have on descending nerve pathways. In the treatment setting, painful conditions will be approached often using a local technique, which is used to influence sensory input; this, in turn, will also affect descending nerve pathways. Therefore, it can be seen that the patient-focused nature of care, together with specificity of treatment, can have potentially strong influences on the patient's pain levels. It is essential that the choice of treatment modality be made in a rational scientific and clinically reasoned way and that changes to treatment are equally made on this basis, only and when a change is required or is necessary.

Care of the patient

Every health professional has a statutory duty of care to the patient (Health Professions Council 2003a). This implies that they must act in the best interests of the patient. They must respect the confidentiality of patients, keep their own professional knowledge and skills up to date, act within the limits of their knowledge, skills and experience and maintain proper and effective communication with patients. They must also obtain informed consent to give treatment (which implies full discussion and consultation with the patient), keep accurate records of patients, carry out duties in an ethical way and behave with integrity and honesty.

Informed consent

Informed consent has been defined as "a voluntary decision made by a sufficiently competent or autonomous person on the basis of adequate information and deliberation to accept or reject some proposed course of action, which will affect 'him or her'." (Gillon 1986, cited by Singleton & McLaren 1995, p. 104). Alternatively, informed consent has been described as 'the voluntary or revocable agreement of a competent individual to participate in a therapeutic or research procedure based on adequate understanding of its nature, purpose and implications' (Sim 1986, p. 584). Sim (1996) believes that informed consent can be analysed into four elements, each of which should be present to a satisfactory degree if consent is valid. These elements are depicted in Figure 9.6.

Disclosure in this context means that the clinician must fully explain the intended interventions, their possible benefits and possible risks but also give information on possible alternative

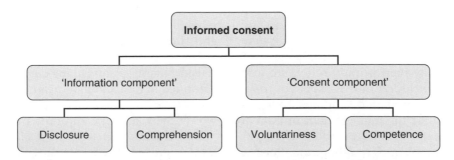

Figure 9.6 The elements of informed consent (from Sim 1996, with permission).

treatments. The clinician must also ensure that the patient has understood the information given, i.e. that comprehension has occurred. 'Voluntariness' relates to the fact that the patient should give consent without undue pressure, influence, or coercion and 'competence' refers to the patient's ability to reach a rational autonomous decision.

Patient care in the context of informed consent relates directly to clear accurate communication and the establishment of an effective therapeutic relationship.

Many hospital departments have standard consent forms and procedures for gaining consent and the reader is referred to Sim's (1996) article and to their own clinical governance departments for more local information on informed consent.

The patient's comfort

The patient's comfort during the examination and treatment session is of paramount importance to their confidence in the clinician, in their treatment and their ability to relax during treatment. Comfort is also likely to have an impact on the outcome of treatment. Comfort can be assured by ensuring that the patient's privacy is respected, i.e. screening of the patient's cubical or ensuring that body parts are adequately covered – and also that the treatment area is as private as possible and that the patient is not inhibited in their discussions with the clinician by fear of being overheard when discussing perhaps sensitive issues.

Physical support should always be given for areas of the body being treated or examined, for example, using adequate pillows for the head and neck and positioning joints in a supported and facilitatory position for treatment; nose holes in hydraulic plinths can be uncomfortable for some patients and a small face towel folded under the forehead can help to reduce this discomfort.

It is essential to ensure that adequate heating is present in treatment areas if the outside temperature is cold and to ensure that good ventilation is available when the weather outside is very warm; this is particularly the case when patients are undertaking exercise. It is also important to ensure that lighting is sufficient for the needs of the clinician and also for the patient's needs, particularly if the patient is elderly and especially if they need to read information booklets, fill in outcome measures and consent forms and the like.

All positions for examination and treatment should be safe, comfortable and should facilitate examination and/or treatment processes. Clinicians should respect patients' preferences for treatment positions; for example, there are some patients who cannot lie flat, perhaps because of a cardiac problem, where treatment positions need to be modified accordingly.

Accuracy of treatment

It is essential to ensure that treatment is applied as accurately as possible. It is important always to reassess signs and symptoms during and after each treatment session. Accuracy relates to all aspects of the treatment application and dose.

Dosage and frequency of treatment

The frequency of appointments, i.e. how often treatment should be applied, is sadly under-researched. Anecdotally, it may be that treatment should be frequent enough so that changes resulting from treatment can be assessed. In this way other activities carried out by the patient between appointments is kept to a minimum and helps prevent a confusing clinical picture (Maitland et al 2001).

Daily treatment may often be preferable where symptoms are severe but not irritable; but daily treatment may be too much where symptoms are severe and irritable, in which case treatments once or twice a week may suffice. In essence, the dosage and frequency of treatment must be guided by individualized examination findings. Often clinicians will apply a short session of treatment directly after examination and assessment has taken place and then the patient may be seen the next day in order to assess what effect the treatment has had. The frequency of treatment can then be judged by the clinician in discussion with the patient, having assessed what the initial reaction to treatment has been.

Caution must be exerted with patients who believe that the more the treatment hurts the better, and a thorough explanation to the patient of how treatment works and is best applied in painful states is helpful here.

The response to treatment between individuals is variable; some patients achieve full recovery while others do not respond. There is a need in the short term to extend neuromusculoskeletal research in order to develop a better classification or profile of patients who respond to certain modalities (Jull & Moore 2002).

Appropriate dosages of treatment are also under-researched. We know little of what dosage or treatment leads to the best outcome of care (Jull & Moore 2002). Closer investigation of dosage of treatment is required but until this research is available clinicians are best advised to treat each patient on an individual basis and be guided by presenting signs and symptoms at all stages.

Settings for treatment

Treatment should take place only where adequate facilities for examination and treatment are available. A private treatment cubical is most appropriate for individual hands-on treatment sessions, while a gymnasium or laboratory setting with appropriate instrumentation may be better for muscle re-education treatments, for example, when using biofeedback or diagnostic ultrasound imaging.

Choice of treatment/technique

Treatment must be chosen specifically to manage the presenting dysfunction, i.e. there must be specificity in all treatments. For example, if a painful joint condition exists a pain-relieving modality should be applied. The technique or modality chosen will depend on what is deemed to be most appropriate by the therapist in discussion with the patient, taking into account their past experiences and preferences. If mobilization is the chosen modality then it should be applied specifically to relieve pain, not to increase joint

range – although, in relieving pain, joint range may increase as a by-product of pain relief. If joint stiffness is the main problem then mobilizations or exercise should be applied in a specific way in order to increase range of movement, i.e. performed at the end of range. If, after examination, the clinician believes that joint stability is lacking then stabilization exercises may be prescribed. In essence, treatment must be applied specifically to influence signs and symptoms that are present, for example, pain, instability, muscle spasm, muscle weakness, joint stiffness, swelling, functional disability etc. Usually the most profound sign and/or symptom is targeted first and as this problem begins to regress then other modalities may be introduced in order to deal with other symptoms and signs that have now become more prominent. The effect of each modality on the condition can then be assessed carefully before another is added or withdrawn. The use of multiple modalities in a 'scatter gun approach' will lead to difficulty in identifying which modality has been effective.

Importantly, clinicians must be guided by their clinical reasoning skills and not by blind application of inappropriate evidence. Simply because a patient has presented with a named syndrome, for example low back pain, clinicians should avoid the temptation to use lumbar stabilization exercises as a treatment modality. Lumbar spine stabilization exercises are used when there are signs and symptoms present suggesting that this treatment approach may be beneficial (because evidence exists for the benefit of such exercises in a certain group of patients suffering with low back pain (Moore & Petty 2001)). Where there are clear indications of signs and symptoms related to published research then clinicians should use treatments which have positive evidence to support their use.

The preferences of patients and clinicians are important in the choice of treatment modalities; for example, a patient may have in the past experienced a treatment which is now being suggested. Previously, the patient may have found that the treatment was ineffective, distressing or uncomfortable. The clinician in this situation would be wise to find an alternative treatment or discuss the advantages/effects of the original technique very fully with the patient, in order to gain their understanding as to why the choice of treatment appears to be the most advantageous. At this point, and in partnership, the clinician and patient can come to an informed agreement about which modality to use.

The clinician may have particular treatments that they believe can be performed better than others; this may relate to the clinician's height, weight, experience and competence in the use of certain modalities, and these are important considerations in the decision-making process about which modalities to use.

CLINICAL REASONING

It is assumed that the clinician is using clinical reasoning throughout the examination, assessment, treatment and re-assessment processes. In the neuromusculoskeletal field, this has been promoted by Jones (1995), based on the work of Barrows & Tamblyn (1980), and further developed by Edwards (1995), the Barrows & Tamblyn (1980) model focuses on the clinician's activities. The later model by Edwards adds the patient to the scenario and has been termed cooperative decision making between the patient and clinician (Fig. 9.7). The model is adapted here to include the patient–clinician relationship and the overriding effects of the clinician's attitudes, values, beliefs and expectations as well as those of the patient, together with their expressed needs. In addition, the concept of empowerment facilitated by the cooperative nature of information and explanation sharing should not be forgotten.

'Knowledge in the clinical reasoning process refers not only to knowledge in particular areas but also to the organization of knowledge into useful and useable entities' Jones (1995 p. 20). 'Cognition refers to the processes of thinking and includes the syntheses and analysis of information and the testing of working hypotheses

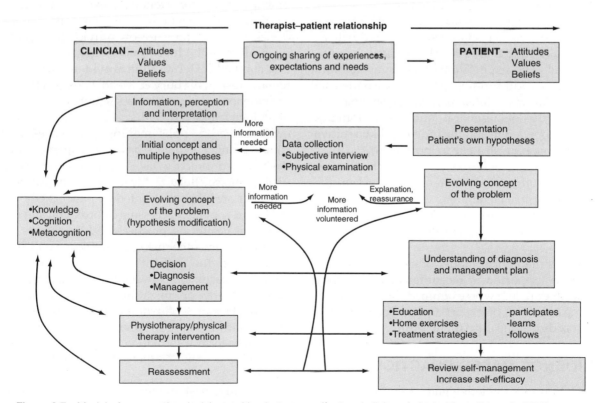

Figure 9.7 Model of cooperative decision making between patient and clinican (adapted from Edwards 1995).

relating to patient information, this includes confirming or disconfirming strategies which actively plays a profound role in knowledge acquisition on behalf of the clinician, hence the close relationship between knowledge and cognition' (Jones 1995, p. 19).

'Metacognition refers to the clinician's ability to think about their own thinking' Jones (1995, p. 19), which becomes more possible the more clinical expertise one has. This expertise can be gained only through clinical experience, during which clinical reasoning involves reflection in action and reflection about action (Schon 1987a). Metacognition refers to thinking about what you are doing, as you are doing it, i.e. when a clinician encounters a problem they engage in a process of critical analysis which then allows them to modify or adapt their practice, or correct their practice until a solution is found. A more detailed explanation of clinical reasoning is to be found in Jones (1995) and Higgs & Jones (1995).

Jones (1995) indicated a number of factors which affect and influence clinical reasoning. There are external factors, which include the patient's needs, expectations, values and beliefs, professional and institutional directives, community needs and expectations and the availability of resources and funding. There are also internal factors relating to clinicians, such as personal values and beliefs, general and local domain-specific knowledge and the individual's cognitive and or reasoning strategies (Jones 1995).

The reader is referred to earlier chapters in relation to domain-specific knowledge in the neuromusculoskeletal areas of muscle, joint and nerve and to the earlier chapter on assessment for practical application of the clinical reasoning process.

Jones's theoretical model of clinical reasoning has been supported by recent research by Doody & McAteer (2002) who examined the clinical reasoning activities of expert and novice therapists in an orthopaedic outpatient setting.

EVIDENCE-BASED PRACTICE

In relation to knowledge gained by the clinician necessary for clinical reasoning the reader's attention is now turned to the concept of evidence-based practice, which, as discussed earlier in this chapter, has gained momentum in the United Kingdom since the Secretary of State for Health's white paper (1998).This Paper indicated that treatment undertaken within the National Health Service should be supported by evidence which is routinely applied.

Evidence-based practice has been variously defined. The definition of Sackett et al (1996) emanates from evidence-based medicine: 'evidence-based medicine is the conscientious, explicit and judicious use of current best evidence in making decisions about the care of individual patients' (Sackett et al 1996, p. 71). This definition has been frequently used; however, it has been adapted by Bury & Mead (1998), acknowledging the individuality of the clinician's expertise and also acknowledging the shortage of strong evidence to support all aspects of the physiotherapist's work at the present time. Their definition is as follows 'Evidence-based practice is the conscientious, explicit and judicious use of current best evidence in making decisions about the care of individual patients, integrating individual clinical expertise with the best available external clinical evidence from systematic research' (Bury & Mead 1998, p. 11).

Evidence-based practice lies within a framework of evidence-based health care, which includes evidence-based policymaking, evidence-based commissioning, evidence-based management, evidence-based practice itself and evidence-based patient choice (Bury & Mead 1998). Increasingly, clinicians are being confronted by patients who are freely and copiously accessing information and evidence on healthcare practices and treatments via the Internet and other media, and this can only help to increase the patient's autonomy and aid informed discussion between the clinician and the patient. Many organizations, for example the National Health Service and the Chartered Society of Physiotherapy, now offer lists of web-based and paper-form information for patients in order to provide a basis for their choices and decision making.

Currently, best evidence refers primarily to high-quality scientific research derived from valid and rigorous research. The strength of evidence is shown in Box 4. Also coming to the fore currently are meta-analyses which are, in fact, analyses and summaries of the data emanating from a series of high-quality randomized controlled trials. As more research is carried out into physiotherapeutic modalities the number of meta-analyses published in this field will increase.

The judicious use of evidence is key here – the evidence above relates largely to high-quality published research work. However, there are available other sources of evidence which must be taken into consideration before treatment is applied, for example:

- clinical experience and expertise of clinicians
- the views of experts in the field
- established practice in health settings
- beliefs and values of the patient and clinician based on previous experiences
- expectation of patients based on information from published sources, other people and intrinsic needs
- information from the clinical examination and assessment procedures using rigorous clinical reasoning procedures
- the patient's preferences for treatment
- clinicians' preferences for the use of specific treatment modalities (Bury & Mead 1998).

Bury & Mead (1998) have usefully defined the steps necessary in carrying out evidence-based practice:

Box 9.4 Hierarchy of strength of evidence (from Bury and Mead 1998, with permission)

I Strong evidence from at least one systematic review of multiple well-designed randomized controlled trials

II Strong evidence from at least one properly designed randomized controlled trial of appropriate size

III Evidence from well-designed trials without randomization, single group pre-post, cohort, time series or matched case-controlled studies

IV Evidence from well-designed non-experimental studies from more than one centre or research group

V Opinions of respected authorities, based on clinical evidence, descriptive studies or reports of expert committees

---

- define the question arising from practice that needs answering
- find the evidence
- critically appraise the evidence
- implement relevant findings into practice
- evaluate the impact on practice.

The implementation of evidence-based practice demands high-level skills on the part of the clinician in the appraisal of literature and research; the clinician must also marry this appraisal with all other sources of evidence, as described above. The eventual choice of treatment should, as mentioned earlier, be fully discussed with the patient.

It is important that clinicians use their clinical reasoning skills in order to identify accurately and precisely the nature of the patient's problem so that they can then define the appropriate clinical question for which evidence must then be found. There is no excuse for clinicians resorting to the use of evidence which is not appropriate for the individual patient under care and their condition. There must be clear indications for the use of evidenced treatment from the patient's clinical picture. Moore & Jull (2000) and Moore & Petty (2001) make this point very strongly.

Despite the agreement among clinicians that research is important in the development of professional practice, there have been a number of reasons for lack of use of evidence by clinicians in the past. These reasons have included: lack of understanding of statistics, lack of access to evidence, conflicting results in research papers, methodological problems in the research processes, lack of replication of studies and poor generalizability of results. In addition, clinicians cited insufficient time available to access evidence, inadequate facilities for the use of evidence-based practice, feeling isolated from colleagues (influencing their confidence in using new evidence and resistance to change in treatments by medical staff) (Metcalfe et al 2001).

It has also been noted that attendance at short courses is a popular form of continuing professional development for clinicians in the neuro-musculoskeletal field, but many short courses are offered without any reference to research underpinning the concepts involved (Turner & Whitfield 1999).

CLINICAL GUIDELINES

Since the evidence-based practice movement began there has been a rapid development of clinical guidelines within a number of health disciplines and within different countries throughout the world. As a result, clinical guidelines are proliferating; for example, guidelines for the management of whiplash-associated disorder and for low back pain are currently under development within the United Kingdom and will sit alongside other already existing guidelines available in other countries. Guidelines for the management of low back pain already exist in Holland and in other countries. It may be essential, however, that individual national guidelines be developed owing to differences in scope of practice, funding arrangements for health care, cultural differences in the population and national differences in health beliefs and values.

Clinical guidelines have been defined by Mann (1996) as 'systematically developed statements, which assist clinicians and patients in making decisions about appropriate treatment for specific conditions'.

The key features of guidelines are that they are based on the best available evidence, which has been appraised and evaluated systematically. Guidelines deal with specific interventions for specific client populations. A systematic process is used to decide who will be involved in the development of guidelines; development often involves experts in the field, patient representatives and, increasingly, other relevant professional groups (Mead 1998). It is suggested that readers obtain up-to-date clinical guidelines from their own professional body in the subject areas that are of most relevance to their own practice. Professional body websites will have full details as to how to access them.

Guidelines – as with all evidence – have to be interpreted and used judiciously, and there may need to be a consensus among clinicians as to how they may be interpreted locally to ensure that all are clear as to the implications of the guideline implementation for their own practice.

EDUCATIONAL SKILLS AND THE CLINICIAN

Educational skills within the role of the clinician have been mentioned throughout this text, and education and advice offered by the clinician has been seen throughout this chapter as key to the therapeutic partnership and mutual patient–clinician understanding. It is also important in helping patients to empower themselves and in potentially developing their self efficacy.

In the main, clinicians deal with adult learners who are well described by Knowles (1983); the education of adult learners will be the key area of concentration here. Where children are attending for treatment parents will often be involved in the educational experiences; therefore, the principles of adult learning will apply but the concept of children's education is beyond the scope of this text. In a qualitative study, Trede (2000) investigated the approaches of physiotherapists to education about low back pain and found that, in a sample of eight physiotherapists who were interviewed in the study, the majority adopted a didactic and clinician-centred approach to patient education. Patients were also interviewed in this study, and Trede concluded that an 'open' patient–clinician relationship is needed in order to encourage dialogue, action and reflection on progress and to ensure that misunderstandings and unrealistic expectations do not occur. Trede (2000) further summarized the components of clinician- and patient-centred approaches to education, as shown in Box 9.5.

Trede (2000) concludes that patients valued a good interpersonal relationship with their clinician as the most effective learning tool.

For details on developing educational skills see Moore et al (1997) (under revision).

As Knowles (1983) has indicated in his theory of adult education, adults as learners see themselves as self-directed and responsible individuals. They possess an accumulation of experiences which are a resource for their own learning, and for that of others (including, in the case of the patient, the clinician). Adult learners are motivated to learn when they perceive that the activity is directly related to their own life tasks, and

---

Box 9.5 Components of clinician and patient-centred approaches to education (after Trede 2000, p. 430–431)

Clinician-centred	Patient-centred
Teaches medical facts	Actively listening to the patient
Predicts and controls problems	Displaying a positive attitude to the patient
Symptom of diagnosis set the scene	Providing technical, factual and counselling support
Listening to patients of low priority	Providing opportunities for patients to learn independently
Planning is done for patients	Planning exercises with the patient
Patients necessarily being compliant	

---

their interests tend to focus on problem solving rather than on abstract content or theory. For example, teaching structural anatomy in patient-education programmes is not the most useful way of facilitating learning in adult patients – they would much prefer to know where their pain is coming from and how to get rid of it!

There are many factors which can affect learning (see Moore et al 1997) but one of the strongest factors is the learning style that suits learners as individuals. The particular learning style which a learner prefers influences the way in which that individual approaches study and the way they think. Learning styles are related to personality but have nothing to do with intelligence levels. In the clinical setting, if the clinician and patient have different learning styles, which are incompatible, then tensions and misunderstandings may arise. Honey & Mumford (1986) identified four learning styles which each have characteristics (Box 9.6).

It is important that clinicians be aware of their own and their patients' learning styles; using the characteristics shown in Box 9.5 will help individuals to define their preferred learning style and then educational events can be adapted accordingly.

Ewles & Simnett (2003) have identified some principles for the education of patients.

PRINCIPLES FOR THE EDUCATION OF PATIENTS

The following is adapted from Ewles & Simnett (2003, p. 246–248):

- Say important things first; patients will be more likely to remember what was said at the beginning of the session.

Box 9.6 Description of learning styles (adapted from Honey & Mumford 1986)

Activists
- involve themselves fully, without bias, in new experiences
- enjoy the here and now, happy to be dominated by immediate experiences
- open-minded, not sceptical
- enthusiastic about anything new
- dash in where angels fear to tread
- like brainstorming problems
- bored with implementation and longer-term consolidation
- gregarious, involve themselves with others
- seek to centre all the activities around them

Reflectors
- like to stand back to ponder experiences, thoughtful
- observe from many different perspectives
- collect data, chew over before coming to conclusions
- tend to postpone reaching conclusions
- cautious, leave no stone unturned
- prefer to back seat in meetings and discussions
- enjoy observing people in action
- listen to others
- adopt a low profile
- have a slightly distant, tolerant, unruffled air

Theorists
- integrate observations into logical theories
- think problems through step-by-step
- assimilate disparate facts into cohesive whole
- tend to be perfectionists
- like to analyse
- tend to feel uncomfortable with subjective judgements
- tend to be detached, analytical and rational

Pragmatists
- keen on trying out ideas, theories and techniques
- positively search out new ideas
- like to experiment
- like to get on with things and act quickly
- tend to be impatient with lengthy open-ended discussion
- essentially practical, like making practical decisions
- respond to problems and opportunities as a challenge

- Stress and repeat key points and emphasize what are the important points; repetition can help.
- Give specific, precise advice and remember to relate to patients' own physical, personal and social circumstances.
- Structure information into categories, i.e. give patients headings and categories and deliver material under these headings.
- Avoid jargon, long words and long sentences.
- Use visual aids whenever possible – for example, leaflets, handouts, models, videos and written instructions.
- Avoid saying too much at once – only two or three key points will be remembered from each session.
- Ensure that your advice is relevant and realistic by discussion with the patient.
- Get feedback from the patients to ensure their understanding.
- Assess whether learning has taken place.

In assessing whether learning has taken place it is important to try to choose a method that is appropriate for the patient and their learning style, their condition and the information and the knowledge you are trying to assess. For example, the clinician could use question-and-answer sessions, gapped handouts or discussion sessions to assess whether the patient has clearly understood all the information necessary for them to participate in their own treatment.

If teaching practical skills, Ewles & Simnett (2003) recommend three stages:

- demonstration by the clinician
- rehearsal by the patient observed by the clinician
- practice by the patient observed by the clinician on a regular basis.

Demonstrations need to be clear, accurate, slow and repeated several times. Again, assessing whether learning has taken place is of paramount importance to ascertain whether the patient has actually grasped what it is necessary for them to learn (see Moore et al 1997).

Obtaining evaluation and feedback on the clinician's personal role as an educator, or of the educational experience that has been provided (see Moore et al 1997), can be very valuable. It is sensible to ask the patient to evaluate both the clinician as an educator and the educational experience that has been provided. Peers can also be helpful in this evaluation, and self-reflection can be very useful. It is important to ask the following questions. What happened? What went well? What could have been improved? How would the experience be beneficially changed for next time? All learning experiences work best if they are planned carefully and in advance. Again, see Moore et al (1997, Ch. 11) for details.

Home exercise programmes

The importance of good-quality teaching in relation to home exercises cannot be overestimated. It is essential that patients who require home exercises are shown how to do these correctly and that an assessment be made regularly as to how effectively the exercises are being undertaken and what effect they are having.

In relation to home management programmes the reader should be aware of issues surrounding the terminology associated with patients responding to agreed/prescribed home management programmes. There are three options: compliance, adherence and concordance. Compliance in the 1980s was a popular term used in medicine; it reported patients' observable actions in carrying out the practitioner's instructions. Sackett & Haynes (1986) defined compliance as the extent to which the patient's behaviour coincides with the clinical prescription, and this makes it a term which is very practitioner-orientated. 'Adherence' has been used interchangeably with compliance for several years Kroll et al (1999), but has implied patient passivity because patients were expected to 'stick' to the practitioner's instructions. The word concordance is being increasingly used as it describes 'unity or the state of being of the same opinion or feeling' (from the Latin concorde, meaning 'of one mind' – Oxford English Dictionary 1996). The term concordance appears to fit well with the concept of patient-focused care.

Because terminology is currently changing, much of the previously published work relates to compliance or adherence and therefore the terms for these studies have been expressed as used by the authors concerned.

According to Meichenbaum & Turk (1987) there are many variables which appear to relate to non-adherence, including personal variables in relation to the patient, disease variables, treatment variables and relationship variables, i.e. variables within the patient–clinician relationship. (see Box 9.7.)

Box 9.7 Factors related to treatment non-adherence (from Meichenbaum & Turk 1987, with permission)

Personal variables (patient)
Characteristics of the individual
Sensory disturbance
Forgetfulness
Lack of understanding
Conflicting health benefits
Competing sociocultural concepts of disease and
    treatment
Apathy and pessimism
Previous history of nonadherence
Failure to recognize need for treatment
Health beliefs
Dissatisfaction with practitioner
Lack of social support
Family instability
Environment that supports nonadherence
Conflicting demands (e.g. poverty, unemployment)
Lack of resources

Disease variables
Chronicity of condition
Stability of symptoms
Characteristics of the disorder

Treatment variables
Characteristics of treatment setting
Absence of continuity of care
Long waiting time
Long time between referral and appointment
Timing of referral
Absence of individual appointment
Inconvenience
Inadequate supervision of professionals
Characteristics of treatment
Complexity of treatment
Duration of treatment
Expense

Relationship variables
Inadequate communication
Poor rapport
Attitudinal and behavioural conflicts
Failure of practitioner to elicit feedback from patient
Patient dissatisfaction

Therefore it is important that clinicians, in building their therapeutic relationship with patients, ensure that these factors are minimized wherever possible in order to increase conformance. Jensen et al (1997) assert that, for a treatment plan to be successfully followed, the patient must choose to do so, they must know when to carry out the plan, they must have the psychomotor skills to perform the plan and they must remain motivated to see the plan through until the problem resolves. Further, Jensen et al (1997) indicate that the clinician must understand the patient's perspectives, motivational factors and their belief systems in order to facilitate change in the patient's behaviour needed to incorporate the treatment plan into their everyday lives. In a study of patient compliance with GP/physicians' instructions, Falvo et al (1980) indicated that patients were more likely to be compliant the more they perceived that the physician gave them explanations and showed concern for them.

Langer (1999) felt that minority populations were being treated by clinicians who were insensitive to patients' cultural norms, and referred to the impact that this may have had on health service use. Langer (1999) asserted that lack of awareness of cultural issues increases social distance, breaks down communication and precipitates misconceptions between minority patients and their health care providers and that this can lead to opportunities for dissatisfaction and non-compliance to increase.

Finally in this section, Friedrick et al (1996) found that exercises learnt only by brochures, without being monitored by a physical therapist, were carried out properly in only one-half of the patients in their study, which appeared to result in fewer improvements in impairment.

It is clear that clarity of written information is highly important, and for those readers wishing to develop written materials for patients the following sources may be helpful: Duman (2003) and Plain English Campaign *www.plainenglish.co.uk*.

MEASUREMENT OF OUTCOME

Throughout treatment, the clinician will assess the outcome of care in terms of the assessment of salient signs and symptoms, and sometimes by utilizing a valid, reliable and sensitive measure of outcome. Sometimes clinicians use a measure of outcome at the beginning of treatment and then again at discharge in order to ascertain improvements in the patient's condition. Sometimes clinicians choose to use measures of outcome regularly throughout the treatment process.

In physiotherapy, a measure of outcome has been defined as 'a test or scale administered and interpreted by physical therapists that has been shown to measure accurately a particular attribute that is of interest to patients and therapists and is expected to be influenced by an intervention' (Mayo 1994, p. 145).

It is important that physiotherapists use measures of outcome that are appropriate to the condition being treated and the patient concerned, i.e. in terms of ethnicity and language abilities.

It is equally important that physiotherapists choose measures of outcome which measure changes in the signs and symptoms that are being targeted by treatment. For example, if pain is predominantly being targeted in treatment, then a measurement of pain should be used – and used at an appropriate time in treatment to reflect the changes that have occurred. The tendency to levy a raft of outcome measures which are designed to measure attributes that are not being specifically targeted by treatment, must be avoided, for example the use of a functional measure when only pain has so far been targeted during treatment is unhelpful and can lead to demoralization of the clinician and the patient when changes do not occur. Some functional changes may occur as a result of a by-product of pain management but functional improvement may not be optimal by the time major pain relief has occurred; therefore it appears obvious that different outcome measures should be used at different stages in the treatment process, reflecting progression of, and changes in, patient–clinician responsibilities and the nature of modalities being used.

The main issues surrounding outcomes are as follows. First, their validity, in other words, does the measure record what it is intended to measure? Second, their reliability, i.e. can the measure

be repeatedly used uniformly when administered on one or more occasions or by one or more raters? Third, is the measure sensitive/responsive, i.e. does the measure of outcome have the ability to detect true changes in the patient's situation over time? Is it sensitive enough to measure the subtle changes that sometimes occur in patients undergoing neuromusculoskeletal therapy? (Hicks 1999).

A wide variety of measures of outcome are available:

- physical measures
- pain scales/questionnaires
- psychological well-being profiling questionnaires
- general health status measures
- self-efficacy measures
- disability measures
- quality-of-life measures
- functional ability measures
- patient-generated indexes
- patient-satisfaction questionnaires
- life-satisfaction and moral questionnaires
- multidimensional measures.

For details of an overview of a number of measures of outcome relevant to neuromusculoskeletal therapy see Cole (1994), Liebenson & Yeomans (1997) and the extensive works by Ann Bowling (2001a, 2001b) on measuring disease and measuring health.

In addition, national physiotherapy/physical therapy professional body websites contain details of recommended measures of outcome. It is important that, as with research evidence, clinicians apply a critical and analytical eye on any proposed measure of outcome and assess the validity, sensitivity and reliability for its use in their own clinical situations. As can be seen, if applied correctly, outcomes are vitally important for measuring the results of healthcare.

CLINICAL AUDIT

In relation to the quality of health care, one of the ways of measuring the quality of the service provided is to measure performance against set standards and then analyse the results. This process is known as clinical audit. Standards to be measured need to be agreed locally or nationally, as does the topic for the audit. Audit is useful in evaluating the process of care, and feedback from audit activities to both departmental staff and individual clinicians can be important in improving practice. Clinical audit can be very important in itself in facilitating the use of evidence-based practice (Buttery 1998). Clinical audit has been defined as 'a clinically led initiative which seeks to improve the quality of outcome and outcome of patient care through structured peer review, whereby clinicians examine their practice and results against agreed standards and modify practice where indicated' (NHS Executive 1996).

Usually, audit is guided by a cycle of events that comprise:

- agreement of guidelines, protocols or standards
- implementation of guidelines, protocols or standards
- assessment by data collection and analysis of compliance of the guidelines, protocols or standards
- agreement of changes in the guidelines, protocols or standards, if required
- implementation of agreed changes in guidelines, protocols or standards (Buttery 1998).

PERSONAL PROFESSIONAL DEVELOPMENT

Readers of this book may be novice practitioners and may be aiming to improve both their cognitive and practical skills and aspiring to becoming expert practitioners. There are many models of expertise available. These include clinical problem solving, knowledge in clinical reasoning, the Dreyfus Model of Skill Acquisition and the Model of Reflective Practice; these models are clearly described by Jensen et al (1999).

The reflective practice model is growing in popularity in the United Kingdom. Donald Schon's work (1987b) has explored how clinicians gain practical knowledge. Schon's theory is that clinicians add to their practical knowledge base

not only through experience but also through a process of reflection, which is triggered by the recognition that a situation is not routine. He (Schon 1987b) believes that there are three processes present in reflection, as shown below:

- initial doubt and perplexity if the situation has been identified as non-routine but problematic (what is going on?)
- questioning the thinking or action that has caused the problematic situation (how did I get here?)
- working for problem resolution by trying new actions (what can I do to resolve the problem?).

Professionals are believed to learn by experience by using reflective enquiry, to think about what they are doing and what worked and what did not work as they were doing it. Patients can also learn by reflective activities.

Brockbank & McGill (1998) have defined reflection as 'the creation of meaning and conceptualization from experience'. It is important that all clinicians avoid clinical stagnation and learn to develop continuously from their clinical experiences. Readers may find the following texts helpful in developing their expertise and capitalizing on their own professional knowledge: Jensen et al (1999) and Higgs & Titchen (2001). In addition, individuals may seek out the opportunity to engage with 'clinical supervision', defined as an enabling process 'defining opportunities for personal and professional growth' (Butterworth & Faugier 1992). Bond & Holland (1998) have further described clinical supervision as an interaction between a supervisee and one or more peers in order to promote professional development through reflection and which is characterized by:

- regular protected time for facilitation of in-depth reflection on professional practice
- an interaction that is facilitated by one or more experienced colleagues with expertise in facilitation
- facilitation of time and venue for the provision of frequent ongoing sessions led by the supervisee's agenda

- an enabling process that permits supervisees to achieve, sustain and develop creatively a high quality of practice through means of focus, support and development
- a reflective process, which permits the supervisees to explore and examine the part they play in the complexities of the events within the therapeutic relationship as well as the quality of their practices
- a life-long learning experience that should continue throughout the practitioner's career, whether they remain in practice or move into management, research or education.

Much more information on clinical supervision can be found in Cutcliffe et al (2001).

Clinical supervision is a concept frequently used in the nursing profession to facilitate post-registration professional development of individual nurses. It is becoming more widespread in use as more hospital trusts in the United Kingdom seek new ways of improving the quality of healthcare delivery and methods of enabling life-long learning in their workforces using their existing in-house expertise and experience.

OVERALL MANAGEMENT OF PATIENTS

In summary, the following are some guidelines for clinicians for the overall management of patients:

- Make treatment and/or overall management patient-focused.
- Ensure that all clinical work falls within professional, local service and national health service-related guidelines for good practice and quality improvement.
- Work within a biopsychosocial model of care.
- Work towards patient autonomy through clinical partnership.
- Ensure that patients have the opportunity to develop an empowered position.
- Facilitate patient self efficacy wherever possible.
- Undertake multimodel patient management within the framework of the patient–clinician relationship.

- Ensure that coping strategies, pain relief and rehabilitation strategies are addressed within overall patient management.
- Base treatment choices on sound, careful and comprehensive clinical reasoning processes, working within the Edwards (1995) cooperative decision-making model.
- Examination and treatment procedures should be carefully undertaken, accurate in application and specific to the patient's background and condition, bearing in mind the patient's needs, expectations and preferences.

Examination should:

- Allow the building of the therapeutic relationship.
- Ensure a full understanding of the patient's condition, how it is manifesting, and how it is affecting the patient.
- Determine how the condition should be approached with respect to treatment.
- Determine exactly what the patient's expectations and needs are in relation to their background circumstances.
- Indicate what, if any, contraindications are present in relation to choice of treatment.
- Help to determine what the likely outcome of treatment will be.

Treatment should be:

- Specific to fulfil the stated aims of treatment.
- Fully discussed with the patient.
- Accurate in its application.
- Applied with frequency and a dosage appropriate to the patient's needs and the manifesting signs of the symptoms.
- Accompanied by the acquisition of informed consent which should be gained as necessary.
- Based on goals agreed with the patient at the start of treatment.
- Inclusive of some form of education or advice to facilitate patients' understanding of their problem, their treatment, their home management and their possible coping strategies.
- Inclusive of patient learning, which should always be assessed and evaluated to ensure that full understanding has taken place.

- Assessed for outcome and goal achievement, both formally and informally, at appropriate points in treatment, which will vary according to the patient's condition. More than one measure of outcome may be appropriate if the patient's condition and treatment is multifactorial.
- Aimed at aiding patient empowerment and self efficacy.
- Modified, progressed, interrupted and/or ceased according to the behaviour of the patient's signs and symptoms, with the therapist using a full range of clinical reasoning skills.
- Based on the best available evidence.
- Accompanied by a self-care or a self-management programme to enhance and continue the effects of treatment. These programmes should be aimed at pain relief and enhancing all other aims of treatment.

Discharge

- Should take place when agreed goals have been reached or are likely to be achieved in the short term by the patient's home management strategy.
- The opportunity for a follow-up appointment should be given to all patients if permissible within the home department's administrative system.

Multidisciplinary working

- As with all areas of practice, the clinician must ensure that they engage fully in communicating, liaising and working alongside the rest of the multidisciplinary team.

Finally, all clinicians should indulge in reflective practice during and after each interaction with a patient in order to improve their knowledge, experience and expertise and to ensure continuing professional development. Individuals and clinical departments may give some thought to adopting a system of clinical supervision in order to maximize reflective practice.

SUMMARY

This chapter has emphasized the need for patient-focused care and has highlighted the facets of care in which patients can and should be involved. It has attempted to show how making patients more of a central focus of care can lead to improvements to the quality of health and improve the outcome of treatment. The specificity of treatment has been shown to be of paramount importance based on the integration of high-quality, cognitive and practical skills which are enmeshed with the concepts of evidence-based practice and the use of clinical guidelines and clinical audit. Finally, the need for a continuous professional development and the role that reflective practice and clinical supervision can have in the development of the practitioner's expertise have been overviewed.

The reader is left with an adapted quotation to reflect upon:

'If you really want to help somebody, first of all you must find them where they are and start there. This is the secret of caring. If you cannot do that, it is only an illusion, if you think you can help another human being. Helping somebody implies your understanding more than they do, but first of all you must understand what they understand. If you cannot do that, your understanding will be of no avail. All true caring starts with humility. You the helper you must be humble in your attitude towards the person that you want to help. You must understand that helping is not dominating, but serving. Caring implies patience as well as acceptance of not being right and of not understanding what the other person understands.'

Kierkegaard (1849)

REFERENCES

Baker S M, Marshak H H, Rice G T, Zimmerman G J 2001 Patient participation in goal setting. Physical Therapy 81(5):1118–1126

Bandura A 1977 Towards a unifying theory of behaviour change. Psychological Review 84:191–215

Bandura A, Walter R H 1963 Social learning and personality development. Thinehart and Winston, New York

Barr J, Threlkeld A J 2000 Patient practitioner collaboration in clinical decision-making. Physiotherapy Research International 5(4):254–260

Barrows H S, Tamblyn R M 1980 Problem based learning: an approach to medical education. Springer, New York

Bond M, Holland S 1998 The surface picture: the development a value of clinical supervision in skills of clinical supervision for nurses, ch 2. Open University Press, Buckingham

Bowling A A 2001a Measuring disease – a review of disease specific quality of life measurement scales, 2nd edn. Open University Press, Milton Keynes

Bowling A A 2001b Measuring health – a review of quality of life measurement scales, 2nd edn. Open University Press, Milton Keynes

Bradshaw J 1972 Concept in social need. New Society 19:640–643

Brockbank A, McGill 1998 Facilitating reflective learning in higher education. Open University Press, Buckingham

Brody D S, Miller S M, Lerman C et al 1989 Patient perception of involvement in medical care: relationship to illness, attitudes and outcomes. Journal of General Internal Medicine 4:506–511

Bury T, Mead J 1998 Evidence based healthcare: a practical guide for therapists. Butterworth-Heinemann, Oxford

Butterworth A, Faugier J 1992 (eds) Clinical supervision and mentorship in nursing. Chapman and Hall, London

Buttery Y 1998 Implementing evidence through clinical audit. In: Bury J, Mead J (eds) Evidence based healthcare. Butterworth-Heinemann, Oxford

Chartered Society of Physiotherapy 2002 Rules of professional conduct, 2nd edn. Lansdowne Press, London

Cole B 1994 Physical rehabilitation outcome measures. Canadian Physical Therapy Association, Ontario

Collins thesaurus 1995 Harper Collins Publishers, Glasgow

Cutcliffe J R, Butterworth T, Proctor B (eds) 2001 Fundamental themes in clinical supervision. Routledge, London

Department of Health 2000 The NHS Plan. The Stationery Office, London

Doody C, McAteer M 2002 Clinical reasoning of expert and novice physiotherapist in an outpatient orthopaedic setting. Physiotherapy 88(5):258–268

Duman M 2003 Producing patient information. Kings Fund, London

Edwards I 1995 Unpublished paper cited by Jones M: Clinical reasoning pain. Manual Therapy Journal 1(1):21

Ewles L, Simnett I 2003 Promoting health – a practical guide, 3rd edn. Scutari Press, London

Falvo D, Woehlke P, Deichman N J 1980 Relationship of physician behaviour to patient compliance. Patient Counselling and Health Education 2(4):185–188

Friedrick M, McErmak T, Maderbacher P 1996 The effect of brochure use versus therapist teaching on patient performing therapeutic exercise and on changes in impairment status. Physical Therapy 76(10):1082–1087

Gillon R 1986 Philosophical medical ethics. John Wiley, Chichester.

Golemann D 1996 Emotional intelligence. Bloomsbury, London, p 43

Golemann D 1998 Working with emotional intelligence. Bloomsbury, London

Grimmer K, Sheppard L, Pitt M et al 1999 Differences in stakeholder expectations in the outcome of physiotherapy management of acute low back pain. International Journal for Quality in Healthcare 11(2):155–162

Health Professions Council 2003a Standards of proficiency. Health Professions Council, London

Health Professions Council 2003b Standards of conduct, performance and ethics. Health Professions Council, London

Heaton J, McMurray R, Sloper P, Nettleton S 2000 Rehabilitation and total hip replacement: patients' perspectives on provision. International Journal of Rehabilitation Research 23:253–259

Hicks C 1999 Research methods for clinical therapists, 3rd edn. Churchill Livinstone, Edinburgh

Higgs J, Jones M (eds) 1995 Clinical reasoning in the health professions. Butterworth-Heinemann, Oxford

Higgs J, Titchen A (eds) 2001 Practice knowledge and expertise in health professions. Butterworth-Heinemann, Oxford

Hoff B 1982 The Tao of Pooh. Mandarin, London, p XIV

Honey P, Mumford A 1986 The manual of learning styles. Printique, London

Jensen G M, Gwyer J, Hack LM, Sheppard K F 1999 Expertise in physical therapy. Butterworth-Heinemann, Boston

Jensen GM, Lorish C 1994 Promoting patient cooperation with exercise programmes: linking research theory and practice. Arthritis Care Research 7:181

Jensen GM, Lorish C, Sheppard KF 1999 Understanding patient receptivity to change. Teaching for treatment adherence. In: Sheppard K F, Jensen GM (eds) Handbook of teaching for physical therapists. Butterworth-Heinemann, Boston

Jette A 1994 Physical disablement concepts for physical therapy research and practice. Physical Therapy 74:380

Jones M 1995 Clinical reasoning and pain. Manual Therapy Journal 1(1):17–24

Jones M, Edwards I, Gifford L 2002 Conceptual models for implementing biopsychosocial theory in clinical practice. Manual Therapy Journal 7(1):2–9

Jull G, Moore A P 2002 What is a suitable dosage of physical therapy treatment? Manual Therapy Journal 7(4):181–182

Kalauokalani D, Cherkin D C, Sherman K J et al 2001 Lessons from a trial of acupuncture and massage for low back pain. Spine 26(13):1418–1424

Kierkegaard S 1849 The sickness unto death. Penguin books, London (Translation from Danish by Hannay A D.)

Knowles M 1983 The modern practice of adult education from pedagogy to androgogy. In: Tight M M (ed) Adult learning and education. Croom Helm in association with the Open University, London, ch 2, p 53–70

Kroll T, Barlow J H, Shaw J 1999 Treatment adherence in juvenile rheumatoid arthritis. Scandinavian Journal of Rheumatology 28(1):10–18

Labonte R 1989 Community and professional empowerment. Infermiere Canadienne 85(3):23–28

Langer N 1999 Culturally competent professionals in therapeutic alliances enhance patient compliance. Journal of Health Care for Poor and Underserved 10(1):19–26

Liebenson C, Yeomans S 1997 Outcomes assessment in musculoskeletal medicine. Manual Therapy Journal 2(2):67–73

Maitland G D, Banks K, English K, Hengeveld E 2001 Communication in Maitland vertebral manipulation, 6th edn. Butterworth-Heinemann, Oxford, p 1–24

Mann T 1996 Clinical guidelines: using clinical guidelines to improve patient care within the NHS. Department of Health, London

May S J 2001 Patient satisfaction with management of low back pain. Physiotherapy Journal 87(1):4–19

Mayo N 1994 Outcome measures or measuring outcome. Physiotherapy Canada 46(3):143–147

Mead J 1998 Developing disseminating and implementing clinical guidelines. In: Bury T, Mead J (eds) Evidence based healthcare – a practical guide for therapists. Butterworth-Heinemann, Oxford, p 162–181

Meichenbaum D, Turk D C 1987 Facilitating treatment adherence. Plenum, New York

Metcalfe C, Lewin R, Wisher S et al 2001 Barriers to implementing the evidence base in four NHS therapies. Physiotherapy 87(8):433–441

Moore A P, Jull G 1997 Editorial. Manual Therapy Journal 2(3):121–122

Moore A P, Jull G 2000 Editorial: fads and fashion. Manual Therapy Journal 5(4):197–256

Moore A P, Jull G 2001 Editorial: The art of listening. Manual Therapy Journal 6(3):129

Moore A P, Jull G 2002 Editorial: reflections on the musculoskeletal therapists multifaceted role and influences on treatment outcome. Manual Therapy Journal 7(3):119–120

Moore A P, Petty N J 2001 Editorial: evidence based practice – getting a grip and finding a balance. Manual Therapy Journal 6(4):195–264

Moore A, McQuay H, Gray J A M eds 1995 Evidence based everything. Bandalier 1(12):1

Moore AP, Hilton R, Morris J et al 1997 The clinical educator – role development. Churchill Livingstone, Edinburgh

Neistadt M 1995 Methods of assessing clients' priorities: a survey of adult's physical dysfunction settings. American Journal of Occupational Therapy 49(5):428–436

NHS Executive 1996 Clinical audit in the NHS. Using clinical audit in the NHS: a position statement. DOH, London

NHS Executive 1999 Continuing professional development quality in the NHS. DOH, London

NHS Executive 2000 Meeting the Challenge a Strategy for Allied Health Professionals. DOH, London

Pearsall J, Trumble B (eds) 1996 Oxford English Reference Dictionary, 2nd edn. Oxford University Press, Oxford

Petty N J, Moore A P 2001 Neuromusculoskeletal examination and assessment – a handbook for therapists, 2nd edn. Churchill Livingstone, Edinburgh

Richardson K E, Moran S 1995 Developing standards for patient information. International Journal of Healthcare Quality assurance 8(7):27–31

Rodwell C M 1996 An analysis of the concept of empowerment. Journal of Advanced Nursing 23:305–313

Rollnick S, Mason P, Butler C 1999 Health behaviour changes, a guide for practitioners. Churchill Livingstone, Edinburgh

Rose M, Klenenman L, Atkinson L, Slade P 1992 A comparison of three chronic pain conditions using the fear avoidance model of exaggerated pain perception behaviour. Research and Therapy 21(4):409–416

Sackett D C, Haynes RB 1986 Compliance with therapeutic regimes. John Hopkins University Press, Baltimore

Sackett D L, Rosenberg W M C, Gray J A M, Haynes R B 1996 Evidence based practice: what is it and what it isn't. British Medical Journal 312:71–72

Schon D 1987a Educating the reflective practitioner. Physical Therapy 70:566–577

Schon D 1987b Educating the reflective practitioner. San Francisco, Jossey Bass

Secretary of State for Health 1997 The NHS Modern and Dependable. NHS Executive, London

Secretary of State for Health 1998 A first class service. Quality in the new NHS. NHS Executive, London

Sigrell H 2001 Expectations of chiropractic patients: the construction of a questionnaire. Journal of Manipulative and Physiological Therapeutics 24(7):440–444

Sigrell H 2002 Expectations of Chiropractic treatment: what are the expectations of new patients consulting a chiropractor and do chiropractors have similar expectations. Journal of Manipulative and Physiological Therapeutics 25(5):300–305

Sim J 1986 Informed consent, ethical implications for physiotherapy. Physiotherapy 72:584–587

Sim J 1996 Informed consent and manual therapy. Manual Therapy Journal 1(2):104–106

Singleton J, Mclaren S 1995 Ethical foundations of health care. Mosby, London.

Stewart M, Roter D 1989 Communicating with medical patients. Sage Publications, New York

Swage T 2000 Clinical governance in healthcare practice. Butterworth-Heinemann, Oxford

Trede F V 2000 Physiotherapists' approaches to low back pain education. Physiotherapy 86(8):427–433

Turner P, Whitfield T W A 1999 Physiotherapists' reasons for selection of treatment techniques. A cross sectional survey. Physiotherapy Theory and Practice 15:235–246

Waddell G, Bircher M, Finlayson D, Main C J Symptoms and signs: physical disease or illness behaviour. 1984 British Medical Journal (Clinical Research Edition) 289:739–741

Index

Page numbers in bold type refer to illustrations and tables.